The Renal System

SYSTEMS OF THE BODY
The Renal System
BASIC SCIENCE AND CLINICAL CONDITIONS
THIRD EDITION

Amanda Mather
MBBS, PhD, FRACP
Clinical Nephrologist
Royal North Shore Hospital
St Leonards, NSW, Australia

Vincent W. Lee
MBBS, PhD, FRACP
Clinical Associate Professor of Medicine
Westmead Hospital
Westmead, NSW, Australia

All of Discipline of Medicine, University of Sydney, Australia

Series Editor
Stephen Hughes
BSc, MSc, MBBS, FRCSEd, FRCEM, FHEA
Consultant in Emergency Medicine, Broomfield Hospital
Senior Lecturer in Medicine, School of Medicine, Anglia
Ruskin University
Chelmsford, UK

For additional online content, visit ExpertConsult.com

ELSEVIER

First edition 2003
Second edition 2010

Notices

Practitioners and researchers must always rely on their own experience and knowledge in evaluating and using any information, methods, compounds or experiments described herein. Because of rapid advances in the medical sciences, in particular, independent verification of diagnoses and drug dosages should be made. To the fullest extent of the law, no responsibility is assumed by Elsevier, authors, editors or contributors for any injury and/or damage to persons or property as a matter of products liability, negligence or otherwise, or from any use or operation of any methods, products, instructions, or ideas contained in the material herein.

ISBN: 978-0-7020-8292-4

Publisher: Jeremy Bowes
Content Project Manager: Fariha Nadeem
Design: Margaret Reid
Illustration Manager: Anitha Rajarathnam
Marketing Manager: Deborah Watkins

Copyedited by Editage, a unit of Cactus Communications Services Pte. Ltd.
Typeset by TNQ Technologies Pvt. Ltd.

Printed in Scotland

Last digit is the print number: 9 8 7 6 5 4 3 2 1

Working together
to grow libraries in
developing countries

www.elsevier.com • www.bookaid.org

Most students now study medicine through a form of integrated curriculum. These courses blend basic science with exposure to clinical medicine from an early stage. These students have the good fortune to be left in no doubt, from the outset, why they are studying medicine. I teach in a medical school that delivers a fully integrated curriculum and I can compare it with the traditional model according to which I received my early medical education. That comparison is very favourable.

Unlike many other texts, the *Systems of the Body* series has been designed very specifically to support an integrated approach to learning medicine. Our carefully selected panel of authors drawn from across the English-speaking world have combined basic science with clinical application. Links to clinical skills, clinical investigation and therapeutics are made clear throughout.

The aim is to offer highly accessible guidance for all student types and stages. It will be invaluable to those who are approaching the subject for the first time or who may have found a topic challenging when using other more traditionally configured resources – as well as greatly assist all students wishing to excel as their course progresses. The clear layout and writing style, together with detail that informs without overwhelming, go a long way to supporting students. It may also provide welcome reminders to postgraduates facing their own examinations.

Whatever curriculum you follow, wherever you are in the world, and whichever stage you are at, we know that the *Systems of the Body* volumes will serve as great places to start when learning something new and enable you to effectively piece together the essential components of each major body system, in a modern clinical context.

Good luck!

Stephen Hughes, MSc MBBS FRCSED FRCEM FHEA
Senior Lecturer in Medicine
Anglia Ruskin University
Chelmsford, UK
and
Consultant, Emergency Medicine
Broomfield Hospital
Chelmsford, UK

Medical students, and indeed many practising doctors, have generally regarded learning about the normal kidney and its diseases as one of the more difficult areas in medicine. Many of the underlying concepts of normal structure and function may seem rather abstract, and the classification and manifestations of disease states can be confusing.

One of the reasons for this perceived difficulty in studying the kidney may be that the component disciplines have traditionally been presented largely in isolation from each other, so that the relationships between normal and abnormal structure and function, and the relevance of basic scientific descriptions to clinical problems, has not been made clear.

Like others in the Systems of the Body series, this book aims to guide beginning medical students in learning about the kidney by adopting a closely integrated approach. Each chapter is based around a clinical case scenario, and the process of working through the patient's problems leads to the exploration of a variety of relevant material drawn from the basic and clinical sciences as required. For example, in the first chapter, the presentation of a child with a probable urinary infection leads to consideration of the normal anatomy of the urinary tract and developmental abnormalities that may predispose to urinary infection. At the same time, aspects of microbiology, antibiotic pharmacology, and modalities for imaging the urinary tract are dealt with in context.

By this means, most of the important basic sciences relevant to understanding the structure, function and diseases of the renal system are covered at a level appropriate to medical students in the first part of their course. The approach taken complements the philosophy of problem-based learning (PBL), which is being adopted by ever increasing numbers of medical schools throughout the world, though it should be equally useful to students enrolled in more conventional programs. Indeed, the book should in no way be seen as short-circuiting the process of self-directed learning, which is at the heart of PBL-based courses, and it is expected that students will also consult conventional discipline-based textbooks and the medical literature to expand the horizons of their understanding of the subject-matter of the book.

In order to acknowledge that many students using this text will have had little clinical experience at this early stage of their course, we have provided a Glossary to define unfamiliar clinical terms used in the book (other than words which are explained within the context of the relevant chapter). Such terms are shown in bold in the text on their first occurrence.

While there are many developments in basic renal science and many clinical conditions involving the kidney, which are not covered in this introductory book, we feel confident that students who master the material we have included here will be in a good position to take the study of the kidney further in their later undergraduate and postgraduate training.

Since this text first appeared, there have been many developments in basic science relevant to renal function and some important advances in therapeutics and clinical care. However, the core knowledge structures that underpin the study of this system at a medical student level have not fundamentally changed; hence the design and essential content of the book has not been greatly altered for this third edition.

The authors have taken care to update information in some areas and to add some new illustrations. Summaries have been added for each chapter, along with "Clinical skill boxes" to enhance learning about commonly used procedures such as urinalysis. Questions relevant to each chapter have been reintroduced, usually adapted from those used in the first edition. Some 'Interesting facts' relating to the material in the main text have been added in a number of places, in keeping with this feature of other volumes in the Systems of the Body series. Worksheets on selected concepts of difficulty (nephron transport processes and approach to glomerulonephritis) have been added in the "e-book" of this publication. Finally, sections on the approach to history and examination of a patient with suspected kidney disease are outlined. Included in the "e-book" is a video of how to do a "renal" examination.

It is hoped that this new edition will continue to be found useful by medical students around the world.

ACKNOWLEDGEMENTS

It is a pleasure to acknowledge the enthusiasm and assistance of the publishers in producing this volume in the Systems of the Body series.

We particularly want to acknowledge the inspiration and writing of our colleagues Michael Field, Carol Pollock and David Harris, who wrote the first two editions of this book, and their trust in us to update this third edition. They have mentored us throughout our careers and we owe them an enormous debt of gratitude.

In particular, we want to recognise the leadership of Jeremy Bowes, Commissioning Editor, and Stephen Hughes, Series Editor, and the helpfulness and attention to detail of Fariha Nadeem and Kim Benson, Project Development Managers.

A number of our colleagues assisted by offering suggestions for improving the text or by providing material for the illustrations. We are grateful for contributors to the previous editions whose contributions still form a part of this edition: Dr. George Kotsiou, of the Royal North Shore Hospital, Sydney, contributed to the microbiology sections of Chapter 1, while various photographic images were provided by colleagues at Concord Hospital, Westmead Hospital, Royal North Shore Hospital and the Department of Pathology, University of Sydney. For the third edition, specific thanks are due to Dr. Danielle Delaney (Department of Urology, Sydney Children's Hospital) for assistance with Chapter 12 and to Dr. Chow Heok P'ng (Department of Anatomical Pathology, Westmead Hospital), Associate Professor Ming Wei Lin and Dr. Logan Gardner who provided valuable assistance with the renal biopsy material. We would also like to extend our gratitude to Jennifer Li, Scot, Kathy Kable, and Sasha Cohen for the video of the renal examination, and the radiology department from Royal North Shore Hospital for radiology images in Chapter 8.

Finally, we would like to thank our families and colleagues for their support- always and particularly during the period in which this book was being written.

CONTENTS

8

DIABETIC NEPHROPATHY AND CHRONIC KIDNEY DISEASE 99

9

KIDNEY FAILURE AND REPLACEMENT OF RENAL FUNCTION 111

10

HYPERTENSION AND THE KIDNEY 123

11

PREGNANCY AND THE KIDNEY 135

12

URINARY TRACT OBSTRUCTION AND STONES 147

13

RENAL MASSES, CYSTS, AND URINARY TRACT TUMOURS 157

14

DRUGS AND THE KIDNEY 167

INTRODUCTION TO THE RENAL SYSTEM

1

Chapter objectives

After studying this chapter, you should be able to:

1. Describe the structure and embryological origins of the major anatomical components of the urinary tract, namely, kidneys, ureters, bladder, and urethra.

2. Understand the clinical distinction between upper and lower urinary tract infections.

3. Describe the organisms commonly associated with urinary infections and the mechanisms which make these organisms uropathogenic.

4. Describe the underlying factors associated with complicated urinary tract infections.

5. Select the most appropriate imaging techniques for the urinary tract when structural abnormalities are suspected.

6. Understand the principles of treatment of upper and lower urinary tract infections.

7. Describe the anatomical abnormalities and complications occurring in patients with vesicoureteric reflux.

8. Describe the approach to history and examination of a patient with kidney disease.

Introduction

The kidneys are highly specialised organs that function to regulate the volume and chemical composition of the body fluids. In carrying out this function, they excrete most water-soluble waste products in urine. Once the urine is formed, it is collected and stored in the bladder. The bladder then empties intermittently during the process known as micturition.

When the normal processes of embryological development are disturbed, defects may develop in the structure of the urinary tract that interfere with the normal production and flow of urine. As a consequence, urinary tract infection (UTI) may occur and may be the initial clue that a structural abnormality of the urinary tract exists. This chapter, illustrated by the case of such an infection in a child, will introduce the basic structure and development of the kidneys and urinary tract and discuss the common problem of UTI (see Case 1.1:1).

Normal anatomy of the urinary tract

The urinary tract is made up of the kidneys, ureters, bladder, and urethra (Fig. 1.1). The kidneys are normally considered to be the upper urinary tract, whereas the remaining structures may be considered to be the lower urinary tract. There are normally two kidneys, each placed retroperitoneally in the posterior abdominal wall on either side of the spine at the level of the upper lumbar vertebrae. Each kidney is 10 to 14 cm in length in adults and is surrounded by a fibrous capsule within perirenal fat. The renal hilus on the concave medial aspect of the kidney is the point of entry for the arteries, veins, and nerves and exit for the urine drainage system. The urine formed by the kidney initially drains into the renal pelvis, which may be considered as the dilated portion of the ureter which links the kidney to the bladder. The urine in the renal pelvis is propelled by peristaltic action along the length of the ureter into the bladder. The ureters run medially and insert into the posterior base of the bladder, with the terminal end of the ureter tunnelled submucosally to form the vesicoureteric junction. The normal intrinsic musculature of the bladder surrounding the oblique course of the intravesical segment of the ureter is thought to be responsible for ureteric competence during bladder emptying, thus preventing the reflux of urine from the bladder back into the ureter. Abnormalities in the development of this intravesical segment are thought to predispose to the development of vesicoureteric reflux (VUR; see later in this chapter).

The bladder is an elastic organ consisting of connective tissue and smooth muscle, known as detrusor, loosely arranged in outer longitudinal, middle circular and inner longitudinal layers. This muscle arrangement results in the bladder's ability to empty during contrac-

Case
1.1
Urinary tract structure and infection: 1

A febrile child

Tommy Baron is a 2-year-old boy who presents with a fever up to 39°C of 24-h duration. Although initially complaining of abdominal pain and being unable to be comforted, he is now clearly ill, with lethargy and diffuse abdominal tenderness. His blood pressure is normal for a child his age at 70/40 mmHg. The examination is otherwise unremarkable. Urinalysis shows blood +++, protein ++ and is positive for leucocyte esterase (markers of white cells) and nitrites (markers of bacterial action).

We can infer from this information that Tommy is systemically unwell, with infection being the likely problem. The urinary abnormalities suggest that the urinary tract is the source of sepsis.

To understand the structural basis of this illness, we should initially familiarise ourselves with the anatomical components of the urinary tract. We can then consider whether Tommy is likely to have any abnormality that may predispose him to infection.

tion. The dome of the bladder is covered by the parietal peritoneum and is in apposition to other organs in the pelvis. The proximal urethra lies between the bladder neck and the pelvic diaphragm and functionally consists of two sphincter mechanisms composed of both smooth and striated muscles. In women, the pelvic diaphragm is responsible for most of the sphincter mechanism. In men, the sphincter mechanism is largely incorporated into the prostate, with minimal sphincteric function incorporated into the bulbar and penile urethra.

The kidneys and ureters are bilateral and paired, whereas the bladder and urethra are centrally placed and form a single structure. As a general principle, damage to a single kidney has minimal impact on the overall renal excretory function, provided the remaining kidney is normal. However, structural abnormalities of a single kidney or ureter may still predispose to infection and may be relevant to Tommy's presentation, as will be discussed later in the chapter.

Structure of the kidney

The functional renal tissue, known as the renal parenchyma, is loosely divided into the cortex and medulla. Each kidney contains about one million functional units, or nephrons, each consisting of a glomerulus and a tubule (Fig. 1.2). All nephrons have their glomeruli located in the cortex, which comprises the outer one-third of the kidney. Approximately 15% of nephrons arise in the deepest part of the cortex (the juxtamedullary area). The inner two-thirds of the kidney consists

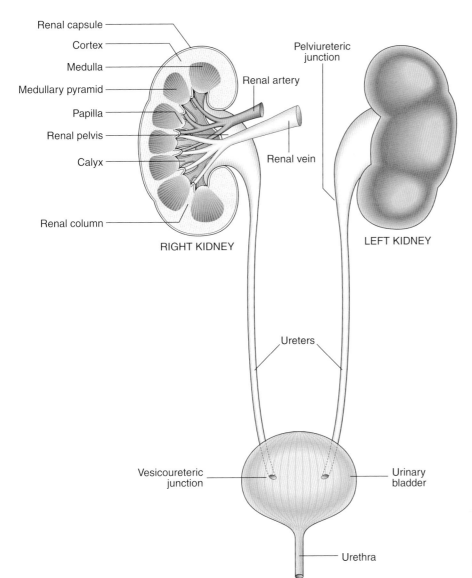

Renal capsule
Cortex
Medulla
Medullary pyramid
Papilla
Renal pelvis
Calyx

Renal column

RIGHT KIDNEY

Pelviureteric junction
Renal artery

Renal vein

LEFT KIDNEY

Ureters

Vesicoureteric junction

Urinary bladder

Urethra

Fig. 1.1 Principal anatomical components of the urinary tract, including features seen on a cut surface of the kidney.

of dark, striated areas known as pyramids, and the intervening renal columns, which together comprise the renal medulla. The apices of the pyramids are the renal papillae which project into the calyces, which are cup-like structures joining within the kidney to form the renal pelvis.

The glomerulus consists of a network of capillaries which invaginates the blinded end of the associated tubule, forming the Bowman's capsule. From this arises, in succession, the proximal tubule, the descending and ascending limbs of the loop of Henle, the distal tubule (including an early convoluted segment, a short connecting segment, and a late segment), the cortical collecting duct, the outer medullary and, subsequently, the inner medullary collecting duct, which opens at the tip of the renal papilla into the renal pelvis. At least one renal artery supplies each kidney, but often multiple renal

arteries are present. Each renal artery typically divides into five segments which subsequently branch up the sides of the pyramids, forming the interlobar arteries. At the junction of the medulla and cortex, the interlobar arteries divide into arcuate arteries. These then divide into interlobular arteries, giving rise to the afferent arterioles, which feed into the glomeruli. The vessels emanating from the glomeruli are known as the efferent arterioles. The majority of efferent arterioles form a capillary network surrounding the proximal tubules within the cortex. However, the juxtamedullary glomeruli give rise to long, meshed capillary networks, the vasa recta, which participate in the countercurrent mechanism of urinary concentration in the kidney (see Chapter 3).

The functional anatomy of the nephron, as it relates to glomerular filtration and tubular function, will be covered in Chapter 2.

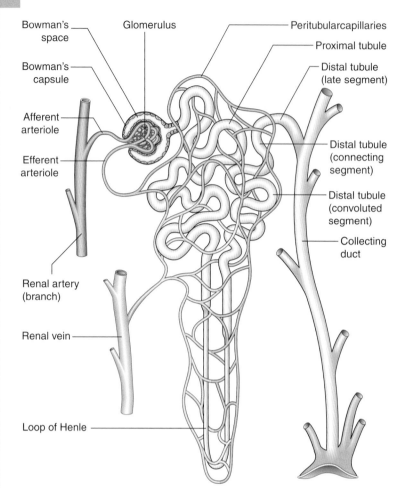

Bowman's space
Glomerulus
Peritubularcapillaries
Proximal tubule
Bowman's capsule
Distal tubule (late segment)
Afferent arteriole
Distal tubule (connecting segment)
Efferent arteriole
Distal tubule (convoluted segment)
Collecting duct
Renal artery (branch)
Renal vein
Loop of Henle

Fig. 1.2 Microscopic anatomy of the nephron showing a relationship between vascular and tubular structures. Note that the anatomical arrangement of the juxtaglomerular apparatus is not illustrated here (see Chapter 2).

Innervation of the urinary tract

The neurological supply to the kidney is largely involved with the regulation of vasomotor tone and hence renal blood flow. Sympathetic fibres originate in the lower splanchnic nerves and travel through the lumbar ganglion to the kidney. Stimulation of the sympathetic nervous system reduces renal blood flow by causing intrarenal vasoconstriction. It also enhances sodium reabsorption and stimulates the local renin-angiotensin system (see Chapter 2). However, denervated kidneys continue to function, usually without significant alterations in major functional parameters.

Both sympathetic and parasympathetic nerve fibres supply the ureter. The spinal segments subtending this supply are the L1 and L2 nerve roots. Sympathetic fibres arising from the renal and intermesenteric plexuses supply the upper part of the ureter, the superior hypogastric plexus supplies the middle part, and the inferior hypogastric plexus (lying at the side of the bladder and prostate) supplies the lower part. Vagal fibres supply parasympathetic innervation to the kidney and ureter via the coeliac plexus and pelvic splanchnic nerves.

The bladder and urethra are innervated by both parasympathetic and sympathetic pathways. The parasympathetic fibres arise in the second to the fourth sacral nerve roots. They function to stimulate bladder emptying, vasodilatation and penile erection. The bladder is less densely innervated by sympathetic fibres, which arise from T11-L3 nerve root segments. Stimulation of the sympathetic nervous system decreases bladder tone and inhibits the parasympathetic system. The base of the bladder and the proximal urethra are more richly innervated by sympathetic fibres which facilitate closure of the bladder neck and the proximal urethral sphincter. Drugs which block noradrenergic alpha-receptors (such as the antihypertensive drug prazosin) may inhibit peri-urethral sphincter function, resulting in incontinence. However, these drugs are useful for the relief of bladder outflow obstruction in benign prostatic hypertrophy and the relief of pain caused by ureteric spasm in the presence of an obstructing stone. The pelvic diaphragm is innervated by somatic motor neurones that allow voluntary contraction and relaxation. These neurones arise from the S2-S4 segments. The pelvic diaphragm is largely responsible for maintaining continence.

The bladder distends as urine is drained into it, resulting in the maintenance of low bladder pressures. This distension is essential to prevent urinary incontinence, which will occur if bladder pressures exceed the resistance of the urethral sphincter.

Micturition is therefore a complex process of coordinated stimulation of the parasympathetic nervous system which results in bladder contraction, and inhibition of sympathetic tone which results in sphincter relaxation. Voluntary control of voiding via the somatic nervous system is essential for regular drainage of the urinary tract to occur, as well as for social and hygiene reasons.

Embryology of the kidney and urinary tract

The development in utero of the urinary and reproductive tracts is closely related in both males and females. In the early stages of development, the urinary and genital ducts open into a common tract or cloaca, which is the dilated portion of the hindgut (Fig. 1.3). In males, the urinary and genital systems continue to share a common distal excretory duct system, that is, the distal urethra. However, in females, the primitive excretory duct undergoes regression and does not form part of the reproductive tract in adults.

The foetus produces and excretes urine into the allantoic or amniotic fluid sac, where it is reabsorbed. The excretory function of the kidney is not essential until after delivery. However, if developmental anomalies of the urinary tract occur, they are often detected on foetal ultrasound because of the obstructed passage of urine.

Human kidneys are derived from the sequential development of the embryonic mesodermal kidney structures: the pronephros, mesonephros, and metanephros. The pronephros degenerates in embryos of about 5 mm in length before full embryonic development. The mesonephros functions for a short time in utero as a provisional kidney before largely degenerating into the mesonephric tubule that persists to form part of the ductal system of the male reproductive tract. The metanephros remains and develops into the functional human kidney.

The excretory part of the metanephros develops from the portion of the nephrogenic cord caudal to the mesonephros. The functional human kidney is formed by invasion of the collecting tubules arising from the ureteric bud into the metanephric mesenchyme (see Fig. 1.3). The branching and invasion of the ureteric bud into the mesenchyme is highly structured, showing several repeating patterns of division. As a result of this invasion, each tip of the branching collecting tubule has a 'cap' of approximately 100 mesenchymal cells, which are induced to survive, proliferate, and undergo mesenchymal-epithelial transformation. These mesenchymal cells are effectively stem cells, capable of undergoing differentiation to form the glomeruli and

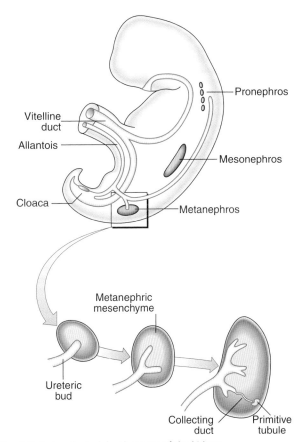

Fig. 1.3 Embryological development of the kidney.

the proximal, loop and distal tubular segments of the nephron. This then joins the collecting tubule derived from the ureteric bud. In addition, the metanephric mesenchyme produces non-epithelial cells that are stromal in distribution. The cells of the mesenchyme and ureteric bud also produce factors which control the growth, differentiation, and migration of endothelial, mesangial, smooth muscle and interstitial cells, as well as the deposition of the extracellular matrix. These nephrons are grouped into lobules, which persist until birth and then generally disappear. However, some lobulation may persist into adult life.

During the development of the metanephros, the kidneys undergo an upward change in position, which is due partly to the cranial growth of the ureter and partly to the diminution of body curvature. Fusion of the lower poles of the kidney during this ascent results in the defect known as horseshoe kidney.

The impact that interference with the normal development of the kidney will have on the kidney and urinary tract depends on the stage of development at which the insult occurs. During the first few weeks of embryogenesis, an injury or insult may result in a congenital absence of the kidney. If the same event occurs during the second or third month of gestation, parenchymal disruption may occur. This results in cystic or hypoplastic

Case 1.1 Urinary tract structure and infection: 2

Tommy's test results

Tommy's blood tests demonstrated a high white cell count of $23.0 \times 10^9/L$* with a neutrophilia (increased neutrophil count) of 85%, suggestive of bacterial sepsis. The overall filtration function of his kidneys was normal, reflected by a serum creatinine concentration of 45 μmol/L. Blood and urine cultures were taken, and he was started on intravenous fluids and antibiotics. His urine culture subsequently demonstrated a pure growth of *E. coli*.

This information confirms the suspicion that Tommy has a urinary infection. We now need to consider the following issues:

1. Is it normal for microorganisms to be present in the urinary tract?
2. What are the factors that protect against organisms entering and infecting the urinary tract?
3. How is urinary tract infection diagnosed?

*Values are outside the normal range; see Appendix.

Table 1.1 Clinical features of acute lower and upper urinary tract infection in adults

Lower urinary tract infection	Upper urinary tract infection*
Dysuria	Systemically unwell
Frequency	Fever and rigors
Suprapubic pain	Loin pain and tenderness
Malodorous urine	Nausea and vomiting
Haematuria	Hypotension or shock
Normal temperature	Features of lower urinary tract infection

*Acute infection of the upper urinary tract is also referred to as acute pyelonephritis.

kidneys or abnormalities of the collecting systems, such as urethral atresia, posterior urethral valves or calyceal distortion. Vestigial tubules derived from metanephric tissue which fail to join the collecting ducts may result in closed secretory loops and form renal cysts. Early separation of the ureteric bud into two or more parts may result in duplex collecting systems. Beyond the fourth month of gestation, an insult is unlikely to affect the pelvicalyceal system, as it is well defined anatomically by this stage.

The genetic and molecular basis of the processes that govern these regulated phases of renal embryonic development remain largely unknown. Several genes, which produce a variety of molecules that may be potential regulators of renal development, have been identified. Disruption of these processes may result in a variety of developmental renal abnormalities.

One consequence of abnormal development of urinary tract structures may be impaired urinary drainage and hence predisposition to infection. This possibility will be explored in relation to a febrile child (see Case 1.1:2).

Infection of the urinary tract

Infection of the urinary tract is one of the most common bacterial infections in both children and adults. The clinical features, diagnosis, treatment, and significance of the infection vary depending on the site of infection and the presence or absence of structural and/or functional abnormalities within the urinary tract. Recurrent urinary tract infection, when complicated by major structural abnormalities, can lead to chronic kidney disease. In the presence of underlying kidney disease, superimposed infection often accelerates functional decline. However, recurrent uncomplicated urinary infection, although common and debilitating, generally has no long-term deleterious consequences.

Asymptomatic bacteriuria

Asymptomatic bacteriuria is defined as the presence of bacteria in the urinary tract in the absence of symptoms attributable to infection. Contamination of urine by organisms normally residing in the female periurethral area at the time of collection is common. Thus, it is generally considered that 'significant bacteriuria' is present when 10^5 or more of the same organisms per millilitre are present in two voided urinary specimens (or in one 'in–out' catheter specimen) in a woman, or in one voided specimen in a man. In general, antibiotic treatment of asymptomatic bacteriuria is only indicated in the presence of factors leading to potentially complicated urinary infections (including pregnancy). In many circumstances, asymptomatic bacteriuria is a recurrent problem and antibiotic therapy may lead to antibiotic resistance that may cause infection to be more difficult to eradicate.

Acute urinary tract infection

Acute infection of the urinary tract can generally be divided on clinical grounds into upper or lower tract infection (Table 1.1).

The clinical presentation of UTI in children is much more variable and is frequently non-specific, as in Tommy's case. Thus, children may present with lethargy, vomiting, fever, poor weight gain, irritability, febrile convulsions, or gastrointestinal symptoms. Hence, the diagnosis should be considered in any sick infant or toddler.

Box 1.1 Underlying factors associated with 'complicated' urinary tract infection

Systemic conditions
Diabetes mellitus
Papillary necrosis (e.g. analgesic nephropathy)
Immunodeficient states (including immunosuppressive drug therapy)

Abnormal drainage of urine
Renal calculi
Urinary obstruction
Vesicoureteric reflux
Pelviureteric junction obstruction
Instrumentation of the urinary tract (including catheters)
Pregnancy

Box 1.2 Microbiological agents causing urinary tract infection

Community-acquired
Escherichia coli
Klebsiella spp.
Proteus mirabilis
Staphylococcus saprophyticus

Hospital-acquired
Escherichia coli
Klebsiella spp.
Citrobacter spp.
Enterobacter spp.
Pseudomonas aeruginosa
Enterococcus faecalis

Coagulase-negative
Staphylococcus spp.
Candida spp. *
* These are yeasts (fungi).

Another basis of classification is whether the infection is 'complicated' (by systemic or anatomical abnormalities; Box 1.1) or 'uncomplicated'.

Lower UTIs are particularly common in women, where they are generally localised to the bladder (cystitis). In adult men, the urethra and/or the prostate may be the primary site of infection. In the latter instances, the presence of a sexually transmitted disease should be considered, particularly if no overt infection is isolated on urine culture (see below).

Upper UTI is defined as an infection involving the kidney. As the renal pelvis is invariably involved in ascending infection, this is also referred to as acute pyelonephritis.

These arbitrary divisions have implications for treatment and prognosis and guide decisions regarding further investigation. If the kidneys and urinary tract are normal anatomically and functionally, infection is unlikely to result in significant kidney impairment, even when persistent and/or recurrent. However, if there is impaired kidney function, reduced systemic resistance to infection, or abnormal drainage of the urinary tract, an infection is likely to become complicated, with the risk of kidney damage, abscess formation, or septicaemia. As dilatation and impaired drainage of the urinary tract are inevitable in pregnancy, all urinary infections in pregnant women should be treated as a potentially complicated infection (see Chapter 11).

Aetiology and pathogenesis of urinary tract infection

There are numerous differences in the clinical features, response to therapy, and prognosis of UTIs according to the age of the patient, site of infection, and whether the infection is complicated or uncomplicated. However, the microbial aetiology of infections is similar throughout the urinary system regardless of the clinical setting.

Bacteria are by far the most common cause of urinary infection, with most other infecting organisms occurring in patients with underlying systemic illness (Box 1.2).

Escherichia coli accounts for approximately 85% of community-acquired and 50% of hospital-acquired urinary infections. However, almost every organism has been associated with UTI, especially in the immunocompromised inpatient population and in those with urological instrumentation. Organisms not traditionally regarded as urological pathogens may also occur in this population in whom natural host defence mechanisms are compromised. These organisms include lactobacilli, *Gardnerella vaginalis*, and mycoplasma species, including *Ureaplasma urealyticum*. Staphylococcal pyelonephritis (almost always *Staphylococcus aureus*) should always raise the possibility of haematogenous spread from distant foci as this is an unusual organism to colonise the periurethra and cause ascending infection.

Most episodes of urinary sepsis are caused by ascending infection, with a small percentage of upper urinary infections arising from the haematogenous (bloodborne) route. The vaginal introitus is normally colonised with a variety of non-virulent streptococci, staphylococci, and lactobacilli which are only occasionally responsible for urinary infection. Gram-negative bacteria which are much more likely to cause urinary infection normally reside in the bowel and colonise the introitus in a proportion of women. Factors thought to be responsible for periurethral colonisation by colonic bacteria and subsequent bacterial entry into the bladder include previous antibiotic therapy, the use of a diaphragm and spermicide for contraceptive purposes, and sexual activity. In

Box 1.3 Virulence factors of uropathogenic *E. coli*

Lower urinary tract

Rapid growth rate
Adhesion to uroepithelial cells (bacterial fimbriae)
Endotoxin production (lipopolysaccharide)

Upper urinary tract

Resistance to serum bactericidal activity
Siderophore and haemolysin production
Resistance to phagocytosis
Persistence of organism within the kidney

many instances, an alteration in sexual activity (either sexual partner or frequency of intercourse) will predispose to urinary infection in women.

Different factors operate to prevent urinary infection at each anatomical level in the urinary tract. The common uropathogens are able to overcome the normal host defence mechanisms that protect against urinary infection. The relative contribution of bacterial virulence factors to infection depends on the site of infection as well as the normality or otherwise of the urinary tract. In the presence of an anatomically abnormal urinary tract, organisms of low virulence may still be able to establish a significant infection. However, this is rarely the case if such organisms infect a structurally normal urinary tract. Under normal circumstances, bacteria introduced into the bladder are rapidly cleared by the constant urine flow, which serves to flush the bladder and dilute its contents. The direct antibacterial properties of the urine and the bladder mucosa, as well as urinary constituents (such as high osmolarity, urea and organic acids), inhibit bacterial growth in the urine. However, the presence of glucose and amino acids may facilitate bacterial growth. Prostatic secretions have bactericidal properties, and white cells within the bladder mucosa participate in local defence against infection.

Bacterial virulence factors have been best studied in *E. coli* (Box 1.3), where a limited number of serotypes have been found to be responsible for the majority of infections. Various antigenic factors have been identified which enhance the urovirulence of a particular strain.

The adherence of *E. coli* to urothelial cells is predominantly determined by bacterial fimbriae, which are filamentous processes projecting from the cell surface. In addition, the capsules of *E. coli* contain specific virulence factors. Capsular antigens possess antiphagocytic activity and are important when tissue invasion occurs. As iron is a necessary bacterial nutrient, mechanisms to chelate and scavenge iron efficiently (siderophores) confer increased pathogenicity. Similarly, bacterial haemolysin production, which facilitates the release of haem, increases iron scavenging and thus virulence.

Urease production by organisms such as *Proteus mirabilis*, *Proteus vulgaris*, and *Staphylococcus saprophyticus* is involved in tissue adherence and splitting urea into

carbon dioxide and ammonia. This urease activity results in urinary alkalinisation and precipitation of magnesium, ammonium, and phosphate. Thus, infection with these organisms often becomes complicated by stone formation (struvite).

Investigation of urinary tract infection

The laboratory diagnosis of UTI depends on microbiological confirmation of infection. This is usually taken to mean a bacterial count of greater than 10^5 colony-forming units (CFU) per millilitre. The technique of collection of the urine specimen is critical and the presence of epithelial cells in the urine sample is suggestive of contamination. In men, the collection of a midstream specimen is usually successful, and contamination is rare. In women, the introitus should be cleaned with saline (not antiseptic as this may inhibit bacterial growth and cause a falsely negative culture result). Midstream urine is collected with the labia spread apart. Collection in infants and children is difficult as adhesive bags are likely to become contaminated. In these circumstances, suprapubic aspiration is a safe alternative that provides a definitive diagnosis. Urine can be stored at 4°C for up to 48 h before culture.

Although the laboratory cut-off for significant infection is regarded as 10^5 CFU/mL, infection may be present when colony counts are between 10^2 and 10^5 CFU/mL, particularly in the case of less common organisms such as gram-positive bacteria and some fungi. Mixed cultures, particularly in the presence of low colony counts in females, are usually the result of contamination.

Because of the delay inherent in microbiological confirmation of UTI, urinalysis is often used as a first-line screen in individuals with symptoms suggestive of urinary infection (Fig. 1.4). Biochemical reagent strips will detect nitrites, which are produced by common uropathogens, and also leucocytes. The finding of pyuria (increased leucocyte excretion) does not always correlate with infection since it may occur with other causes of urogenital inflammation and in normal pregnancy. Microscopic haematuria and proteinuria on urinalysis may be indicative of urinary tract inflammation but are unreliable as markers of infection when additional renal or urinary tract pathological conditions are present. Urine microscopy may demonstrate red cells, white cells, and bacteria characteristic of infection. Evidence of white cell casts is suggestive of renal parenchymal infection. In patients presenting with systemic features of pyelonephritis, septicaemia is possible and, in this clinical setting, blood should be taken for culture.

In otherwise healthy sexually active women, isolated lower urinary infection in the absence of systemic or structural factors predisposing to complicated infection (see Box 1.1) requires no further investigation unless it is recurrent (more than three episodes per year). Urinary infection in males should be regarded as being potentially complicated, and underlying abnormalities of the urinary tract, particularly those causing obstruction of

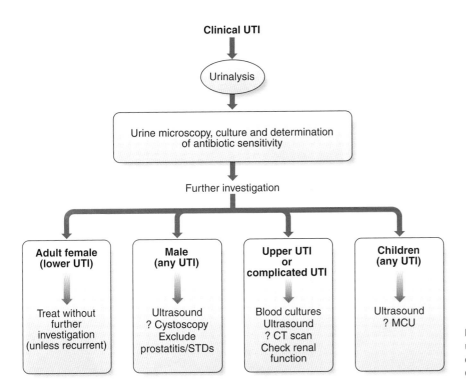

Fig. 1.4 Patterns of investigation in urinary tract infection. MCU, micturating cystourethrogram; STDs, sexually transmitted diseases; UTI, urinary tract infection.

urine flow, should be sought. In younger males, congenital abnormalities of the urinary tract predominate, including VUR and the presence of urethral valves, whilst in older males, bladder neck obstruction caused by prostatic hypertrophy or urethral stricture is more likely. In appropriate male patients, it is important also to exclude active prostatitis or sexually transmitted disease. Further imaging investigations are necessary in cases where structural abnormality in the urinary tract is suspected, as in any child with UTI or any patient with a complicated or upper UTI. (see Case 1.1:3)

Case 1.1

Urinary tract structure and infection: 3

The next step

The severity of the systemic features in Tommy's case suggests that an underlying abnormality of the urinary tract may account for the infection. Indeed, the above discussion would suggest that, if free drainage of the urinary tract existed, infection is unlikely to have taken hold, particularly in a male.

In light of Tommy's age, the most likely underlying cause is a congenital abnormality of the urinary tract. In an older person, acquired abnormalities of the urinary tract are more commonly found. The nature of the structural abnormality is often easily determined by simple imaging of the urinary tract. This raises the issue of what techniques are available to gain a view of the anatomy of the urinary tract in different clinical settings.

Imaging of the urinary tract

Renal ultrasound is the initial screening test used for imaging the urinary tract in children, in men, or in the presence of complicated infection. It will define whether urinary tract dilatation is present and whether the underlying kidney size and parenchymal thickness is normal (Fig. 1.5). The level of obstruction is suggested, but the result may not be definitive, and computed tomography (CT) may be indicated subsequently (Fig. 1.6). CT is rarely indicated in the acute setting of infection but is frequently performed as a follow-up investigation, especially where resolution is slow or incomplete. CT is also the best imaging modality if abscess formation is suspected, both to define the intrarenal mass as well as to monitor the response to therapy.

Intravenous pyelography (IVP) provides a functional and anatomical assessment of drainage of the urinary tract, particularly after correction of obstructive pathologic condition or in the investigation of pelvicalyceal disease (see Fig. 1.9). However, it is now rarely undertaken and has largely been superseded by CT and magnetic resonance imaging (Table 12.2), where these newer modalities are available.

A radionuclide blood flow scan is of use in assessing renal perfusion (see Chapter 10) and avoids exposure to potentially nephrotoxic contrast agents.

Cystoscopy (direct inspection of the interior of the bladder) should be performed if primary bladder or prostate pathology is suspected. It is rarely indicated in patients with urinary infections who have normal upper tracts demonstrated on ultrasound. If impaired bladder

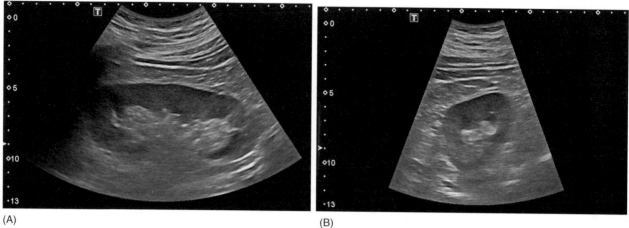

(A)　　　　　　　　　　　　　　　　　　　(B)

Fig. 1.5 Normal renal ultrasound (long axis (A) and transverse axis (B) views).

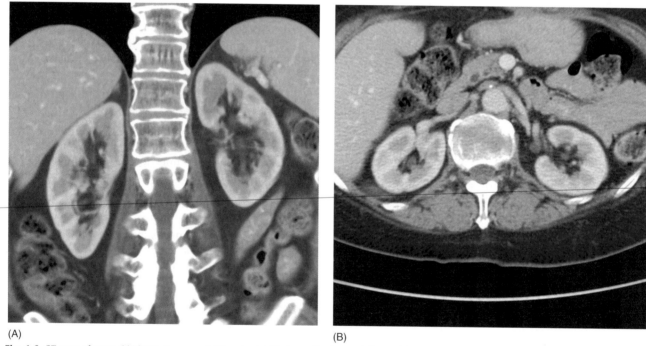

(A)　　　　　　　　　　　　　　　　　　　(B)

Fig. 1.6 CT scan of normal kidneys, in coronal (A) and axial (B) views. Corticomedullary differentiation is enhanced as a result of an injection of contrast agent.

function is suspected, urodynamic studies which record changes in pressure during bladder filling and emptying may be indicated.

All children presenting with urinary infection should be investigated with imaging of the urinary tract since up to 50% will be found to have a urological abnormality. In the majority of these children, VUR (Box 1.4) will be confirmed. In infants who are acutely unwell with pyelonephritis, both ultrasound and micturating cystourethrogram (MCU) should be performed. The MCU demonstrates the presence of backflow of urine from the bladder into the ureters during micturition (VUR). In older children, an MCU is not always considered necessary in the presence of a good quality ultrasound view of the upper urinary tract, with visualisation of the ureteric orifices and ureteric peristalsis. A radionuclide scan using dimercaptosuccinic acid (DMSA) is performed to detect renal parenchymal scarring (Fig. 1.7). This is not generally undertaken within 6 to 12 months of acute pyelonephritis to avoid false-positive results.

Vesicoureteric reflux

Vesicoureteric reflux (VUR) is caused by incompetence of the vesicoureteric junction. In most instances, the defect is a shortness of the submucosal segment because of lateral ectopia (displacement) of the ureteric orifice. This results in loss of the normal valve-like action associated with the oblique path of the terminal segment of the ureter through the bladder wall (Fig. 1.8).

In the majority of infants, VUR presents with a complicating urinary infection. However, signs localising the infection to the urinary tract may not always be present, especially in the very young. In males particularly, infection may not always occur, and more subtle signs of renal damage caused by retrograde urine flow (reflux nephropathy) may be present (see Box 1.4).

If enuresis (bed-wetting) persists until after primary school age (10 years), reflux should be excluded with renal ultrasonography. Enuresis in this setting is caused by the presence of residual urine after voiding as the upper urinary tract empties into the bladder and also by impaired tubular function with loss of the ability to concentrate the urine which leads to increased urine volumes. In adults, enuresis rarely persists but nocturia may be a prominent symptom.

It has recently been recognised that reflux nephropathy is inherited as an autosomal dominant condition. Thus current recommendations advise routine ultrasound in neonates of parents known to have reflux nephropathy independent of the grade of reflux in the affected parent. Recent research also suggests that a small and scarred kidney may be the primary congenital abnormality in at least some cases, with abnormalities of the vesicoureteric junction and associated or secondary development.

The diagnosis of VUR is based on demonstration of reflux on an MCU or real-time ultrasound. There may also be radiological findings of focal scarring in the kidneys, generally at the upper pole, with calyceal clubbing. If more severe VUR is present, the kidney may be diffusely damaged with generalised loss of parenchymal tissue (see Fig. 1.9).

VUR is the commonest underlying cause of hypertension in children and is associated with the presence of renal scarring. VUR may present in adults with moderate to severe hypertension without a history of

---

Box 1.4 Features of vesicoureteric reflux and reflux nephropathy

Vesicoureteric reflux

Ultrasound *in utero* (incidental finding)
Enuresis
Double voiding
Loin pain on micturition
Urinary tract infection
Family screening

Reflux nephropathy

Hypertension
Proteinuria
Renal impairment
Impaired urine concentration *with or without features of vesicoureteric reflux*

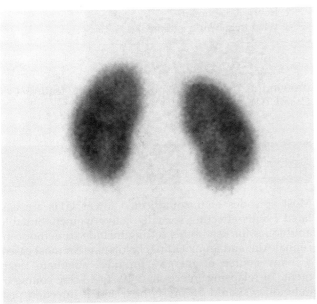

(A)

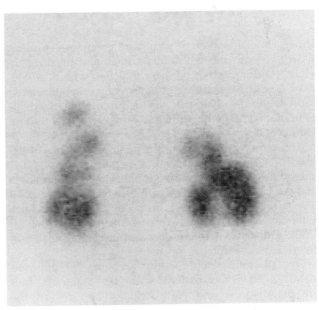

(B)

Fig. 1.7 (A) Normal dimercaptosuccinic acid (DMSA) renal scan; (B) DMSA renal scan showing multiple cortical defects and severe bilateral renal scarring, worse in the upper pole.

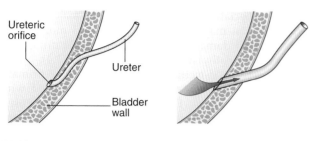

(A) Normal VUJ (B) Refluxing VUJ

Fig. 1.8 Vesicoureteric junction (VUJ): (A) normal; (B) defective, with reflux.

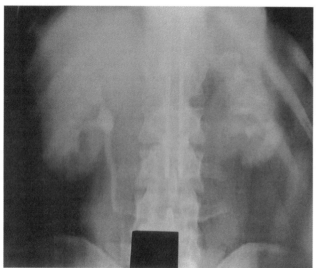

Fig. 1.9 Intravenous pyelogram showing gross scarring of left kidney, with clubbing of calyces' characteristic of reflux nephropathy. Normal right kidney and collecting system.

urinary infection. Renal calculi are commonly present in areas of scarring within the kidney and presumably relate to urinary stasis. Urinary infection with *P. mirabilis* or other urea-splitting organisms may be associated with staghorn calculi but, with appropriate early treatment of infection with antibiotics, this is a relatively rare complication.

Anti-reflux surgery to correct the incompetence of the vesicoureteric junction is not generally recommended unless severe reflux causing upper tract dilatation is present. Corrective surgery is not undertaken after 2 to 3 years of age. It has long been appreciated that once renal parenchymal scarring is present, even in unilateral reflux, anti-reflux surgery does not protect against progressive decline in renal function.

Overall, reflux nephropathy accounts for approximately 2% to 3% of patients with end-stage renal failure in Australia and New Zealand and 5% of the paediatric population with end-stage renal failure. Reflux nephropathy with progressive functional deterioration is characterised by hypertension and persistent

Diagnosis and management

Soon after admission, Tommy underwent renal ultrasonography, which showed that the right kidney was 2 cm smaller than the left, with generalised loss of cortical thickness. The pelvis and ureter were dilated down to the level of the vesicoureteric junction, but no obstruction was demonstrated. The right ureteric insertion into the bladder was laterally placed, and ureteric 'jets' (indicating a normal pulsatile flow of urine from the ureter to the bladder) were not seen. This was taken as evidence of an abnormality of the vesicoureteric junction on that side. No abnormality was observed in the left kidney, pelvis, or collecting system, and a normal left ureteric insertion and ureteric jets were noted.

After starting antibiotics (ceftriaxone), Tommy became afebrile with improved appetite over the ensuing 72 h. Intravenous antibiotics were continued for a total of 7 days, after which he was given oral cefaclor for a further week. Tommy was subsequently maintained on a preventative dose of trimethoprim/sulfamethoxazole at night. A repeat urine culture 3 weeks after his initial presentation was sterile.

It was recommended that his two siblings, aged 5 and 7 years, who were asymptomatic, should undergo urine culture screening and ultrasonography for the detection of vesicoureteric reflux.

It is clear that an underlying anatomical abnormality has contributed to Tommy's infection. Vesicoureteric reflux is one of the commonest congenital abnormalities of the urogenital tract. The following questions are likely to be raised by Tommy's parents and will be discussed:

1. What causes vesicoureteric reflux?
2. How is it diagnosed?
3. What treatment is indicated?

proteinuria, which is a poor prognostic feature (see Case 1.1:4).

Overview: treatment of urinary tract infections

Most episodes of uncomplicated lower UTIs are isolated events affecting sexually active women. Suitable antibiotics for use in this setting include trimethoprim, cephalexin, and amoxicillin/clavulanate. In most cases, a 3-day course of therapy provides adequate treatment. In relapsing infection, a 10- to 14-day course of antibiotics should be prescribed, and if infection persists or recurs, an investigation should be undertaken. Recurrent infection (more than three episodes per year) is best treated with prophylactic low-dose antibiotics.

Urinary tract structure and infection: 5

Follow-up

At review 12 months later, Tommy's urine remains sterile with no proteinuria, and his growth and milestones appear normal. His blood pressure is at the upper limit of normal at 90/60 mmHg. Repeat renal ultrasound is unchanged from that performed during the acute phase of his illness, although the right renal parenchyma is now less oedematous, and the kidney measures 2.5 cm smaller than the left. A DMSA scan is performed, which shows diffuse parenchymal cortical scars in the right kidney but none in the left kidney.

The management plan for Tommy is to maintain the prophylactic antibiotic until he is 5 years of age and then repeat the ultrasound and DMSA scan. In the absence of new scar formation, it is planned that antibiotics will be ceased at that stage. Regular follow-up of blood pressure and urinalyses are advised to detect any increase in urinary protein excretion.

His 7-year-old sister has sterile urine, but renal ultrasonography and subsequent DMSA scan are suggestive of a right upper pole scar. There is no ultrasound evidence of ongoing reflux, with ureteric peristalsis and ureteric jets appearing normal. The management plan is to have 6-monthly urinalyses and a repeat DMSA scan in 1 year. In the absence of infection and progressive renal scarring, her blood pressure and urinalysis will be monitored on a 2–3-yearly basis. The risks of infection in pregnancy and potential for developing hypertension, particularly in pregnancy, are explained to her mother for future information. The remaining sibling is normal.

However, in patients with a clear relation between infection and sexual activity, single-dose therapy after intercourse may be effective. Generally, follow-up cultures are not needed in otherwise uncomplicated urinary infections.

The treatment of acute upper UTI (acute pyelonephritis) is generally performed in a hospital. Intravenous (IV) fluids and empiric antibiotic treatment (e.g. intravenous third-generation cephalosporin such as ceftriaxone, with or without an aminoglycoside such as gentamicin) should be commenced before culture results become available. An appropriate oral antibiotic with good renal parenchymal penetration, such as amoxicillin/clavulanate or norfloxacin, may be substituted when the fever subsides. The total duration of antibiotic treatment is generally 2 weeks. If no significant improvement is observed within 48 h, the diagnosis and choice of antibiotic therapy should be reviewed, and imaging of the kidney undertaken to exclude obstruction or abscess (see Case 1.1:5).

History and examination of the renal system

A suggested approach to taking a history and examination of a person with suspected or known kidney disease is outlined in the clinical skills boxes on these topics in this chapter. There is also a video of a renal system examination available online (https://studentconsult.inkling.com/). The approach to a patient with suspected kidney disease needs to encompass most organ systems of the body – this includes taking a history and performing a physical examination. Whilst this approach does not fall neatly into a systems examination like the cardiovascular or abdominal examination, certain details need to be ascertained to enable a proper assessment. The clinical skills boxes outline a suggested approach. Much of the reasoning behind each of these assessments is outlined in the rest of this book, so we encourage you to review this section regularly.

Clinical skills 1.1 - Taking a history of kidney disease

When taking a history from a patient suspected or known to have kidney disease, it is important to ask about symptoms that may suggest a possible cause, conditions that are risk factors for kidney disease, symptoms caused by kidney disease or complications related to end-stage kidney disease. Try to elicit a time course to distinguish between acute and chronic disease, and with both, it is important to try to understand the impact of this disease on patients' work life, social life, family life, and general quality of life.

Symptoms to suggest a possible cause of kidney disease: haematuria, frothy urine, brown urine (that may suggest myoglobinuria or haemoglobinuria), smelly urine, dysuria or symptoms to suggest obstruction-hesitancy, weak urinary stream, double voiding, incontinence or nocturia. Note that nocturia can also occur because of a lack of urinary concentrating ability which is an early sign of chronic kidney disease itself.

Risk factors for kidney disease: diabetes, hypertension, recurrent UTIs, kidney stones, gout, nephrotoxic medications, autoimmune disease, hepatitis B and C, and HIV. Commonly associated diseases such as cardiovascular disease (heart disease, stroke, peripheral vascular disease), cancer (especially kidney, bladder and prostate), blood dyscrasias (myeloma, lymphoma, leukaemia), and venous and arterial thrombosis

Clinical skills 1.1 - Taking a history of kidney disease – cont'd

should be sought. Ask about a family history of kidney disease, in particular conditions such as polycystic kidney disease and Alport's syndrome (associated with deafness). Also, if the patient has had a kidney biopsy or imaging investigations, this would be useful information as would information with regard to treatments received and discussions about plans for treating end-stage kidney disease, if appropriate.

Symptoms caused by kidney disease: Fluid overload causes shortness of breath, peripheral oedema, or weight gain, whilst dehydration causes thirst, dizziness, and weight loss. Symptoms of anaemia or uraemia include fatigue, anorexia,

nausea, pruritus, metallic taste, restless legs, insomnia, or weight loss. Chest pain worse with inspiration and supine posture are commonly associated with pericarditis, a feature of uraemia, and neuropathic symptoms (e.g. numbness in feet and hands) can be because of a sensorimotor neuropathy seen in people with long standing kidney disease. Abdominal pain may be seen in certain types of kidney disease, such as infected or bleeding renal cyst, renal mass, infection, or bladder distension associated with retention. Bone pain or fractures may be seen. Menstrual disturbances may be seen in moderate to severe forms of kidney disease.

Clinical skills 1.2 - Examination of a patient with kidney disease

Because the kidney system affects most parts of the body in some way, the examination of the renal system is general in nature. Nevertheless, there are some features that need to be specifically checked.

- General inspection: bruising, scratch marks, sallow complexion, haemodialysis access (look for an arteriovenous (AV) fistula on the patient's arms or legs or a temporary line in the neck).
- Take the blood pressure (see the Clinical skills box in Chapter 10) and note other vital signs.
- Peripheral examination: nails (leuconychia, Muehrcke's nails), palmar crease pallor, fistula, scars, uraemic frost.
- Eyes: fundoscopy looking for diabetic or hypertensive retinopathy.
- Face/neck: mucous membranes, assess jugular venous pressure.

- Abdominal exam: inspection looking for scars, Tenckhoff catheter, transplanted kidney, or large mass (polycystic kidney).
- Abdominal exam: palpate for abdominal masses (polycystic kidney) or transplanted kidney. Ballot the kidneys (see the Clinical skills box in Chapter 13) and assess for renal angle tenderness. Auscultate for renal bruits.
- Percuss and palpate for the bladder.
- Ask about weight: increases in weight can be a sign of fluid overload.
- Check for oedema (ankle/sacral) and auscultate the chest for evidence of pulmonary congestion. (See Clinical skills box in Chapter 3)
- Check the urine for blood, protein. Centrifuge the urine and examine the urine under microscopy for casts and dysmorphic red blood cells.

Summary

1. The urinary tract is made up of the kidneys, ureters, bladder, and urethra. The glomeruli and initial parts of the kidney tubule are largely derived from the metanephros. The collecting ducts, derived from the ureteric bud, invade the developing metanephros to form a functional kidney.
2. Upper UTIs usually present with loin pain, whereas lower UTIs present with bladder symptoms such as dysuria and urinary frequency. Both can present with fever and discoloured urine.
3. The most common organisms commonly associated with urinary infections are gram-negative bacteria, with other organisms capable in people with underlying structural abnormalities of the urinary tract. Infection occurs because of an imbalance between 'defence' (hostile environment of urine

because of acidity, high urea levels and others, preservation of normal urinary tract structure) and 'attack', which make these organisms uropathogenic (e.g. fimbriae found on *E. coli* and urease found on *Proteus*).

4. The most appropriate imaging techniques for the urinary tract when structural abnormalities are suspected include ultrasound and CT scan.
6. Treatment of upper and lower UTIs includes antibiotics and supportive treatment with hydration (oral and IV). Upper UTIs often require IV therapy and therefore hospitalisation. An important component of management is the investigation of the underlying cause of UTIs.
7. The approach to history and examination of a patient with kidney disease utilises a thorough systems-based approach.

Self-assessment case study

A 24-year-old woman presents at 28 weeks gestation with frequency and dysuria. On examination, she looks relatively well. She is afebrile, but her blood pressure is elevated at 145/95 mmHg. She has mild suprapubic tenderness but no loin tenderness. Urinalysis and subsequent culture are consistent with UTI, and cephalosporin treatment is prescribed.

Upon review of her antenatal history, asymptomatic bacteriuria had been detected at her booking-in visit at 8 weeks' gestation. This was treated with a 7-day course of antibiotics. A follow-up urine culture was not performed. Her blood pressure had been 140/95 at both 8 and 12 weeks' gestation and 140/90 at 18 weeks. At a visit at 12 weeks' gestation, no urinary infection was detected and urinalysis demonstrated proteinuria +.

Her past history included an episode of kidney infection at age 11 years, at which time a horseshoe kidney was diagnosed. She was told that her kidney functioned normally, and no specific follow-up was recommended. She had enuresis till the age of 12 years, as did her sister, and has had nocturia on a regular basis for as long as she can recall.

After studying this chapter, you should be able to answer the following questions:

Q1. What are the key clinical features suggestive of underlying urinary tract abnormality in this case?

Q2. What tests would have been done to confirm infection in this young woman?

Q3. Is it likely that she currently has a lower or upper urinary tract infection? What factors predispose her to developing a complicated (or upper urinary tract) infection?

Q4. What recommendations would you make about her current treatment and what follow-up investigations would you perform after the delivery of her child?

Self-assessment case study answers

A1. The clinical features suggestive of an underlying urinary tract abnormality are:

- Kidney infection in childhood (and any urinary infection in men or in women who are not sexually active) can suggest the presence of underlying abnormalities in the structure or function of the urinary tract.
- Asymptomatic bacteriuria and subsequent failure to eradicate infection suggests abnormalities in the drainage of the urinary tract. Although this may occur in normal pregnancy, it does not usually result in bacteriuria or infection.
- Nocturia can occur because of failure to empty the urinary bladder adequately (e.g. as occurs in reflux nephropathy) or because of damage to the distal tubules of the kidney resulting in failure to concentrate the urine (see Chapters 2 and 3). This results in an increased volume of urine, often manifesting as enuresis in children and nocturia in adults.
- As structural abnormalities of the kidney are often familial, the presence of symptoms suggestive of a similar problem in her siblings increases the likelihood of an anatomical defect being found.
- The presence of hypertension suggests that renal parenchymal disease may be present.

A2. Infection would initially be suggested by the finding of blood, protein, nitrites, and leucocytes in the urine on urinalysis. An increased white cell excretion normally occurs in pregnancy, and there is also a marginal increase in normal urinary protein excretion. However, the additional abnormalities do not occur unless an infection is present. Urine microscopy would have demonstrated bacteria and red and white cells. Over 10^5 bacteria, which cause a 'pure growth' on urine culture, are normally present in clinically significant infections. However, even smaller numbers of bacteria, when in a pure growth, may be significant.

A3. She is likely to have lower urinary tract infection as dysuria and frequency are bladder and urethral symptoms, and her tenderness localises to the bladder. Classic features of upper urinary infection – fever, loin tenderness, and being generally 'unwell' – are not present. Lower urinary tract infection is more likely to develop into an upper urinary infection in pregnancy because of incomplete bladder emptying and/or partial obstruction of the urinary tract caused by the uterus encroaching on the bladder. Ureteric contraction resulting in pooling of the urine in a dilated urinary tract also occurs in normal pregnancy. The presence of a horseshoe kidney is an additional factor resulting in impaired urinary drainage. Asymptomatic bacteriuria and recurrent infection increase the risk of ascending infection as this may be present without necessarily causing symptoms; pyelonephritis may be an initial symptom.

A4. Because of recurrent infection and the risk of pyelonephritis in pregnancy, which may increase uterine irritability and precipitate premature labour, prophylactic antibiotics should be prescribed. After the urine is rendered sterile with a full 2-week course of oral antibiotics, a single night-time dose of either a cephalosporin or amoxicillin (both of which are safe for the developing foetus) should be administered until after delivery. Routine urine culture is recommended on a monthly basis and, if breakthrough infection occurs, a full course of antibiotics, determined by the sensitivity of the organisms and the safety of the foetus, should be prescribed. Blood pressure should be treated as she is at high risk for pre-eclampsia (exacerbation of hypertension) later in pregnancy. After delivery, her baby should be screened for abnormalities of the urinary tract, and she should be warned that if her baby has an unexplained febrile illness, urine infection should be considered. She should have further renal imaging, but not sooner than 3 months after delivery. If imaging is performed before this time, dilatation of the urinary tract owing to pregnancy rather than because of intrinsic renal disease may complicate the interpretation.

Self-assessment questions and answers

Q1. Can you describe the major anatomical components of the urinary tract?

A1. The major anatomical components of the urinary tract are two kidneys, two ureters, bladder, and urethra. Renal artery, veins, nerves, and the ureter enter (and/or leave) the kidney through the hilum.

Q2. Describe the embryological derivation of the major structures of the kidney.

A2. The glomeruli and initial parts of the kidney tubule are largely derived from the metanephros. The collecting ducts, derived from the ureteric bud, invade the developing metanephros to form a functional kidney. The metanephros also forms the additional components of the kidney, i.e. the mesangial cells, which support the glomerular capillaries, endothelial cells, smooth muscle cells, and matrix components.

Q3. Describe the mechanisms that normally protect the urinary tract from infection.

A3. Urinary infection is normally prevented by the continuous unobstructed flow of urine, and a hostile biochemical environment, i.e. high osmolarity, acidic pH, and high urea concentration. Local host defences also include white cells within the bladder mucosa and prostatic secretions that have bactericidal properties.

Q4. What are the principles of treatment of uncomplicated lower urinary tract infection and upper urinary tract infection?

A4. In lower urinary tract infection, a precipitating cause should be sought (e.g. contraceptive diaphragm use, altered sexual activity) and appropriate advice given. A high fluid intake is recommended and a short course of antibiotics (3 days) is generally sufficient to eradicate infection. Dysuria may be alleviated by alkalinisation of the urine with a bicarbonate-based medication in tablet or solution.

Upper urinary tract infection often requires analgesia, intravenous fluids, and appropriate antibiotic treatment (5 days IV and subsequent oral treatment) for 2 weeks. Imaging of the urinary tract is generally indicated after treatment of an acute infection.

BODY FLUIDS, NEPHRON FUNCTION, AND DIURETICS

2

Chapter objectives

After studying this chapter, you should be able to:

- Describe the normal distribution and composition of body fluids.

- Understand how the clinical syndromes of hypovolaemia and hypervolaemia occur and consider causes and clinical features.

- Use the worksheet found in the accompanying e-book to understand sodium transport mechanisms that are found throughout the nephron.

- Use the worksheet to consider sodium regulation across the nephron and how each part of the nephron plays a different role.

- Use the worksheet to describe the site and mechanism of action of commonly used diuretic drugs.

- Outline some common disturbances of sodium and potassium balance.

Introduction

The main function of the kidney is not 'to produce urine' (this is an inconvenient byproduct rather than a biological necessity) but to regulate the volume and composition of the body fluids within narrow limits. Whilst the best known task performed by the kidney is filtration of the blood by the glomerulus, this is just the first step in a sequence of actions whereby the functional unit of the kidney, the nephron, responds to disturbances in the volume and composition of the circulating fluids by altering the volume and composition of the tubular filtrate. This results in the excretion of urine. In this chapter, we will be exploring the mechanisms by which the nephron is able to alter the composition and volume of the urine in order to maintain the homeostasis of the blood.

Whilst many types of kidney disease can interfere with these nephron processes, significant alterations can be produced even in a person with normal kidneys by pharmacological agents, which interfere with the normal physiological mechanisms operating in the nephron. As illustrated by the case discussed in this chapter, this can have serious implications for the volume and electrolyte composition of the plasma. See Case 2.1:1.

Body fluid and electrolyte distribution

Several features of Joanne's history and physical examination suggest that her total body fluid volume is reduced. First, her symptoms of light-headedness and near-fainting attacks suggest that her cardiovascular system is unable to maintain perfusion of her brain, especially when she is upright. This inference is confirmed on physical examination, where it is found that she has a lowish lying blood pressure which falls further on standing, accompanied by a marked increase in her pulse rate. These features are suggestive of activated sympathetic nervous system responses to maintain her cardiac output in the face of a low circulating fluid volume. Her dry mouth and flaccid skin are suggestive of depletion of mucosal and tissue water, consistent with dehydration.

A summary of clinical features of hypovolaemia (sometimes loosely called dehydration, which strictly refers to a pure water deficit) contrasted with features typically found in hypervolaemia (also called fluid overload) is given in Table 2.1. As will be explained further below, these disturbances come about more through underlying disturbances of body sodium content than from primary changes in body water.

Case 2.1 — Body fluids and nephron function: 1

Fluid and electrolyte depletion

Joanne Smithfield is a 19-year-old woman who presents to her family doctor complaining of weakness and light-headedness. These symptoms have been troubling her for some 6 months, but in the last week, she has become more concerned as she has had several near-fainting episodes at work. These attacks are usually initiated by getting up rapidly from her desk, which makes her feel light-headed until she sits or lies down again. She has also noticed increasing difficulty walking up the stairs in her block of flats, where she lives with a girlfriend on the second floor. She attributes this to weakness in her legs, though she had previously been a strong runner at school.

Joanne's past medical history is unremarkable. Her menarche (commencement of menstruation) was at age 11 years, and her periods have been regular in timing and moderate in volume. She mentioned that she had gained too much weight as an adolescent but considered that this was now 'under control'.

Her family history includes hypertension and heart failure, diagnosed recently in her father, but her mother is well at age 48 years and is a fitness instructor. She has a younger sister who is a keen athlete. Joanne smokes 10 cigarettes/day and drinks a little alcohol after work on some days and on weekends. Her only medications are occasional laxatives when she gets constipated, and 'fluid tablets' to remove puffiness around her ankles which she thinks makes her look unattractive.

On physical examination, Joanne looks well though a little tired. She takes a few moments to stand up from her chair and steadies herself against the wall after doing so. Her tongue and mouth appear rather dry, and her skin feels quite doughy. Her blood pressure is 105/70 lying, 95/70 sitting, 85/65 standing. The pulse rate increases from 85 beats/min lying to 105 beats/min standing. The heart sounds are normal, and the lung fields are clear. Abdominal examination is unremarkable, although some stretch marks are noted. Neurological examination reveals normal cranial nerves but moderate weakness proximally in the upper and lower limbs. Reflexes and sensory testing are normal.

At the end of the examination, Joanne is questioned further about her use of diuretic tablets. She confesses that lately, she has been taking one or two furosemide (frusemide; Lasix) tablets daily, as she finds this helps to keep her weight down and avoid swelling around her ankles and hips. She initially obtained these from her father but subsequently got them from a friend who was prescribed them by her family doctor for premenstrual swelling.

In response to this presentation, we can ask the questions:

1. What physiological disturbances are causing Joanne's symptoms?
2. How might these disturbances have come about?

Table 2.1 Clinical features of hypovolaemia and hypervolaemia

	Hypovolaemia	Hypervolaemia
Symptoms	Thirst	Ankle swelling
	Dizziness on standing	Breathlessness
	Weakness	Abdominal swelling
Signs	Low JVP	Oedema
	Postural hypotension	Raised JVP
	Tachycardia	Pulmonary crepitations
	Dry mouth	Pleural effusion
	Reduced skin turgor	Ascites
	Reduced urine output	Hypertension
	Weight loss	(sometimes)
	Confusion, stupor	Weight gain

JVP, jugular venous pressure.

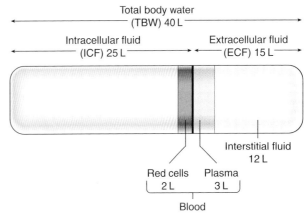

Fig. 2.1 Compartments of distribution of total body water. Approximate volumes (in litres) are shown for an average adult.

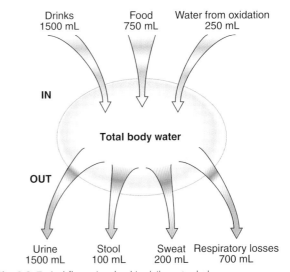

Fig. 2.2 Typical fluxes involved in daily water balance.

Since we suspect that something has depleted Joanne's body of fluid, we need to ask this question: how is water normally distributed within the body, and what is the composition of the fluid in different body compartments?

Body fluid compartments

The total body water content for a typical adult is approximately 60% of the lean body mass, that is, about 40 litres in an average 70 kg man. This can be determined by studying the dilution of marker substances which are known to distribute into all compartments of the body water.

The most familiar fraction of body fluid, namely the blood, represents a relatively small compartment of the total body water. Indeed, Fig. 2.1 shows that some 62.5% of the total body water is actually located inside cells (the intracellular fluid or ICF), whilst 37.5% is in the extracellular fluid (ECF) compartment. Furthermore, the plasma component of the blood accounts for a relatively small part (around 20%) of the ECF, with the remainder being distributed as interstitial fluid (ISF) within the various organs and tissues of the body but outside the cells. It can also be seen from Fig. 2.1 that the blood is actually composed in part of ECF (the plasma component) and in part ICF (the red cells).

In a normal individual, the volumes in the various body fluid compartments are remarkably constant in the face of somewhat variable water intake from one day to another. This constancy, an example of the homeostasis of the body's internal environment, is dependent on several finely tuned regulatory mechanisms which will be outlined in this and the next chapter and in other books in this series. In brief, a state of equilibrium (or balance) is achieved such that the net intake of water, largely by the mouth under normal circumstances, is matched by the total losses through the skin, lungs, gut, and kidneys. Typical volumes involved in these fluxes on a daily basis are shown in Fig. 2.2. It is important to understand that the major control mechanism for adjusting water loss

from the body to match daily water intake resides in the kidney. The kidney has a highly regulated capacity to vary the daily output of urine, whilst losses from the other sites are largely fixed.

Body fluid composition

There are important differences in the solute composition of the various compartments of body fluid, and these have major implications for normal cell metabolism and for the normal function of the circulatory and neuromuscular systems.

The major features of the chemical make-up of the ICF and the ECF (the latter having two major subdivisions, the plasma and the ISF) are shown in Fig. 2.3.

In brief, the main distinction between the ICF and the ECF is that the dominant cation in the ECF is sodium (Na$^+$), whilst in the ICF, it is potassium (K$^+$). Chloride and bicarbonate make up most of the balancing anions in the ECF, whilst in the ICF, the principal negative charges are carried by phosphate and other organic

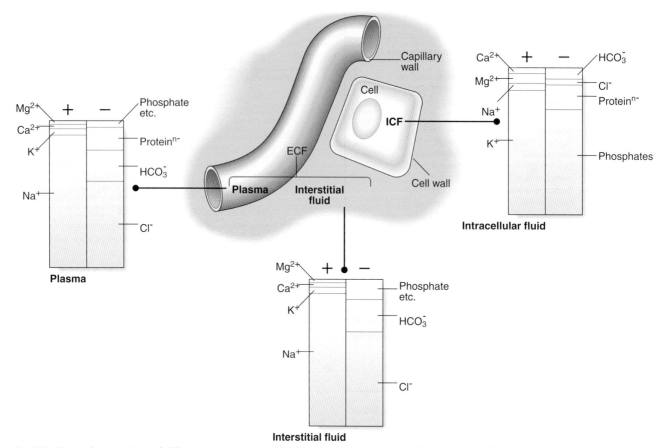

Fig. 2.3 Chemical composition of different compartments of body water. ECF, extracellular fluid; ICF, intracellular fluid.

anions. In addition, there is an important contribution to the intracellular anion pool from negative charges on the many cellular proteins contained in that compartment. There is normally a zero net flux of water across the cell membrane, that is, the ECF and ICF are in 'osmotic equilibrium'.

The mechanism for establishing and maintaining this substantial gradient for cations between the interior and exterior of cells is the membrane-bound sodium-potassium 'pump' (Na,K-activated ATPase). This ubiquitous active transport carrier uses energy derived directly from the hydrolysis of ATP to extrude three sodium ions from the cell for every two potassium ions it takes up from the ECF. The pump itself is thus 'electrogenic' and contributes towards generating the inside-negative membrane potential of the cell. A more significant contribution, however, comes from the back-diffusion of intracellular potassium ions to the cell exterior through potassium channels present in the cell membrane.

The significance of the gradient for Na and K maintained across cell membranes in all body tissues is profound. First, high intracellular K concentrations are essential for the normal operation of many enzyme systems which drive cell metabolism. Second, the basis of electrical excitability of neuromuscular and cardiac membranes is the presence of steep concentration gradients for Na^+ and K^+ across these membranes. Third, the

capacity of epithelia which line interfaces between the body and the exterior, to carry out net transepithelial solute transport depends on the maintenance of Na^+ and K^+ gradients in cells of these tissues. In the last case, however, the pump units are asymmetrically distributed in opposing cell membrane surfaces (illustrated for the kidney later in this chapter).

Another important distinction is that existing between the composition of the plasma and ISF components of the ECF. As shown in Fig. 2.3, the main difference here is that the plasma, but not the ISF, contains a substantial concentration of proteins comprising both serum albumin as well as a spectrum of globulins.

The mechanism for maintaining this protein differential within the subsections of the ECF is the presence of a permeability barrier at the capillary wall, which largely prevents the movement of proteins out of the capillaries under normal circumstances.

The significance of this protein concentration gradient is that it makes an important contribution to the balance of forces across the capillary wall (specifically to the colloid osmotic – or oncotic – pressure of the plasma), favouring fluid retention within the capillaries, thus maintaining an adequate circulating plasma volume. The effect of disturbance of this gradient will be illustrated in the discussion of oedema states in Chapter 6 of this volume.

Box 2.1 Causes of hypovolaemia and hypervolaemia

Hypovolaemia

- **Gastrointestinal sodium loss**
  e.g. vomiting, diarrhoea, nasogastric suction
- **Skin sodium loss**
  e.g. excessive sweating, burns
- **Renal sodium loss**
  e.g. diuretics, mineralocorticoid deficiency, tubulointerstitial disease
- **Internal sequestration**
  e.g. bowel obstruction, peritonitis, pancreatitis, crush injury
- **Haemorrhage**

Hypervolaemia

- **Iatrogenic**
  e.g. salt loading (oral or intravenous)
- **Renal sodium retention in generalised oedema states**
  e.g. congestive cardiac failure, cirrhosis, nephrotic syndrome
- **Renal sodium retention in renal failure**
  e.g. acute and chronic kidney disease (usual case)
- **Renal sodium retention in primary mineralocorticoid excess**
  e.g. Conn's syndrome (note no oedema)

Central importance of sodium for stability of the circulation

From the above discussion, it is clear that sodium is the dominant ionic species in the ECF since, together with its accompanying anions, it accounts for over 95% of the solute present in this fluid compartment. This is equivalent to saying that sodium is responsible for nearly all of the osmotic activity in the ECF (the 'oncotic' pressure attributable to plasma proteins, referred to above, is much smaller, though it is important as a differential osmotic force across capillary membranes). Thus, when water is added to the body, the amount held in the ECF is largely determined by the body's sodium content since the great majority of sodium ions are confined to the ECF compartment.

It is therefore apparent that factors which deplete the body of sodium will be associated with a low ECF volume (and hence of circulating plasma), whilst sodium retention is associated with expanded ECF volume. A summary of the causes of hypovolaemia and hypervolaemia based on sodium disturbances is given in Box 2.1. Note that pure disturbances in body mechanisms for regulating water itself are relatively uncommon causes of these conditions but are more likely to produce changes in plasma sodium concentration and osmolality (see Chapter 3).

Functional anatomy of the nephron

In fundamental terms, the kidney provides a site of interface between the circulating blood and the outside

Case 2.1 Body fluids and nephron function: 2

A probable culprit

So far, we can deduce from the cardiovascular clues in the history and physical examination that Joanne has probably experienced a reduction in the circulating component of the ECF, namely, the plasma. The dryness of her mouth and laxity of her skin suggests that other tissue fluid compartments are also depleted of water.

Whilst several causes for this situation may be considered, in this case, we have the information that she has been taking a drug which is intended to cause the kidneys to excrete higher than normal volumes of urine, causing her total body water content to be reduced.

Several new questions now arise related to the role of the kidney in the origin of Joanne's problem, namely:

a How does the kidney normally make urine?
b How has the diuretic drug interfered with these processes to lead to body fluid depletion?

world. At this interface, several regulatory processes occur which allow for a finely tuned response by the kidney to signals concerning the volume and composition of the circulating plasma. The urine that is excreted from the body is therefore a by-product of these processes, necessary to maintain homeostasis of plasma volume and composition.

As outlined in Chapter 1, the functional unit in which these interchanges are carried out within the kidney is the nephron. It is a microscopic structure consisting of a glomerulus, or 'small ball' of capillaries derived from the renal arterial supply, closely associated with an elongated tube-like structure (the tubular system) which is lined by a single layer of epithelial cells. In brief, the glomerulus is responsible both for filtering blood to form an ultrafiltrate and for ensuring that various proteins and cells are excluded from the filtrate. The renal tubule is responsible for modifying the filtrate to ensure that the final product of urine contains the correct amount of electrolytes and water to maintain plasma homeostasis.

As shown schematically in Fig. 2.4, we must consider three global aspects of glomerular and tubular function to understand the function of the kidney, as outlined below, and thereby understand how different types of pharmacological interventions and pathological processes impact the function of the kidney.

Glomerular filtration

Glomerular filtration is the process whereby a clear fluid is produced from the blood perfusing the glomerulus at the beginning of each nephron. This ultrafiltration process occurs largely as a result of the hydrostatic pressure in the arterial tree generated by the heart and is described in more detail in Chapter 5. The ultrafiltrate so produced contains electrolytes and small

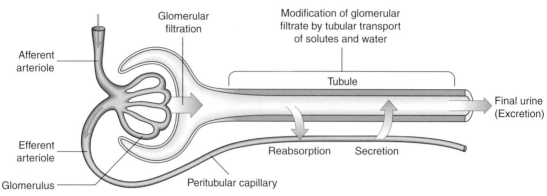

Fig. 2.4 Functional anatomy of the nephron.

solutes in plasma-like concentrations and constitutes the 'primary' fluid from which the final excreted urine is derived.

Glomerular filtration barrier

The glomerular filtration barrier is a three layered interface between the blood in the glomerular capillaries and the tubules. This barrier ensures that blood cells and macromolecules such as proteins are excluded from the ultrafiltrate and remain in the blood. This barrier and pathological processes that can interfere with its function, resulting in blood or protein in the ultrafiltrate and ultimately the urine, is explored in more detail in Chapter 6.

Tubular modification of ultrafiltrate

The renal tubule alters the volume and composition of the glomerular filtrate by transport processes carried out along the length of the tubular system. The single layer of epithelial cells that lines the renal tubules is responsible for fine-tuning the ultrafiltrate such that fluid and electrolytes that are required are reabsorbed back into the bloodstream and those that need to be excreted remain or are secreted into the urine.

The ultrafiltrate that enters the renal tubule is virtually free of large proteins and blood cells but has an electrolyte composition and osmolality similar to plasma. The task of the renal tubule is to ensure that the volume and composition of urine are appropriate to maintain homeostasis of the volume and composition of the plasma. This is done by appropriately altering the ultrafiltrate by transport processes carried out along the length of the tubular system. The dominant modification overall is the reabsorption of the great majority (over 99%) of the filtered fluid, together with most of its solute content (notably sodium). However, some electrolytes and many 'foreign' organic molecules undergo transport *into* the tubular fluid, a process called secretion. The final urine excreted from the kidneys reflects the net effect of all these tubular transport processes.

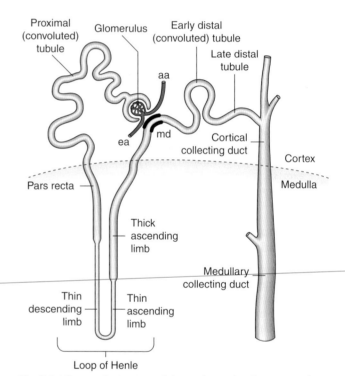

Fig. 2.5 Microscopic structure of the nephron, showing names of successive tubular segments. Refer to Fig. 1.2 for details of vascular elements. aa, afferent arteriole; ea, efferent arteriole; md, macula densa.

Nephron segments

A more anatomically detailed view of the tubular structures comprising the nephron is given in Fig. 2.5. Each of the kidney's one million nephrons has its glomerulus located in the renal cortex (see Chapter 1). Blood is delivered through a series of branches of the renal artery until it enters each glomerulus via an afferent arteriole. After breaking up into the capillary loops constituting the glomerulus, the blood emerges via an efferent arteriole which itself gives rise to the network of peritubular capillaries. These eventually join to take the blood away from the kidney via the renal vein. The vascular structures are shown in more detail in Fig. 1.2.

The segments of the tubular system attached to each glomerulus are named, in order, the proximal tubule, the loop of Henle, the distal tubule, and the collecting duct. Each segment consists of a single layer of specialised epithelial cells adapted to perform particular transport functions. As we explore these segments, it will become clear how the structure and layout of the segments as well as their specialised epithelial cells are designed to allow for their unique functions.

The **proximal tubule** is some 2 to 3 mm long. It forms several turns, or convolutions, before descending in a straight segment (pars recta) down into the outer medulla. Its cells are characterised by a prominent brush border consisting of numerous elongated processes arising from the apical (lumen-facing) cell membrane. Many mitochondria lie between the extensive invaginations of the basolateral (blood-facing) membrane.

The **loop of Henle** descends from the outer medulla a variable distance into the inner medulla, going deepest for loops arising from nephrons having their glomeruli located in the inner cortex (the juxtamedullary nephrons). It consists of a thin descending limb and, after a hairpin turn, a shorter thin ascending segment, both of which comprise flat cells with few mitochondria and little membrane amplification. The cells of the thick ascending limb, in contrast, are larger and contain abundant mitochondria and extensive basolateral infoldings, suggestive of a role in active ion transport.

The **distal tubule** starts within the cortex at the point where the thick ascending limb passes by the glomerulus of the related nephron, where it forms the macula densa (see later in this chapter). The early part of the distal tubule is convoluted, with metabolically active cells. After a short connecting segment, the late distal tubule is straight and joins with similar segments from adjacent nephrons to form the **cortical collecting duct**, with which it has structural and functional similarities (and indeed a common embryological origin from the ureteric bud; see Fig. 1.3).

The **medullary collecting duct** arises in continuity with the cortical collecting duct as it crosses the corticomedullary junction. The lumen becomes progressively wider as it passes towards the tip of the **renal papilla**, where it empties into the calyces and the renal pelvis.

Sodium transport

An appreciation of the mechanisms involved in handling sodium in the nephron is of crucial importance in understanding how our patient's body fluid depletion has come about. As mentioned previously, over 99% of the fluid filtered are normally reabsorbed along the tubular system of the nephron, and this is largely related to the reabsorption of a similar proportion of filtered sodium. Assuming a plasma Na^+ concentration of 140 mmol/L and a glomerular filtration rate (GFR) of 144 L/day, the amount of sodium passed into the filtrate is 140 × 144, which equals 20,160 mmol/day. For a person consuming some 100 mmol of sodium per day in the diet, daily balance with

Table 2.2 Sodium reabsorption in successive segments of the nephron

Tubular segment	Sodium reabsorption (%)
Proximal tubule	65
Loop of Henle (thick ascending limb)	25
Distal tubule	
Early (convoluted segment)	6
Late (initial/cortical collecting duct)	2–3
Medullary collecting duct	<1

Amounts reabsorbed at each site are expressed as a percentage of the filtered load of sodium.

regard to sodium requires the excretion of only 100 mmol Na/day into the final urine (neglecting the very small losses through the gut and skin). This represents just 100/20160) or 0.5% of the sodium contained in the glomerular filtrate, so we conclude that 99.5% of the filtered sodium load must be reabsorbed by the tubules.

The segments in which this reabsorptive activity occurs have been defined by micropuncture experiments in animal models. Microscopic amounts of fluid are sampled from different points along the nephron, and their composition is compared to that of the filtered fluid. Table 2.2 shows the estimated contributions by successive tubular segments under normal conditions, which have been deduced by these experiments.

In the following sections, an outline of the cellular mechanism of sodium reabsorption in each of these segments will be provided. You will also discover how the reabsorption of sodium is often linked to movements of other electrolytes, often in a very specific way. Before we look at each section, refer to Fig. 2.6 for an overview of a tubular epithelial cell and general transport processes that can occur in different cell types.

As we work through the segments, you may wish to fill in the key features of each segment in sheet 1 and the transport processes of each segment in sheet 2 in the accompanying e-book.

Proximal tubule

Much of the cortical tissue mass in the kidney consists of proximal tubules, and these are the most metabolically active cells in the kidney. This activity is directed primarily towards the reabsorption of nearly 70% of the sodium contained in the tubular fluid, together with associated solutes and water.

The mechanisms involved in this reabsorptive process are complex and will only be outlined here. A model for the operation of a typical cell in this tubular segment has been developed, as shown in Fig. 2.7. Compare this to Fig. 2.6 and refer to this cell outline as we examine how the proximal tubule achieves its task.

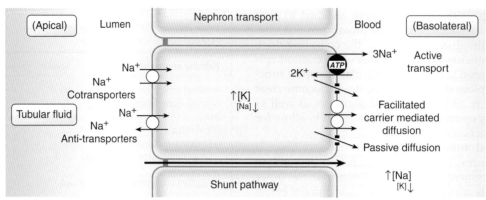

Fig. 2.6 Tubular epithelial cells line tubules and can be considered the interface between the lumen of the tubules where the tubular fluid flows and the renal interstitium where blood vessels lie. The apical side of the cell refers to the inner or luminal portion of the tubule and is where the tubular fluid run from segment to segment. The basolateral side of the cell is on the exterior of the tubule and faces the interstitium of the kidneys and blood vessels that run through the interstitium. Transport processes are either active where energy is required to transport substances against their concentration gradient or passive where no energy is expended, and substances are transported down a concentration gradient. The Na/K-ATPase pump is an example of active transport and uses energy to set up a concentration gradient such that the intracellular concentration of Na is low in comparison to the tubular fluid, thereby allowing transport of Na into the cell. This movement of Na is then often linked to the secondary active transport of other substances either into the cell (Na cotransporter) or back to the tubular fluid (Na anti-transporter). On the blood side of the cell, substances may passively diffuse down their concentration gradient or are facilitated to return to the bloodstream. In some segments, a shunt pathway exists between the cells that allows for bulk water flow or electrolyte flow. Note that the symbol conventions for the tubular epithelial cells are: open circles represent carrier molecules without direct linkage to ATP hydrolysis. Blackened circles are carriers with such linkage. Gaps in cell membranes represent ion channels. The arrow between cells indicates the paracellular shunt pathway.

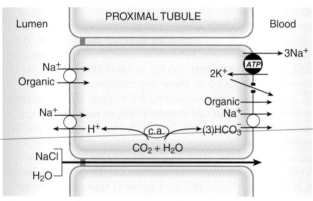

Fig. 2.7 Principal transport properties of a proximal tubule cell. Note that the potassium ions taken up by the basolateral sodium-potassium pump 'recycle' across that membrane via a potassium channel. See text for detailed description. c.a., carbonic anhydrase.

The primary active transport step underlying absorption of sodium and, secondarily, other solutes and water is the Na,K-dependent ATPase located along the basolateral (blood-facing) membrane of the proximal tubular cells. This pump lowers the sodium concentration inside the cell to around 5 to 10 mmol/L, thereby creating a marked electrochemical gradient for the entry of sodium from the tubular fluid (where it is present in plasma-like concentrations) across the apical cell membrane into the cell. Located in this membrane are several carrier proteins through which sodium entry is coupled with the transport of other solutes, which themselves move against their electrochemical gradient (or 'uphill') by what is termed secondary active transport. In other words, by creating an electrochemical gradient that allows sodium to run down the concentration gradient into the cell, there is also the opportunity to move other electrolytes up their concentration gradient coupled to the sodium reabsorption process.

Two types of such carriers are particularly important in the proximal tubule. One group mediates the cotransport of a variety of organic solutes from the luminal fluid in conjunction with sodium, and are responsible for almost complete reabsorption of these organic molecules. In this group are several carrier molecules, each with specificity for a different substance, for example, a sodium–glucose cotransporter, a family of related sodium–amino acid cotransporters, and a sodium–phosphate cotransporter. SGLT2 (sodium glucose cotransporter 2) inhibitors have been developed as a treatment for type 2 diabetes by increasing the excretion of glucose. They have a small diuretic effect related to an osmotic diuresis because of increased glucose in the urine and a small natriuretic effect related to inhibition of Na reabsorption.

Interesting facts

Phlorizin, a substance found in the bark of apple trees, inhibits both **SGLT1 and SGLT2 transport proteins**. In the 1930s, it was found to cause glycosuria and reduce plasma glucose levels, but because of its effects on SGLT1, its effects are not limited to the kidney resulting in side effects that excluded its use in humans. However, its discovery led to the understanding of the SGLT transport proteins and ultimately to the development of SGLT2 inhibitors, which target SGLT2, found exclusively in the kidney.

A second carrier type mediates the countertransport of an absorbed sodium ion with a hydrogen ion produced within the epithelial cell. This sodium-hydrogen exchanger (NHE-3) is one of a family of such proteins having widespread ramifications for cellular acid–base metabolism and is important in the mechanism of proximal bicarbonate reabsorption (see Chapter 4). Acetazolamide is another diuretic that acts in the proximal tubule by inhibiting carbonic anhydrase (CA) and thereby impacting on the function of the NHE-3 exchanger. As the diuretic effect is small and the potential toxicities prohibitive (in particular metabolic acidosis), this drug tends not to be used for its diuretic properties but rather to inhibit CA in other parts of the body, such as in the eye in glaucoma.

Whilst these and other mechanisms for the movement of sodium into the proximal tubular cells from the luminal fluid are well documented, they can account for only a fraction of the total reabsorptive flux of sodium which occurs across the epithelium in this segment. More than half of this sodium movement appears to occur between adjacent epithelial cells through what is termed the 'shunt' pathway. A component of this flux is driven by transepithelial electrical gradients, but some sodium and other ions are carried across the tubular wall by 'solvent drag', pulled in the bulk flow of water, which is known to occur through the intercellular pathway. This water flux itself is driven partly by the small but significant osmotic (and oncotic) gradients established across the proximal tubular wall along its length and partly by a small hydrostatic pressure gradient favouring fluid movement from the tubular lumen into the peritubular capillaries.

Therefore, we can summarise the transport properties of the proximal tubule:

- The process occurs almost isotonically, that is, the osmolality of the tubular fluid falls only very slightly below that of the plasma along the length of the tubule. This is because Na reabsorption and water reabsorption (because of a very high water permeability across the proximal tubular cell layer) is happening concurrently, maintaining a similar osmolality along the proximal tubule.
- This segment is responsible for 65% Na reabsorption.
- Sodium reabsorption is associated with complete reabsorption of filtered glucose and amino acids (when plasma concentrations are normal) and almost complete reabsorption of bicarbonate and phosphate ions because of the two main transport processes outlined above.
- Because of the high energy requirement of this very metabolically active segment, reabsorption of all solutes and water is very sensitive to metabolic poisons.
- There is a low electrical potential difference across the tubular epithelial wall.
- Sodium transport is inhibited by acetazolamide and SGLT2 inhibitors.

Thick ascending limb of the loop of Henle

The thick ascending limb segment is responsible for reabsorption of a further 25% of the filtered load of sodium and, together with the thin descending limb, contributes importantly to the build-up of the medullary interstitial concentration gradient which is essential in the mechanism for ultimate concentration of the urine (see Chapter 3).

Studies of the mechanism of ion transport in the thick ascending limb have given rise to the cell model shown in Fig. 2.8. As in the proximal tubule, the primary active transport step is the Na,K-ATPase located on the basolateral cell membrane. In this cell, however, sodium entry from the luminal fluid across the apical cell membrane is via a different mechanism than that operating in the proximal tubule. Here, one sodium ion, one potassium ion and two chloride ions interact with a carrier protein molecule embedded in the apical cell membrane ('the triple cotransporter', or NKCCT). It is this carrier whose function is blocked by loop diuretics such as furosemide (frusemide), which therefore results in the inhibition of the reabsorptive activity of this segment. Note that the movement of sodium into the cell via this carrier is electrochemically 'downhill' but is coupled through the action of the carrier to the uphill transport of chloride and potassium. Of the potassium accumulated inside the cell, some are transported out of the cell across the basolateral membrane, in part coupled with chloride, resulting in net reabsorption of potassium across the epithelium. However, a component of intracellular potassium recycles through a potassium channel in the apical cell membrane into the lumen, where it becomes available for re-entry into the cell through the triple cotransporter. It should be noted that there is a considerable flux of cations such as sodium, potassium, calcium, and magnesium across this epithelium via the shunt pathway between adjacent cells, driven largely by the lumen-positive transepithelial potential difference.

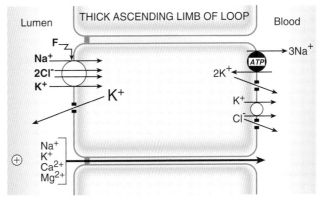

Fig. 2.8 Principal transport properties of a cell in the thick ascending limb of the loop of Henle. The ⊕ indicates that the transepithelial electrical potential difference is positive in the lumen relative to the blood side. The carrier marked F is the molecular target of the diuretic furosemide and related drugs. Symbol conventions as in Fig. 2.7. See text for detailed description.

As will be explained in the next chapter, the segment plays a vital role in building the concentrating capacity of the renal medulla. It is therefore a critical portion of the nephron not only for net electrolyte reabsorption but in contributing to the regulation of the osmolality of the body fluids. All of these processes are disrupted by agents such as loop diuretics which interfere with the operation of this segment.

Again, we can summarise the transport properties of the thick ascending limb, which include the following:

- Extensive transepithelial reabsorption of sodium and chloride is accompanied by smaller fluxes of potassium, magnesium, and calcium.
- This nephron segment is impermeable to water under all conditions resulting in dilution of urine (see Chapter 3).
- The combination of the water-permeable thin descending limb of the loop Henle and the water-impermeable thick ascending limb of the loop of Henle contribute to the medullary concentration gradient involved in the concentration of urine (see Chapter 3).
- A small lumen-positive transepithelial potential difference normally exists across this segment which contributes to the reabsorption of calcium and magnesium.
- Transport of all ions across this segment is powerfully inhibited by loop-acting diuretic drugs such as furosemide.

Early distal tubule

The cell model which has been developed to explain the operation of this segment is shown in Fig. 2.9. Again, the primary active transport step is the operation of the Na,K-ATPase in the basolateral membrane. There is again a passive gradient for sodium to enter the cell from the luminal

fluid across the apical cell membrane, and in this segment, this uptake step is mediated by a sodium–chloride cotransport carrier molecule (called the NCT), in which one sodium and one chloride ion are taken up simultaneously. It is this carrier whose function is blocked by the thiazide diuretics and related molecules, resulting in the loss of unreabsorbed sodium chloride into the urine.

Whilst no significant potassium fluxes occur across this cell segment, transepithelial calcium reabsorption does occur by the mechanisms shown in Fig. 2.9. This involves uptake of calcium across the apical cell membrane via a calcium channel, with extrusion of calcium across the basolateral membrane via a sodium-calcium countertransport carrier, driven by the passive inward movement of sodium from the ECF. Thus, during thiazide action, sodium entry into the cell is inhibited, resulting in a lowering of intracellular sodium by the continued action of the basolateral Na,K-ATPase. This in turn increases the activity of the basal sodium-calcium exchanger, resulting in lower cell calcium and thus enhanced entry of calcium through the apical membrane, and hence across the epithelium. This may explain the apparent paradox of treatment with thiazide diuretics during which sodium excretion is increased, but calcium excretion is decreased, although other mechanisms (such as enhanced calcium reabsorption with sodium in the proximal tubule secondary to mild hypovolaemia after thiazide action) may also be involved.

The fact that this tubular segment is impermeable to water under all conditions means that it acts as a site of dilution of the luminal fluid, that is, removal of electrolytes but not water lowers the luminal osmolality. This will be further explored in Chapter 3.

We can therefore summarise the transport properties of the early distal tubule (or distal convoluted tubule) to include the following:

- Sodium is reabsorbed with chloride but with little net potassium movement.
- Water permeability is very low under all conditions, resulting in dilution of urine (see Chapter 3).
- A further component of filtered calcium is reabsorbed.
- Sodium transport is inhibited by thiazides and related drugs.

Cortical collecting duct

The late segment of the distal tubule has similar transport properties to the earliest part of the collecting duct system, formed where two distal tubular segments join together. These properties continue until the collecting duct leaves the cortex to become the medullary collecting duct.

The cell mechanisms which have been proposed to account for the transport properties of the cortical collecting duct are shown in Fig. 2.10. There are two distinct cell types defined histologically in this segment, mediating different transport functions.

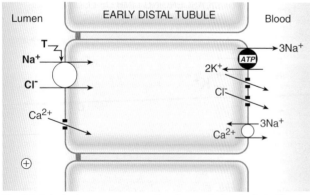

Fig. 2.9 Principal transport properties of an early distal tubule (distal convoluted tubule) cell. The lumen is electrically positive with respect to the blood side. The carrier marked T is the molecular target of thiazides and related diuretic drugs. Symbol conventions as in Fig. 2.7. See the text for a detailed description.

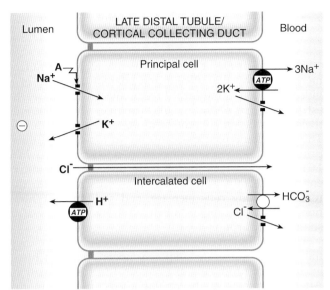

Fig. 2.10 Principal transport properties of the cells of the late distal tubule/cortical collecting duct. The lumen is electrically negative with respect to the blood side. The channel marked A is the site of action of the diuretic amiloride. Symbol conventions as in Fig. 2.7. See text for detailed description.

The principal cells are the site of sodium reabsorption and potassium secretion. Again the primary active transport step driving these processes is basolateral Na,K-ATPase. Sodium enters the cell from the luminal fluid down its electrochemical gradient, passing in this instance through a channel called the epithelial sodium channel (ENaC). This step generates a lumen-negative diffusion potential. Potassium accumulated in the cell moves into the luminal fluid through an apical potassium channel, down its electrochemical gradient. This cell type is also known to be a target for the action of aldosterone, which enters the cell from the blood, and interacts with a receptor molecule located in the cytoplasm. The hormone-receptor complex undergoes translocation into the nucleus, after which transcription and translation of aldosterone-induced proteins occurs, resulting in activation of all the transport steps undertaken by this cell. In addition, this cell contains basolateral membrane receptors for circulating vasopressin, the action of which results in increased transepithelial water transport in this segment in order to concentrate the urine (see also Chapter 3).

The intercalated cells are involved in acid–base regulation. The alpha intercalated cells are the site of acid secretion into the lumen within this tubular segment. This is mediated by an active hydrogen pump, the H⁺-ATPase, located on the apical cell membrane, which translocates hydrogen ions from the cell cytoplasm into the lumen. These hydrogen ions are generated within the cell by the action of CA, which catalyses the formation of carbonic acid from water and carbon dioxide. This disassociates into a hydrogen ion which is secreted into the lumen and a bicarbonate ion which enters the ECF across the basolateral membrane in exchange for chloride via an anion countertransporter ('anion exchanger 1'). This process of acid

secretion is also activated by aldosterone. Beta intercalated cells are responsible for bicarbonate secretion and will be discussed in greater detail in Chapter 4.

This nephron segment is sensitive to several transport inhibitors. Amiloride blocks the epithelial sodium channel in the principal cells. This results not only in inhibition of sodium reabsorption but also greatly reduces potassium and acid secretion, which are partly dependent on the negative lumen potential generated by sodium reabsorption. Spironolactone blocks the binding of aldosterone to its cytoplasmic receptor, thereby interfering with the activation by aldosterone of sodium reabsorption, potassium secretion and acid secretion.

It should be mentioned that, under unusual metabolic conditions, namely potassium depletion and alkalosis, this nephron segment is able to adapt its transport functions to mediate potassium reabsorption and bicarbonate secretion (respectively), though these processes are not active under normal dietary and metabolic conditions.

Consequently, the transport properties of this nephron segment include the following:

- There is reabsorption of some 2% to 3% of the filtered sodium load, accompanied in part by chloride reabsorption, potassium secretion, and acid secretion into the lumen.
- All of these transport processes are stimulated by the circulating steroid hormone aldosterone.
- Water permeability of this segment is variable, being increased by circulating antidiuretic hormone (vasopressin).
- There is an appreciable lumen-negative transepithelial potential difference.
- Sodium reabsorption in this segment is inhibited by amiloride and spironolactone; when these drugs are present, secretion of both K and H is reduced.

Before we move onto considering how these transport processes are regulated, try drawing each of the segments yourself and use the nephron outline in the e-book material to summarise the transport process of each segment, where diuretics act in each section and predict the metabolic consequences of having a patient on one of these diuretic agents.

Regulation of sodium transport

Several mechanisms interact to ensure that sodium excretion by the kidney is appropriately matched to changes in sodium intake and the ECF volume. These mechanisms require the precisely balanced operation of various sensory systems which detect changes in the ECF volume (and related parameters) and several effector mechanisms capable of altering the kidney's sodium excretion rate.

The **sensing mechanisms** include:

- Volume receptors in the cardiac atria and intrathoracic veins.

- Pressure receptors in the central arterial tree and the afferent arterioles within the kidney.
- Tubular fluid NaCl concentration receptors within the distal nephron (the macula densa).

The intrathoracic volume receptors respond to reduced distension by signalling to the brainstem that central venous volume has fallen, resulting in activation of effector mechanisms to restore the volume and pressure within the circulation. The opposite responses take place during ECF volume expansion. In addition, during volume expansion, the increased stretch of the cardiac atria directly results in the release of atrial natriuretic peptide (see below). Other afferents arise from arterial baroreceptors in the aortic arch and carotid sinus, and these give signals paralleling those of the volume receptors in most circumstances. The operation of the intrarenal baroreceptors and the macula densa is explained below in the section on the renin–angiotensin–aldosterone (RAA) system.

The **effector mechanisms** involved in adjusting renal sodium excretion are summarised in Table 2.3.

Of the **neurohumoral mechanisms**, the most important is the RAA system. As illustrated in Fig. 2.11, this system is activated by stimuli leading to the release of renin, an enzyme contained within specialised smooth muscle cells in the walls of the afferent and efferent arterioles. The principal stimuli to its release are as follows:

- Reduced perfusion pressure in the afferent arteriole.
- Increased sympathetic nerve activity in fibres innervating the afferent and efferent arterioles.

- Decreased sodium chloride concentration flowing through the distal tubule.

The inset in Fig. 2.11 shows the anatomical arrangements whereby the afferent and efferent arterioles of a given nephron come into direct contact with the earliest part of that nephron's distal tubule, where the epithelial cells become modified to form the macula densa. This juxtaglomerular apparatus brings together the three principal stimuli promoting renin release: thus, when ECF volume is low, the pressure distending the afferent arteriole falls, sympathetic nerve discharges to the renin-containing cells increase, and sodium concentration in the distal tubular lumen falls because of activated sodium reabsorption in earlier tubular segments.

The renin released into the circulation acts to cleave the peptide substrate angiotensinogen (manufactured in the liver), producing angiotensin I in the circulation. After passage through capillary beds, notably in the lungs, this is cleaved by angiotensin-converting enzyme into angiotensin II. This octapeptide is the central mediator of the RAA system, having multiple actions:

- It directly acts to vasoconstrict small arterioles.
- It directly stimulates proximal tubular sodium reabsorption.
- It causes the zona glomerulosa cells of the adrenal cortex to release the steroid hormone aldosterone.

As described earlier in this chapter, aldosterone acts to stimulate salt reabsorption in the cortical collecting duct

Table 2.3 Effector mechanisms involved in the regulation of renal sodium transport

Effector system	Site of action	Net effect of activation
Neurohumoral mechanisms		
Renin–angiotensin–aldosterone system	PT (angiotensin II), causing increased Na reabsorption CCD (aldosterone), causing increased Na reabsorption	Decreased Na excretion
Sympathetic nervous system/catecholamines	PT (noradrenaline; norepinephrine), causing increased Na reabsorption	Decreased Na excretion
Atrial natriuretic peptide	Glomerulus, causing increased GFR PT, causing decreased Na reabsorption MCD, causing decreased Na reabsorption	Increased Na excretion
Brain Natriuretic Peptide	PT, causing decreased Na reabsorption	Increased Na excretion
Prostaglandins	Glomerulus, causing increased GFR TAL and CCD, causing decreased Na reabsorption	Increased Na excretion
Haemodynamic-mechanical mechanisms		
GFR changes	Glomerulus	Increased GFR causes increased Na excretion
Peritubular physical forces (hydrostatic and oncotic pressures in the peritubular capillaries)	PT	Increased filtration fraction causes decreased Na excretion

Note that the table excludes several mediators of altered sodium transport whose physiological role is not well established.
CCD, cortical collecting duct (including late distal tubules forming initial collecting duct); GFR, glomerular filtration rate; MCD, medullary collecting duct; PT, proximal tubule; TAL, thick ascending limb of the loop of Henle.

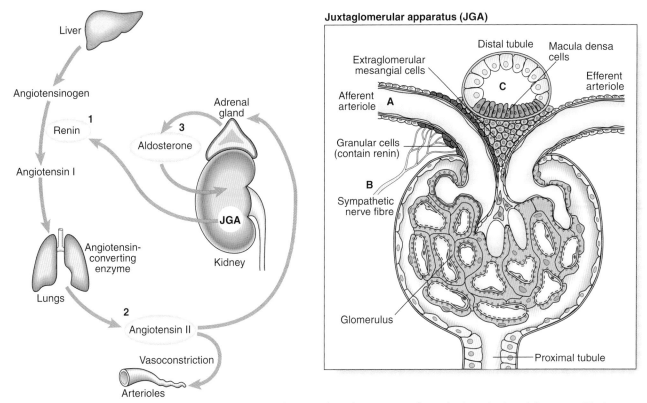

Fig. 2.11 The renin–angiotensin–aldosterone system. The numbers 1–3 show the sequence of steps in the activation of the system. The inset shows the juxtaglomerular apparatus (JGA) with the three major stimuli acting as triggers for renin release: A, fall in pressure in afferent arteriole; B, release of noradrenaline (norepinephrine) by sympathetic nerve endings on granular cells; C, fall in NaCl concentration in the distal tubule. Note that angiotensin II has several additional actions not shown on this figure (see text).

of the nephron, hence reducing sodium and water excretion from the kidney. The net effect of these actions is to restore blood pressure and ECF volume towards normal, thereby decreasing the stimulus, which leads to the activation of the system.

The sympathetic nervous system is also involved in the response to hypovolaemia, not only by acting as a stimulus for renin release, described above, but also by releasing noradrenaline (norepinephrine) around the proximal tubular cells, where it directly stimulates tubular sodium reabsorption. In addition, sympathetic activation vasoconstricts the afferent arteriole, reducing GFR and further limiting sodium and fluid losses.

Most of the other humoral mechanisms involved in sodium regulation lead to an increase in sodium excretion, thereby playing an important role in defending against volume expansion during periods of high salt availability.

Atrial natriuretic peptide is released from the cardiac atria when they undergo stretch during high volume states. It circulates as a peptide containing 28 amino acids and has numerous actions contributing to enhanced sodium excretion:

- The GFR is increased via an action of atrial natriuretic peptide to dilate the afferent arterioles.
- Sodium reabsorption by the proximal tubule and medullary collecting duct is inhibited.

- Secretion of renin and aldosterone is reduced, further switching off sodium-retaining systems.

Another mediator of sodium excretion during volume expansion is the natriuretic hormone released from the brain (pre-pro B-type natriuretic peptide (BNP), which is cleaved to BNP and N-terminal proBNP (NT-proBNP)) during these conditions. It is known to have ouabain- or digoxin-like properties in that it inhibits Na,K-ATPase in both vascular smooth muscle and renal epithelial cells. In the former, the result is an increase in intracellular sodium and calcium concentrations leading to vasoconstriction, whilst in the kidney, the effect is inhibition of sodium reabsorption, promoting natriuresis (increased sodium excretion). Natriuretic peptides undergo enzymatic degradation by neutral endopeptidases called neprilysin.

A variety of other intrarenal mediators are involved in inhibiting sodium reabsorption under certain physiological conditions, and of these, the most important clinically is the intrarenal prostaglandin (PG) system. Locally acting prostaglandins, PGE^2, in particular, are known to enhance glomerular filtration and decrease sodium reabsorption in the thick ascending limb of the loop of Henle and in the cortical collecting duct, the net effect being enhancement of sodium excretion. Other systems which have been implicated in sodium transport regulation include dopamine, kinins, adenosine/ATP, nitric oxide, and endothelin.

The role of these mediators under physiological conditions is incompletely defined at the present time.

Another important system involved in the response to major (5%–10%) changes in circulating volume is antidiuretic hormone. This effector peptide acts both to increase water reabsorption from the nephron and to vasoconstrict blood vessels, with little direct effect on sodium balance. It will be described in more detail in Chapter 3.

Haemodynamic and mechanical mechanisms are also involved in the maintenance of sodium balance. Changes in GFR are involved in mediating the actions of some of the neurohumoral mechanisms outlined above. Minor minute-to-minute changes in GFR are usually not a determinant of sodium excretion, largely because of the phenomenon of glomerulotubular balance: this describes the proportional adjustment of proximal reabsorption to shifts in GFR, minimising the net excretory effect of such changes. During wider swings in circulating blood volume, proximal tubular reabsorption is thought to be altered by changes in the physical forces affecting sodium and fluid reabsorption from the proximal tubule, namely the hydrostatic and oncotic pressures in the peritubular capillaries.

Before we continue with Joanne's case, use sheet 4 in the eBook to consider the different mechanisms and sites of sodium regulation across the nephron and which effector mechanisms would be activated in high or low effective circulating volume. Now, look at Case 2.1:3 and let's discuss Joanne's biochemistry results.

Looking first at Joanne's urea, creatinine and urate results, we note that the urea and urate are elevated, whilst the creatinine is within the normal range. As will be discussed further in Chapter 5, creatinine acts as a marker of the glomerular filtration rate (GFR), and the fact that it is not significantly elevated suggests that the GFR has not fallen greatly (though a small rise in creatinine within the normal range cannot be excluded). The increase in plasma urea is consistent with hypovolaemia since urea is handled by the kidney both by filtration and by partial reabsorption within the nephron, the extent of which is increased during low volume states (several other factors can influence the plasma urea, as described in Chapter 5).

The increase in plasma urate (the anion base of uric acid) is also suggestive of volume depletion. This nitrogenous breakdown product of nucleic acid metabolism is freely filtered at the glomerulus but undergoes extensive reabsorption from and secretion into the proximal tubule, usually resulting in a final excretion of some 10% of the filtered urate load. However, during volume contraction, the forces promoting increased proximal tubular sodium and fluid reabsorption also increase the absorptive component of proximal urate transport, resulting in elevated plasma urate concentration. Indeed, in susceptible individuals, this can result in an attack of gout because of uric acid crystallisation in joint tissues and the resulting inflammation. In addition, the transport protein responsible for transporting loop and thiazide diuretics into the tubular lumen is also responsible for urate secretion. This competitive inhibition of urate secretion is also responsible for the increased risk of gout seen on these diuretics.

Joanne's electrolyte results show that the sodium and chloride concentrations are normal, whilst the potassium concentration is reduced and the bicarbonate concentration is elevated. It is important to recognise that the normal sodium concentration does not reflect normal total body sodium, as indeed we have concluded that she has been partially depleted of sodium because of the action of the diuretic. The normal concentration simply reflects the fact that, in this instance, water loss from the ECF has been roughly proportionate to sodium, resulting in no net change in the ECF sodium concentration or osmolality. Disturbances of sodium concentration may be seen during diuretic treatment when loss of sodium and water is not proportionate, as discussed in the next chapter.

To understand the origin of hypokalaemia, we need to review mechanisms regulating potassium balance.

Potassium transport

Potassium is freely filtered at the glomerulus, and like sodium, some 65% of the filtered amount is reabsorbed in the proximal tubule. Again paralleling sodium, about 25% more is reabsorbed in the thick ascending limb of the loop of Henle. Whilst no potassium is transported

---

| Case 2.1 | **Body fluids and nephron function: 3** |

Biochemistry results

We can now understand that Joanne's symptoms and signs of volume depletion have resulted from the action of the furosemide tablets she had been taking, resulting in inhibition of sodium reabsorption in the loop of Henle, and hence negative net sodium balance.

Further investigation included the following biochemistry results:

Sodium 136 mmol/L
*Potassium 2.7 mmol/L
Chloride 95 mmol/L
*Bicarbonate 32 mmol/L
*Urea 10.5 mmol/L
Creatinine 0.12 mmol/L
*Urate 0.48 mmol/L.

These results lead us to the following question:

How have the abnormalities in her biochemical profile come about?

*Results outside the normal range; see Appendix.

in the early (convoluted) distal tubule, in the late distal tubule joining the cortical collecting duct, potassium is actually transported into the tubular fluid by secretion. This secretory step is carried out by the mechanisms illustrated in Fig. 2.10 – the principal cell of the cortical collecting duct.

Under conditions of low potassium intake, the extent of secretion may be minimal, resulting in a net fractional excretion of potassium of some 10% of the filtered load. During potassium depletion, net reabsorption from the cortical and medullary collecting duct can even occur, resulting in fractional excretion rates as low as 5%. More commonly, however, under normal dietary conditions or during potassium loading, potassium secretion can be stimulated such that the final urine contains 20% or more of the filtered potassium amount.

The factors regulating the extent of potassium secretion in the cortical collecting duct segment include:

Circulating factors
- high plasma aldosterone concentration
- high plasma potassium concentration
- high plasma pH

Luminal factors
- high sodium delivery rate
- high luminal flow rate
- negative lumen potential difference

Aldosterone acts as the key regulator of potassium balance, in parallel with its role in sodium metabolism but mediated by a quite different feedback mechanism. As shown in Fig. 2.12, a high plasma potassium concentration resulting from increased dietary potassium or other reasons directly stimulates the zona glomerulosa cells of the adrenal cortex to secrete aldosterone, which, by increasing potassium secretion into the distal nephron, leads to increased potassium excretion, thereby reducing the high plasma potassium. This is the main negative feedback mechanism responsible for maintaining the plasma potassium within the range 3.5 to 5.0 mmol/L.

Of the luminal factors, the rate of delivery of sodium and fluid from the earlier nephron segments is an important determinant of potassium secretion because of their influence on the transport processes of the cortical collecting duct.

From the above, it can be seen why a diuretic drug acting to inhibit the loop of Henle sodium reabsorption would lead to potassium depletion. The following factors may be involved:

- The potassium normally reabsorbed across the thick ascending limb is lost into the urine.
- The sodium not reabsorbed in the loop passes through to the distal tubule and cortical collecting duct, where it is available for increased exchange for potassium through the principal cell mechanisms.
- The volume depletion resulting from diuretic action stimulates aldosterone (via renin and angiotensin), further amplifying potassium secretion.

Hypokalaemia can be caused by a variety of other disturbances, as shown in Box 2.2. Note that in some cases, the low ECF potassium concentration results largely from a shift into the larger ICF pool. When external losses do occur, this may be from either the gastrointestinal tract or the kidney. Frequently, losses occur from both systems since, when there is a reduction in ECF volume, aldosterone promotes potassium

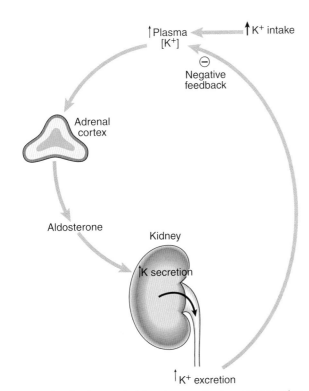

Fig. 2.12 Feedback control of the plasma potassium concentration.

Box 2.2 Causes of hypokalaemia

- **Redistribution into cells**
  e.g. alkalosis, catecholamines, insulin excess, hypokalaemic periodic paralysis
- **Inadequate K intake**
  e.g. starvation, inadequate replacement after an operation
- **Increased external K losses**
  Gastrointestinal tract:
  e.g. vomiting, diarrhoea, laxative abuse, villous adenoma of rectum
  Kidney:
  e.g. high mineralocorticoid activity (hyperaldosteronism, steroid therapy), diuretics, renal tubular acidosis, congenital tubular transport disorders (Bartter's and Gitelman's syndromes)

secretion in the kidney and hence increases urinary potassium excretion.

The increase in plasma bicarbonate in Joanne's case reflects a mild metabolic alkalosis, largely owing to the enhancement of hydrogen ion secretion resulting from increased sodium delivery through the cortical collecting duct segment, as outlined above. Again, enhancement of this step by high levels of aldosterone serves to aggravate this loss of acid.

Pharmacology of diuretic agents

This chapter has introduced the mechanisms of action of several commonly used diuretic drugs. For completion, a summary of the major agents in clinical use, together with their principal properties and actions, is given in Tables 2.4 and 2.5.

An important generalisation about most of the drugs used as diuretics is that they act on the mechanism for sodium uptake from the luminal fluid across the apical cell membrane in a particular tubular segment. This gives rise to the specificity of their site of action, given that the apical uptake step is mediated by different mechanisms in each segment, as described earlier. In contrast, the sodium exit step from the base of the cells is the same in each tubular segment, namely the Na,K-ATPase pump.

One group of diuretic drugs not shown in the accompanying tables is osmotic diuretics. These substances are freely filtered and are not reabsorbed by any part of the tubular system. Their action is thus not site-specific in that they entrain fluid osmotically within the tubular lumen and therefore limit the extent of sodium reabsorption in multiple segments. The principal clinical example of such an agent is mannitol, which must be given by intravenous infusion, and may be used to achieve short-term diuresis in conditions associated with cell swelling, such as cerebral oedema.

All the other diuretic drugs detailed in the tables (except spironolactone) must be delivered into the luminal fluid in appreciable concentrations to affect the apical sodium transport mechanisms. Delivery to the site of action is achieved partly by filtration, but there is an important component of active secretion of the diuretic molecules across the proximal tubular epithelium, mediated by the transport mechanisms available to secrete weak organic acids and bases in this nephron segment. This is of particular importance in determining the pharmacokinetics of these drugs since most are strongly protein-bound in the plasma, a property which itself leads to a very low delivery rate into the tubule by glomerular filtration alone.

More background information concerning the action of CA inhibitors and the effects of diuretics on concentrating and diluting capacity is given in the subsequent two chapters of this volume.

Table 2.4 Summary of sites and mechanisms of action of the principal classes of diuretic drugs

Site	Drug class	Prototype drug	Mechanism of action
Proximal tubule	Carbonic anhydrase inhibitors	Acetazolamide	Prevent $NaHCO_3$ reabsorption by limiting H^+ formation
Thick ascending limb of the loop of Henle	'Loop' diuretics	Furosemide (frusemide)	Block apical Na, K, 2Cl cotransporter
Early distal tubule	Thiazides and related drugs	Chlorothiazide	Block apical Na, Cl cotransporter
Late distal tubule/cortical collecting duct	a. Sodium channel blockers b. Aldosterone antagonists	a. Amiloride b. Spironolactone	a. Block apical Na channel b. Block aldosterone receptor in the cytoplasm

---

Table 2.5 Effects of diuretics on renal electrolyte and water excretion

Diuretic class	Na excretion*	K excretion	Anion excreted	Concentrating capacity[†]	Diluting capacity[†]
Carbonic anhydrase inhibitors	5	Increased	HCO_3^-	Increased	Increased
Loop blockers	20	Increased	Cl^-	Decreased	Decreased
Thiazides	6	Increased	Cl^-	No change	Decreased
K-sparing drugs	2	Decreased	Cl^-/HCO_3^-	No change	No change

*Maximum percentage of the filtered load of Na excreted into the urine during diuretic action.
[†]Effect of the diuretic on the capacity of the kidney to concentrate and dilute the urine (see Chapter 3).

Box 2.3 Adverse effects of diuretic drug use

'Physiological' side effects

Hypovolaemia
Hyponatraemia
Hypokalaemia*
Metabolic alkalosis*
Hyperuricaemia
Hypomagnesaemia*
Hypocalcaemia (loop-acting drugs only)
Hypercalcaemia (thiazide drugs)

Metabolic side effects

Glucose intolerance/hyperglycaemia
Hyperlipidaemia

Miscellaneous side effects

Hypersensitivity reactions
Acute pancreatitis/cholecystitis (thiazides)
Impotence

The effects shown apply chiefly to the loop and early distal acting drugs.

*These effects are not seen with drugs acting in the cortical collecting duct; these may cause the opposite side effects (hyperkalaemia and metabolic acidosis). Carbonic anhydrase inhibitors may cause hypokalaemia with metabolic acidosis.

Interesting facts

An extract from the foxglove plant, now known to contain digitalis, a cardiac glycoside related to digoxin, was used in the 18th and 19th centuries as a treatment for oedema (then called dropsy) in the belief that it acted on the kidney as a diuretic agent. It is now known that the diuretic action results instead from an improvement in the force of cardiac contraction caused by the drug, with a consequent increase in cardiac output, renal perfusion and hence GFR.

Clinical use of diuretics

The two most common indications for diuretic prescription are in the treatment of hypertension (see Chapter 9) and in the reduction of ECF volume in oedematous states (see Chapter 6).

Diuretic use is frequently complicated by several adverse effects, which are summarised in Box 2.3. These fall broadly into three categories: physiologically predictable side effects (including abnormal plasma electrolyte concentrations), metabolic side effects (including effects on glucose and lipid metabolism, where the mechanism is poorly defined), and allergic or idiosyncratic reactions. The latter are most prominent with drugs in the sulphonamide class, including CA inhibitors, furosemide and thiazides.

Regarding the physiologically predictable side effects, it is useful to consider the specific sodium transport mechanism that a particular diuretic blocks and predict how this would manifest clinically. For instance, as we have seen with Joanne's case, a loop diuretic that blocks the triple cotransporter in the ascending loop of Henle is likely to result in hypovolaemia (because of sodium and water loss), hypokalaemia and metabolic alkalosis (because of increased delivery of sodium to the collecting duct with an increase in sodium reabsorption via the ENaC channels and subsequent increase in excretion of potassium and bicarbonate) and increase in magnesium and calcium excretion (because of interference in the shunt pathway).

Before we continue, have a look at the worksheet in the e-book and see if you can predict the physiological side effects of each of the main classes of diuretics based on where they act.

There are several indications for the rational prescription of combinations of diuretic drugs. First, to reduce an unwanted electrolyte effect such as hypokalaemia induced by one class of agents (loop and early distal drugs), simultaneous treatment with a potassium-sparing drug such as amiloride can lead to a more neutral net effect on potassium balance whilst maintaining adequate diuretic action. Second, in resistant oedema associated with advanced disease of the heart or kidneys, it is sometimes appropriate to coadminister drugs acting at multiple sites along the nephron to counter the 'resistance' which may develop to one agent because of compensatory enhancement of sodium reabsorption by more distally located segments. In these circumstances, the prescriber must take particular care to avoid complications resulting from uncontrolled losses of fluid and electrolytes by careful clinical and laboratory monitoring.

In general, the following summarises the guidelines for diuretic use under most conditions:

- Use the minimum effective dose.
- Use for as short a period of time as necessary.
- Monitor regularly for adverse effects.
- Use only for appropriate indications.

Concerning the last point, Joanne's use of diuretics for cosmetic or weight control purposes is clearly inappropriate.

Principles of fluid and electrolyte replacement therapy

The key steps in correcting a disturbance in body fluid and electrolyte composition are:

1. Cessation or reversal of the causative disturbance.
2. Replacement of estimated deficits.
3. Provision of ongoing maintenance requirements.

Where the dominant clinical problem relates to an inadequate circulating blood volume, the chief goal is to restore the circulation by supplying fluid that will be held preferentially in the circulating compartment of the ECF, that is, the plasma.

Three basic types of replacement fluid are available for clinical use:

- Electrolyte-free sugar solutions (e.g. 5% D-glucose in water).
- Isotonic solutions of sodium salts (e.g. 0.9% sodium chloride, which is 150 mM NaCl or normal saline or lactated ringers).
- Isotonic salt solutions containing colloid macromolecules (e.g. semi-synthetic gelatins or concentrated albumin). However, semi-synthetic gelatins have been shown to increase the risk of acute kidney injury and anaphylaxis and therefore have limited use nowadays.

The effectiveness of each of these solutions in restoring circulating volume can be deduced by reference to Fig. 2.3. Using first principles, considering 1 L of each solution infused into a vein, the approximate distribution of volume would be as follows:

- The 5% dextrose solution would distribute approximately as does total body water, given that glucose is taken up freely by most cellular tissues. This would result in a minimal expansion of the circulating blood volume since the entire plasma, and red cell volume is only about 12.5% of the total body water.
- A litre of normal saline or lactated ringers would remain largely confined to the ECF, but of this, only some 20% would remain in the plasma, the rest moving into the ISF compartment.
- A litre of colloid-containing solution would be largely retained in the plasma compartment since the oncotic effect of the colloid macromolecule would serve to hold the added fluid inside the capillary endothelial barrier.

The urgency of fluid replacement and the choice of fluid used depends on the clinical circumstances, including the rate of development and nature of the deficit, assessed by clinical and biochemical parameters. Many cases of mild or chronic fluid and electrolyte deficiency can be corrected by simple measures involving cessation of the causative disturbance and oral replacement of fluid and electrolytes found to be deficient. In more acute or severe situations, intravenous therapy

---

Case 2.1 — Body fluids and nephron function: 4

Treatment

The clinicians caring for Joanne considered that her circulation was significantly affected by her prolonged diuretic use and that a period of intravenous therapy would be the most effective way of restoring her circulation and potassium levels. She was admitted to hospital, and the diuretics were ceased. She was given 1 L of normal saline intravenously every 12 h for 48 h, with 30 mmol potassium chloride added to each litre.

Her symptoms rapidly resolved, and her plasma biochemistry normalised. She received counselling about the importance of refraining from further use of diuretic medications and was given support and advice about her perceived weight and swelling problems. Her family doctor was involved in following her up in these matters.

will be necessary. In either case, attention also needs to be given to prevent recurrence of the initiating disturbance (see Case 2.1:4).

Summary

1. Changes in volume status relate to changes in total body sodium.
2. The ability to assess a patient's 'hydration status' can be difficult but is important to practice.
3. The nephron is responsible for adjusting the volume and composition of the ultrafiltrate to maintain homeostasis of the blood volume and composition.
4. Sodium transport is crucial in this process and occurs via different mechanisms in each of the segments of the nephron.
5. Regulation of sodium transport is intricate and occurs via neurohumoral mechanisms (the most important being the renin-angiotensin system) and haemodynamic mechanisms.
6. Diuretics are used to alter sodium transport processes and thereby increase sodium and water excretion.
7. It is important to understand the side effects of diuretics, which can largely be predicted by understanding the nephron transport processes that occur in each segment of the nephron.

Clinical skills 2.1 - Assessing hydration

We often hear that patients are 'overloaded' or 'dehydrated', but how is this determined? Both are clinical diagnoses requiring careful assessment of the patient. Blood tests tend not to be useful, and patients can become clinically dehydrated and fluid overloaded long before the blood tests become abnormal, such is the ability of the body to maintain the composition of its fluids.

First, one can ask, 'are you thirsty?' Look at the mucous membranes. Is the mouth dry? Is the tongue dry? Check whether the patient has been receiving oxygen which may affect their oral hydration. Now, look at the soft tissues. Are the eyes sunken in their orbits? – this is a late sign and is more commonly seen in children. Next, gently pinch a fold of skin over the back of the hand on one side. Do the tissues spring back and regain their normal shape, or does the skinfold remain pinched? If the latter, then this is loss of skin turgor and the patient may be dehydrated or it may be related to older age.

Check the jugular venous pulse. You may already know how to do this if you have studied the cardiovascular sys-

tem. Sit the patient up at 45 degrees and turn the head gently to the left. Look at the right side of the neck. Are neck veins visible and distended? Can venous pulsation be seen? If so, measure the height of the uppermost point above the sternal angle where pulsation is observed, but be sure that you are not simply seeing prominent carotid pulsation. The jugular venous pulse is triphasic and looks quite different.

Look at the ankles. Is pitting oedema present? This is elicited by gently pressing the thumb into the soft tissues over the shin just above the ankle. If an indentation remains, pitting oedema is present. In some cases, this may also be observed over the sacrum.

Listen to the lung bases. Bilateral basal crepitations may be heard if the patient is fluid overloaded.

Finally, check the urine output and weight. These may be useful to track over time in the assessment of fluid status and response to treatment.

Self-assessment case study

A 43-year-old woman is referred to the electrolyte clinic for further evaluation. She recently saw her family doctor complaining of weakness and tiredness, and a routine biochemical check revealed low plasma potassium (*2.6 mmol/L). She has been generally well in the past, though always prone to light-headedness, especially in hot weather. She has recently experienced weakness on sustained use of her upper limbs, such as when hanging out the washing. She takes no regular medications and denies irregularities of bowel function.

Her physical examination shows a tired-looking woman with mild weakness affecting especially the proximal muscles of the arms and legs. The mouth appears rather dry, though the skin is unremarkable. Jugular venous pressure is not visible, with the patient reclining at 45 degrees. The blood pressure is 105/70 lying and 90/65 standing, and pulse rate is 100 beats/min in both positions.

At the time she is seen in the referral clinic, she is accompanied by the following biochemical profile:

*Sodium 131 mmol/L
*Potassium 2.6 mmol/L
*Chloride 96 mmol/L
*Bicarbonate 33 mmol/L
*Urea 9.2 mmol/L
Creatinine 0.11 mmol/L.

Urine electrolytes ('spot' sample):
Sodium 48 mmol/L
Potassium 26 mmol/L.

After studying this chapter, you should be able to answer the following questions:

1. In this patient, the urine calcium excretion was found to be very low. In which segment of the nephron would you predict that there was an inherited or acquired functional defect?
   A. Early distal tubule
   B. Proximal tubule
   C. Ascending limb of the loop of Henle
   D. Descending limb of the loop of Henle
   E. Cortical collecting duct
2. If this was related to diuretic use, the most likely diuretic would be?
   A. Loop diuretic
   B. SGLT2 inhibitor
   C. Thiazide diuretic
   D. Spironolactone
   E. Carbonic anhydrase inhibitor

*Values outside the normal range; see Appendix.

Self-assessment case study answers

A1. Early distal tubule
   The clinical presentation is consistent with that of either ascending limb of the loop of Henle or early distal tubule inhibition. Hypokalaemia, alkalosis and high urinary Na/K results could be consistent with either location. However, low

urinary calcium excretion suggests inhibition of the early distal tubule.
   A2. Thiazide diuretic
   Thiazide diuretics inhibit the Na-Cl cotransporter in the early distal tubule.

WATER BALANCE AND REGULATION OF OSMOLALITY

3

Chapter objectives

After studying this chapter, you should be able to:

1. Define the normal range for plasma osmolality.

2. Outline the mechanisms by which the kidney can concentrate the urine (during underhydration) and dilute the urine (during overhydration).

3. Explain the feedback mechanisms for the control of plasma osmolality and the role of vasopressin (antidiuretic hormone).

4. Outline the differential diagnosis of polyuria and explain some mechanisms involved in conditions associated with impaired capacity to concentrate the urine.

5. Give a differential diagnosis of hypernatraemia.

6. Describe the mechanisms involved in conditions involving impaired ability to dilute the urine.

7. Give a differential diagnosis of hyponatraemia.

8. Use the worksheet found in the accompanying e-book to understand the roles of the nephron segments in urinary dilution and concentration.

Introduction

The previous chapter was largely concerned with the mechanisms whereby the kidney regulates body sodium balance. The point was made that the volume of the extracellular fluid (ECF) is largely determined by body sodium content, and hence adjustments to the renal sodium excretion rate have a major bearing on the ECF volume. We explained that, for the most part, alterations in tubular sodium transport are accompanied by parallel movements of water (though not necessarily in the same tubular segment) such that no net change in body fluid osmolality generally results from these adjustments.

In this chapter, we consider the mechanisms whereby water is handled by the kidney, independent of movements of sodium. These principles will give rise to an understanding of how the kidney can concentrate the urine by retaining water or dilute the urine by excreting water as circumstances demand. It will also lead to an understanding of the origin of the clinical problems of polyuria, hypernatraemia, and hyponatraemia (see Case 3.1: 1).

Causes and assessment of polyuria

In principle, a high urine flow rate may be produced either by a primary increase in solute excretion or a primary increase in water excretion.

Polyuria caused by solute diuresis results from the delivery of a high load of solute through the nephron, either as a result of filtration of a poorly reabsorbed solute or of blunted reabsorption of a solute normally transported out of the tubular fluid. (Note that increased glomerular filtration rate (GFR) per se is not a common cause of polyuria, largely because of glomerulotubular balance; see Chapter 2). The first mechanism applies to the osmotic diuresis produced by infusions of mannitol, which cannot be reabsorbed from the nephron and hence traps water osmotically within the tubular lumen, resulting in a high urine flow rate. Osmotic diuresis can also occur during disease states, notably in uncontrolled diabetes mellitus. In this case, increased plasma glucose concentrations result in the filtration of a glucose load greater than that which can be reabsorbed by the proximal tubule glucose reabsorption mechanism (saturation of the sodium-glucose cotransport carrier), leading to glycosuria accompanied by increased water flow because of the osmotic effect of the glucose trapped in the lumen. This mechanism accounts for the polyuria and dehydration encountered in newly presenting or uncontrolled diabetes mellitus. A broadly similar mechanism is occasionally seen during the development of chronic kidney disease, where high levels of urea have a diuretic effect.

The second mechanism for solute diuresis is that produced by commonly used diuretic drugs, which act to block the specific mechanisms for sodium reabsorption

---

Water balance and regulation of osmolality: 1

A case of polyuria

Robert Underwood is a 46-year-old man who presents to a doctor in a suburban medical centre complaining of passing large volumes of urine, which is virtually colourless ('like water'), accompanied by excessive thirst. He claims to be drinking 5 or more litres of water per day and passing similar volumes of urine. These symptoms have been troubling him for several weeks. He denies a history of similar complaints in the past and has never been diagnosed with diabetes. He has no known kidney disease and states that his general health has been good, although he has had some 'emotional problems' over the years. The family history is unremarkable. He says he is an ex smoker and does not drink alcohol at all.

On examination, he seems a little agitated but otherwise looks quite well. The skin, lips and mouth appear rather dry, but the blood pressure is normal at 130/80, the pulse 84 beats/min. The rest of the examination is normal. A urine specimen is obtained, which is a very pale colour, and on urinalysis, proves to be negative for glucose, blood, and protein. This specimen, as well as a sample of blood, is sent to the pathology laboratory.

The questions that arise in considering this case are:
1. What might be causing his polyuria and thirst?
2. What determines how concentrated the urine is under normal conditions?

---

in discrete segments of the nephron (see Chapter 2). Polyuria of this cause is most prominent soon after the commencement of the diuretic drug.

Water-based or dilute polyuria has a quite different mechanism and can arise in one of two ways. First, a high intake of water will lead directly to a high output of dilute urine through mechanisms to be described in this chapter. Whilst a history of excessive water drinking might be expected in this situation, covert overdrinking is sometimes encountered in patients with psychiatric disturbances (psychogenic polydipsia). An alternative mechanism for polyuria associated with dilute urine is when the primary disorder involves the kidney's inability to concentrate the urine normally. The physiological defects giving rise to this condition, known as diabetes insipidus, will be detailed further below.

Table 3.1 illustrates some differential features in the diagnostic approach to polyuria. Of particular interest in this case and for the subject matter of this chapter is the differentiation between the two forms of water diuresis. While in both forms the urine is dilute with low osmolality, in the case where the diuresis is being driven by high water intake, the plasma would be expected to have a low osmolality, resulting directly from excessive water reabsorption from the gut. In the case of impaired urinary concentration mechanisms, the plasma osmolality would

Table 3.1 Diagnostic approach to polyuria

Type	Examples	Plasma	Urine
Solute	Uncontrolled diabetes mellitus (solute = glucose)	Increased osmolality, hyperglycaemia	High osmolality, glycosuria
	Furosemide (frusemide) therapy (solute = NaCl)	Normal osmolality*	Variable osmolality, high Na
Water	Psychogenic polydipsia	Low-normal osmolality	Low osmolality
	Impaired urine concentration (central or nephrogenic DI)	High-normal osmolality	Low osmolality

*The plasma osmolality and sodium concentration may be normal, low, or high during loop diuretic therapy, depending on the water intake. DI, diabetes insipidus.

be high since the primary problem is excessive loss of water from the ECF into the urine (See Case 3.1: 2).

Reminder Box

Osmolality refers to the number of osmoles of a solute in a kilogram of solvent, while osmolarity refers to the number of osmoles of a solute in a litre of solvent. In a solution, osmolarity is slightly less than osmolality because the total solvent weight in osmolality excludes the weight of any solutes, whereas the total solution volume in osmolarity includes solute content (i.e. the denominator when measuring osmolality is less than the denominator for the same solution when measuring in osmolarity). In plasma, there is minimal difference between the two measurements, but clinical laboratories measure readings in units of osmolality (mosm/kg). By reference to Table 3.1, Mr. Underwood's polyuria cannot be attributed to glucose or sodium as solutes but is a water diuresis. Since the plasma sodium and osmolality are above the normal range, we can deduce that his problem arises from impaired urine concentration mechanisms rather than forced water drinking.

Renal mechanisms for urine concentration

It is obvious that there is a wide range in the normal intake of water and also in the normal loss of water through the lungs, skin, and gut (these three being sources of 'insensible' water loss). However, despite this, under normal circumstances, the osmolality of the plasma is tightly regulated around a mean of 290 mosm/kg, the normal range being within 5 mosm/kg either

Case 3.1 Water balance and regulation of osmolality: 2

Biochemistry results

The results of Mr. Underwood's biochemistry become available the following day. These are shown below:
*Sodium 154 mmol/L
Potassium 4.2 mmol/L
*Chloride 114 mmol/L
Bicarbonate 30 mmol/L
*Urea 11.5 mmol/L
*Creatinine 130 μmol/L
Glucose 4.5 mmol/L
*Osmolality 312 mosm/kg

Urine biochemistry

Sodium 26 mmol/L
Glucose 0 mmol/L
Osmolality 80 mosm/kg

The questions now are:

1. What pattern of polyuria is suggested by these results?
2. What further history or investigations are appropriate? (*Results outside the normal range; see Appendix.)

way. The homeostatic maintenance of this set point for plasma osmolality implies that the kidney is capable of adjusting the rate of water excretion over a wide range by generating dilute urine when water is abundant or by generating concentrated urine when water is scarce. As illustrated in Fig. 3.1, this corresponds in the first case to excretion of urine with an osmolality below 300 (50 mosm/kg being the most dilute urine possible), or in the second case to the production of urine with maximum water extracted (resulting in a typical maximum osmolality around 1200–1400 mosm/kg). We will first look at how the process of concentration is achieved.

In overview, there are two broad requirements for the kidney to be able to produce urine more concentrated than the plasma (Fig. 3.2). First, a zone must be created within the renal medulla where the tissue fluid osmolality is high. Second, the tubules forming the final segment of the nephron must conduct the urine through this concentrated zone, where water reabsorption can occur passively by osmosis (given that these segments can be made permeable to water). The first of these requirements is achieved by the operation of the loop of Henle as it dips into the renal medulla, while the second requirement is fulfilled by the collecting ducts as they pass from the cortex through the medulla on their way to deliver final urine to the renal pelvis. The mechanism whereby the water permeability of the collecting ducts can be increased where appropriate is through the action of circulating vasopressin (antidiuretic hormone; ADH). We will now explore these two processes in more detail.

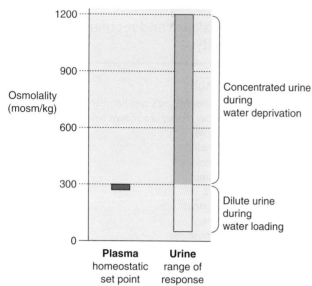

Fig. 3.1 Range of osmolality in plasma and urine.

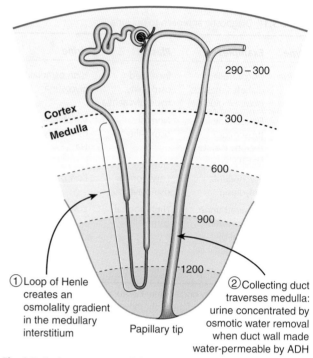

Fig. 3.2 Basic components of the urinary concentrating mechanism. Figures show osmolality of the tissue fluid (in mosm/kg) in different zones of the kidney. The loop of Henle sets up the tissue fluid osmolality gradient within the renal medulla, and the collecting duct traverses this gradient. ADH, antidiuretic hormone.

Countercurrent multiplication by the loop of Henle

The principle whereby a loop structure can generate a longitudinal gradient of concentration (from the top ends of the loop to its bend) is illustrated in Fig. 3.3. Here the descending and ascending limbs of the loop are shown to be parallel and adjacent, with an intervening layer of tissue fluid lying between them. Flow in the two limbs is said to be countercurrent, in that fluid entering the descending limb (from the end of the proximal tubule) flows downward, while the flow in the adjacent ascending limb is upward, being delivered at the top into the early distal tubule. A second property of the model is that the walls of the descending limb are permeable to water, while those of the ascending limb are impermeable to water. The third and key property of the system is that the walls of the ascending limb contain a pump mechanism capable of removing sodium chloride from the lumen and adding it to the surrounding interstitial fluid such that a gradient of 200 mosm/kg can be created across the tubular wall at any point. For clarity, the final effect of operating such a system in a steady state is built up as a series of discontinuous steps in the diagram.

The flow step shows the effect of introducing some fluid from the proximal tubule into the descending limb (shown with an osmolality of 300 mosm/kg for convenience) and the effect this would have of displacing fluid in the loop in each stage of the model. The second step shows the effect of activating the pump in the ascending limb, creating the 200 mosm/kg gradient across its wall. The third step shows the effect of water movement by osmosis out of the descending limb such that the fluid in that limb attains the same osmolality as the tissue fluid surrounding the ascending limb. It can be seen that the sequential effect of admitting more fluid into the descending limb and then activating the pump once more is to multiply the effectiveness of the thick ascend-

ing limb's pump mechanism in creating an area of high osmolality around the turn of the loop. In reality, the system operates continuously, resulting in the steady state situation shown in Fig. 3.4.

There are three important consequences of the operation of this system. First, the fluid leaving the ascending limb of the loop ends up being quite hyposmolar (100 mosm/kg) compared to the fluid entering it. Second, the osmolality near the bend of the loop is raised several folds above the osmolality of the entering fluid. Third, there is ultimately a continuous gradient of tissue osmolality from the 300 mosm/kg pervading near the top of the loop (in the renal cortex) to the 1200 mosm/kg achieved around the turn of the loop of Henle (although not all of this is because of salt accumulation; see below). This provides the environment through which the collecting ducts pass from the cortex through the medulla, providing an opportunity for water extraction from the collecting ducts by osmosis, given that their water permeability is sufficiently high.

From the above model, it can be deduced that three factors would increase the concentrating power achieved by the operation of the loop, namely:

1. An increased length of the loop.
2. An increased capacity of the pump in the thick ascending limb.
3. A reduced flow rate through the loop.

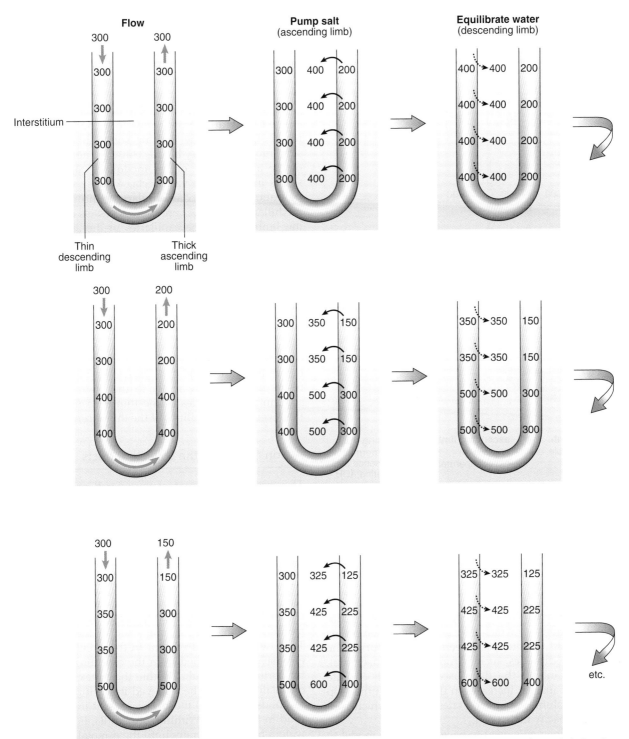

Fig. 3.3 Discontinuous model for the operation of the loop of Henle as a countercurrent multiplier. Figures are osmolality (mosm/kg). See the text for a detailed description.

Interesting facts

The role of the loop of Henle in water conservation is illustrated by the comparative anatomy and physiology of different mammalian species. In desert-dwelling rodents, such as the marsupial mouse of central Australia, the renal papilla is particularly elongated, containing very long loops of Henle, which allow concentration of the urine up to osmolalities greater than 9000 mosmol/kg.

Variations in the length of the loop underlie the differences in the urinary concentrating capacity between

WATER BALANCE AND REGULATION OF OSMOLALITY

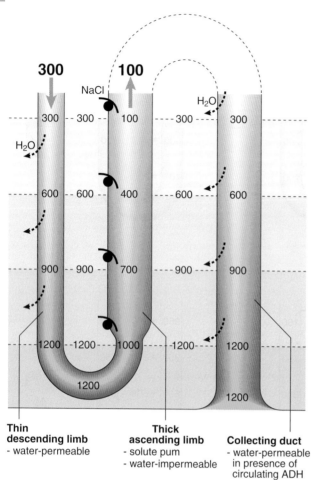

Thin descending limb
- water-permeable

Thick ascending limb
- solute pum
- water-impermeable

Collecting duct
- water-permeable in presence of circulating ADH

Fig. 3.4 Key properties and final outcome of the loop of Henle function. The collecting duct properties are those during water deprivation when maximal urine concentration is being achieved. Figures are osmolality (mosm/kg). Note that in the thin descending limb and the collecting duct there is actually a small (5–10 mosm/kg) osmolality gradient between the lumen and the adjacent interstitium (which is higher) to make water move, as shown. ADH, antidiuretic hormone.

different mammalian species, related to the water availability in the habitat to which they are adapted. Variations in the power of the pump are seen clinically during the action of loop diuretics, such as furosemide (frusemide), which act to inhibit the thick ascending limb's solute reabsorptive capacity. Increases in flow through the loop are seen in volume-expanded states, during which concentrating capacity is reduced.

Several refinements need to be added to the model to describe the actual situation in the mammalian kidney more fully.

First, the osmolality gradient within the medulla is not solely comprised of sodium chloride. Indeed, about half of the interstitial osmolality is contributed by urea. This relatively abundant small organic solute is 'trapped' within the renal medulla because of the different permeability of segments of the nephron to urea (being high in the thin descending and ascending limbs of the loop, deep

within the medulla and in the medullary segment of the collecting duct when ADH is present, but low in the thick ascending limb and cortical distal tubule). Thus, under antidiuretic conditions, urea recycles from the medullary collecting duct (out) to the turn of the deep loops of Henle (in), adding to the inner medullary osmolality.

Second, it is clear that a capillary blood supply that crossed the kidney from cortex to medulla would allow for dissipation of the built up solute gradient by diffusion into the capillary blood. This does not occur because of the arrangement of the medullary capillaries themselves in loops, the vasa recta, which parallel the configuration for the juxtamedullary nephrons. Thus, while medullary solute does enter these vessels in the descending limb, it exits the capillaries in the ascending limb, while water moves in the opposite direction in each case (countercurrent exchange). Since, however, in the steady state, the operation of the loop of Henle results in the loss of more solute than water from the tubular lumen, it follows that the vasa recta must remove more solute than water during their passage through the medulla.

A third refinement of the model is that it can be shown that countercurrent multiplication occurs even in the deepest hairpin part of the loop within the inner medulla before the start of the thick ascending limb. The mechanisms involved here relate to the high water but low sodium permeabilities of the thin descending limb and the reverse permeabilities of the thin ascending limb.

Action of ADH in the collecting ducts

The second component of the overall process involved in concentrating the urine is the action of ADH, also known as vasopressin (see also Systems of the Body: The Endocrine System). This peptide, which is released from the posterior part of the pituitary gland during conditions of water deprivation, acts to increase the water permeability of all segments of the collecting duct, from its earliest parts within the cortex (including the initial segments formed from the late distal tubules) through to the medullary segment as it traverses the outer and inner medulla on the way to emptying at the renal papilla. Thus, when ADH is present in the circulation, water is extensively reabsorbed from the collecting ducts in both the cortex and medulla. Within the cortex, the maximum osmolality that can be achieved in the luminal fluid corresponds to the 300 mosm/kg present in the interstitial fluid in the cortex. Within the medulla, however, further water abstraction occurs until the osmolality of the urine in the terminal parts of the inner medullary collecting duct can reach the maximum osmolality achieved by the countercurrent mechanism at the tip of the renal papilla, namely about 1200 mosm/kg in men. This reabsorbed water is carried away by the capillaries forming the vasa recta, thus leaving the medullary interstitial osmolality gradient intact.

During states of overhydration, when ADH levels are low (see below), the urine remains dilute since fluid

Box 3.1 Conditions required for urinary concentration and dilution

To concentrate the urine
- Adequate solute delivery to the loop of Henle
- Normal function of the loop of Henle
- Antidiuretic hormone (ADH) release into the circulation
- ADH action on the collecting ducts

To dilute the urine
- Adequate solute delivery into the loop of Henle and early distal tubule
- Normal function of the loop of Henle and early distal tubule
- No ADH in the circulation

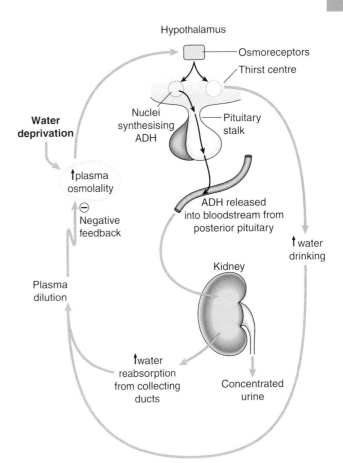

Fig. 3.5 Feedback control of plasma osmolality.

emerging from the ascending limb of the loop is already hypotonic (see Fig. 3.4). It can be rendered somewhat more dilute by further removal of sodium chloride during passage through the distal tubules and collecting ducts which, under these conditions, are relatively impermeable to water. Hence the urinary osmolality can be lowered from the 100 mosm/kg emerging from the loop to as low as 50 mosm/kg under maximum water diuresis. In fact, considerable water recovery does occur from the medullary collecting ducts during water diuresis since, although the water permeability is relatively low, the osmolality gradient favouring water reabsorption is high.

In summary, Box 3.1 shows in simple form the factors required to achieve a concentration of the urine on the one hand and dilution of the urine on the other. The implications of interfering with these factors for the development of disturbed water balance during clinical conditions is discussed later in this chapter. For the moment, it might be noted that loop diuretics clearly have the capacity to impair the kidney's ability to both concentrate and dilute the urine, while the thiazide diuretics, affecting only the component of urinary dilution which occurs in the early distal tubule within the cortex, interfere with the maximum dilution of the urine but not with the mechanism for urinary concentration.

Feedback control of plasma osmolality

During conditions of water deprivation, plasma osmolality tends to rise. This osmolality change is detected by specialised neural cells in the hypothalamus called osmoreceptors, which on shrinking, convey electrical signals to adjacent hypothalamic structures, with two parallel outcomes. First, sensation of thirst is stimulated, leading the individual to seek and ingest water actively. Second, cells within the supraoptic and paraventricular hypothalamic nuclei are activated to synthesise ADH, which is transferred bound to a carrier protein neurophysin down specialised axons terminating in the poste-

rior pituitary gland where it is released into the capillary blood. The ADH added to the circulation in this way reaches the kidney, where it acts to increase the water permeability of the collecting duct epithelial cells, resulting in enhanced water reabsorption from the tubular fluid. This, combined with a greater intake of water stimulated by thirst, serves to bring the plasma osmolality down towards normal, whereupon osmoreceptor activity reduces and the water-retaining mechanisms are deactivated (Fig. 3.5).

The reverse sequence of events occurs after ingestion of a large volume of water. The plasma is initially diluted slightly as the water is reabsorbed from the gut. This results in a fall in osmolality, which leads the osmoreceptor cells to reduce their activity, following which thirst is suppressed and ADH release is inhibited. These two measures lead to production by the kidney of dilute urine of high volume, as tubular fluid diluted within the loop of Henle becomes further diluted as it passes through distal nephron segments, which remain impermeable to water in the absence of ADH. As the water load is rapidly excreted, plasma osmolality returns towards normal and baseline conditions are restored.

Fig. 3.6 shows the relationship between the plasma osmolality and the concentration of ADH released into

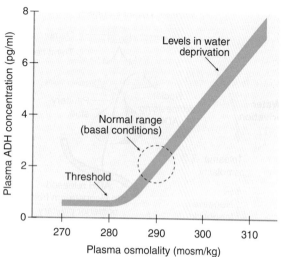

Fig. 3.6 Relationship between plasma osmolality and plasma concentration of ADH. ADH, antidiuretic hormone.

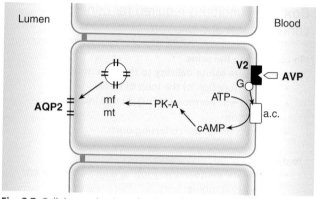

Fig. 3.7 Cellular mechanism of action of ADH in the collecting duct. ADH, antidiuretic hormone; a.c., adenyl cyclase; AQP2, aquaporin 2; AVP, arginine vasopressin (ADH); G, G protein; mf, microfilaments; mt, microtubules; PK-A, protein kinase-A; V2, vasopressin 2 receptor

the plasma. It can be seen that the threshold for release of ADH is around 280 mosm/kg, only slightly below the normal set point for plasma osmolality (290 ± 5 mosm/kg). A steep linear rise in circulating ADH results as osmolality passes above 290, while ADH release is virtually zero below 280 mosm/kg.

Two factors make the ADH system very effective in the short-term regulation of plasma osmolality. First, ADH is a small peptide (nine amino acids) which has a very short half-life in the circulation so that its action is not unduly prolonged following its release. Second, the release of ADH from the hypothalamus in response to osmoreceptor signals and its action within the kidney are extremely rapid events, such that the system tracks minute-to-minute changes in the osmolality of the plasma, correcting them towards the norm without undue delays.

A variety of non-osmotic stimuli may also cause secretion of ADH, independent of the plasma osmolality. Thus, haemodynamic changes associated with a fall in circulating plasma volume are potent triggers for ADH release. These disturbances are signalled to the brainstem via the volume and pressure sensors located in the central circulation (see Chapter 2), and the result is an independent input into the ADH secretory cells in the hypothalamus, resulting as before in ADH release into the circulation. While stimuli such as hypovolaemia and hypotension can lead to very high levels of ADH in the plasma, the sensitivity of the system to these changes is less than to alterations in plasma osmolality. Thus, while a 1% rise in plasma osmolality is sufficient to trigger a rise in ADH secretion, a 5% to 10% decrease in blood volume or blood pressure is required to provoke its secretion. Changes of this order do occur, however, in states of circulatory collapse. In addition, other non-osmotic stimuli such as pain, nausea and stress may also provoke ADH release, while alcohol inhibits it.

Mechanism of ADH action in the kidney

Fig. 3.7 shows the cellular events involved in the action of ADH in increasing the water permeability of the collecting duct. The ADH in the circulation binds to a specific receptor, named the V2 receptor, which is located on the basolateral membrane of the collecting duct epithelial cells. Through an intermediary G protein, this results in the activation of the membrane-bound enzyme adenyl cyclase, which catalyses the conversion of cellular adenosine triphosphate (ATP) to cyclic adenosine monophosphate (AMP). This second messenger is responsible for activating protein kinases within the cytoplasm, which leads to the phosphorylation of certain proteins involved in the activity of cytoskeletal elements (myofilaments and myofibrils) located in the apical cell cytoplasm. These appear to mobilise vesicles lying below the apical cell membrane, which contain preformed water channels comprising the specific channel protein aquaporin 2 (AQP2). The movement of these vesicles into the apical cell membrane results in the addition of AQP2 channels into that membrane, greatly increasing its water permeability. The relatively dilute tubular fluid is now able to move down an osmotic gradient through the cell cytoplasm and into the interstitial fluid and plasma across the basolateral membrane (the water permeability of which is because of the presence of aquaporins 3 and 4).

Two other intrarenal actions of ADH have been defined, both of which amplify its capacity to cause concentration of the urine. First, there is evidence that ADH can increase the activity of the sodium chloride reabsorptive mechanism located in the thick ascending limb of the loop of Henle; and second, ADH increases the permeability of the inner medullary collecting duct to urea. Both of these actions lead to an intensification of the medullary interstitial concentration gradient.

Finally, it is important to mention here that ADH has a separate action, mediated by a different receptor (the V1 receptor, involving intracellular calcium mobilisation), by which it promotes vasoconstriction of arterioles throughout the body. This vasoconstrictor action of the hormone increases the blood pressure in the central circulation at the same time as its renal tubular actions serve to retain water. Both actions therefore counteract the circulatory collapse associated with hypovolaemia or dehydration.

Failure to concentrate the urine

We can return now to an analysis of Robert Underwood's apparent failure of urine concentrating capacity. It follows from the above discussion that failure of the normal urine concentrating mechanism may result from any of the causes listed in Table 3.2. It is usually quite straightforward to exclude the first causes, involving either established renal failure or the presence of loop diuretics, either of which can lead to inadequate generation of the medullary concentration gradient by the loop of Henle. It is less easy, however, to distinguish whether impaired concentration results from failure to manufacture or release ADH from the brain (hypothalamic or central diabetes insipidus) or from the failure of ADH to act appropriately on the renal collecting duct cells (nephrogenic diabetes insipidus).

Both indirect and direct methods for distinguishing between these two conditions are available. First, as shown in Fig. 3.8, a water deprivation test can be performed. In this test, the subject is initially well hydrated such that the urine osmolality is quite low. Urine osmolality is monitored as the patient is observed closely during a period of water deprivation. While the normal subject will develop increased urine osmolality after some 9 to 12 h of water deprivation as a result of endogenous ADH release, in neither form of diabetes insipidus (DI) will substantial urine concentration occur. Administration of an exogenous dose of ADH at this point will produce a urine concentrating response in the patient with central DI, where there is a lack of hypothalamic hormone synthesis, while the patient with nephrogenic DI will have a negligible response, reflecting impaired collecting duct capacity to respond to the hormone. Fig. 3.9 shows where these two classes of patients would appear on the plasma osmolality versus plasma ADH concentration graph. As the plasma osmolality rises, the patient with central DI is unable to raise the near-zero levels of ADH in the plasma appreciably, while the ADH concentration rise in nephrogenic DI may be within the normal range. With the short half-life and pre-analytic instability of ADH in serum, plasma ADH measurements are not routinely utilised. A related peptide to ADH, copeptin, is now being used to aid in the diagnosis of the various hypotonic polyuric states.

The causes of central DI include tumours, trauma, irradiation, or cerebrovascular accidents, which destroy the relevant regions of the hypothalamus or the pituitary stalk or the posterior pituitary itself. Inflammatory conditions such as sarcoidosis can occasionally produce the same effect. Causes of nephrogenic DI, in contrast, include either inherited or acquired problems with the collecting duct ADH response mechanism shown in Fig. 3.7. Inherited conditions have been defined in which there is

Table 3.2 Failure of urinary concentration

Mechanism	Clinical example
Failure to generate medullary concentration gradient:	
Poor solute delivery to the loop of Henle	Low GFR (chronic kidney disease)
Impaired action of the thick ascending limb of the loop of Henle	Loop diuretic therapy (furosemide [frusemide])
Failure of ADH effect:	
No ADH released	Central DI (hypothalamic/pituitary lesion)
No ADH action in the kidney	Nephrogenic DI (collecting duct cell dysfunction)

ADH, antidiuretic hormone; DI, diabetes insipidus; GFR, glomerular filtration rate.

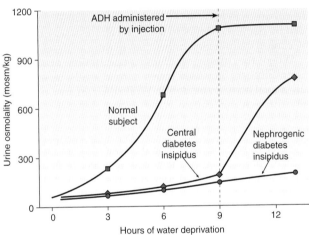

Fig. 3.8 Urinary osmolality versus time during a water deprivation test. Characteristic patterns are shown for a normal subject and for patients with central and nephrogenic diabetes insipidus. ADH, antidiuretic hormone.

faulty structure and impaired function of either the V2 receptor protein on the basolateral membrane or of AQP2 water channels in the apical membrane. Acquired forms of nephrogenic DI can occur when the collecting duct system is affected by infection or obstruction or where there is interference with the intracellular steps after generation of cyclic AMP, preventing aquaporin translocation into the apical membrane. Examples of this latter mechanism include nephrogenic DI during hypokalaemia, hypercalcaemia, and lithium therapy (see Case 3.1: 3).

Differential diagnosis of hypernatraemia

A useful generalisation is that disturbances in ECF sodium concentration reflect primary alterations in body water content. In contrast, as discussed in Chapter 2, primary

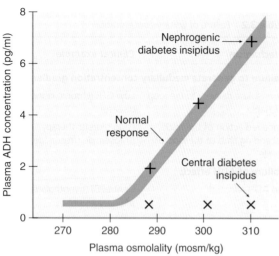

Fig. 3.9 Position of patients with central and nephrogenic diabetes insipidus on the plasma ADH versus plasma osmolality graph. ADH, antidiuretic hormone.

disturbances in body sodium content are usually accompanied by parallel changes in the ECF volume status, detected by clinical examination rather than plasma analysis.

When the plasma sodium concentration (and hence osmolality) are increased above normal levels, there is usually a total body water deficit. While this can arise occasionally through inadequate water intake alone, the cause is usually excessive loss of water from the body. As shown in Box 3.2, in some settings, this water loss is accompanied by a degree of salt loss, although the water loss in these cases is disproportionately greater. This may occur through the kidney, as for example, during diuresis induced by osmotic agents or loop-acting drugs (in water-restricted patients), through the skin (during excessive sweating), or via the gut (during colonic diarrhoea, especially in children).

Water loss unaccompanied by electrolyte depletion does occur in DI, where there is a failure of the normal operation of the ADH system. As described above, this may occur because of hypothalamic failure to synthesise ADH (central DI) or through renal tubular insensitivity to ADH present in the circulation (nephrogenic DI).

Less commonly, hypernatraemia can result from sodium loading, with either normal or reduced body water content. This is an unusual occurrence and may occur during enteral or parenteral alimentation with hyperosmotic solutions or during the administration of dietary or therapeutic supplements containing high salt content.

Note that whatever the underlying cause, sustained or severe hypernatraemia must reflect an impaired thirst mechanism, such as that associated with brain damage or stroke and/or impaired availability of, or access to, water. When thirst mechanisms and water availability are not limiting, the subject will normally drink sufficient water to keep the osmolality from rising very high.

It is clear from the above analysis that the finding of hypernatraemia itself gives no guide as to the total body sodium status. This must be independently assessed using clinical clues, including history and a physical

Case 3.1 Water balance and regulation of osmolality: 3

The diagnosis

Mr. Underwood's history, physical examination, and biochemical results were reviewed, looking for clues to one of the known mechanisms for impaired urinary concentration. Severe kidney disease was excluded by the virtually normal plasma creatinine concentration, and loop diuretics had never been prescribed or taken by the patient.

Initially, investigations were directed towards excluding the possibility of central DI by arranging for an assay of plasma copeptin level at a time when the patient was dehydrated and hyperosmolar, as at presentation. A cerebral computed tomography (CT) scan was also organised, looking for evidence of structural damage in the area of the hypothalamus or pituitary fossa.

At this point, however, the patient volunteered that he had been receiving psychiatric treatment for 1 month, following his presentation in an agitated and hypomanic state. He had started on lithium carbonate tablets, 500 mg BD, and therapy was currently being stabilised in conjunction with his psychiatrist. Indeed, a plasma lithium concentration of 0.9 mmol/L had recently been obtained by his psychiatrist, with whom contact was now made.

A diagnosis of lithium-induced nephrogenic DI was therefore made. Consistent with this, the plasma copeptin concentration result later came back in the high-normal range, appropriate for the elevated plasma osmolality. The cerebral CT scan proved to be normal.

In this situation, management consists of several steps: the patient was advised to always maintain an adequate water intake but not drink more than his thirst demanded. If indeed the psychiatric judgement was that lithium therapy should be continued, given its efficacy in controlling the mood swings of bipolar affective disorder, close monitoring of the resultant plasma lithium levels was recommended to maintain the serum lithium within and at the lower end of the recommended therapeutic range (0.4–0.8 mmol/L). Finally, if polyuria and thirst persisted and were troublesome to the patient, a trial of amiloride or thiazide therapy could be considered.

examination seeking signs of hypovolaemia or hypervolaemia (see Chapter 2).

Failure to dilute the urine

The reverse scenario of that described in the previous sections of this chapter occurs when the ECF becomes hyposmolar because of impairment of the mechanisms normally involved in excreting excess ingested water; that is, in diluting the urine. As summarised in Box 3.1, this process requires adequate delivery of filtrate through the segments of the nephron capable of lowering the osmo-

Box 3.2 Differential diagnosis of hypernatraemia

Water deficit with proportionately smaller sodium deficit
- Renal: osmotic or loop diuretic (during water restriction)
- Extrarenal: skin (excessive sweating); gut (colonic diarrhoea)

Water deficit alone
- Renal: central or nephrogenic diabetes insipidus

Sodium loading with normal or reduced body water
- Enteral or parenteral alimentation
- Intravenous or oral salt administration

Note that in all cases, there is usually some blunting of the normal thirst mechanism and/or restricted access to water.

Box 3.3 Differential diagnosis of hyponatraemia

Sodium deficit with relative water retention
- Renal: thiazides and loop diuretics (during water drinking), adrenocortical failure
- Extrarenal: gut (e.g. vomiting)

Water retention alone
- SIADH: ectopic antidiuretic hormone (ADH) secretion from tumour, lung disease, CNS disease, drugs
- Hypothyroidism

Sodium retention with relatively greater water retention
- Generalised oedema states: congestive cardiac failure, cirrhosis, nephrotic syndrome
- Chronic kidney disease

Water intake overwhelms maximal urinary dilution
- Psychogenic polydipsia
- Forced water drinking

SIADH, syndrome of inappropriate ADH secretion.

lality of the luminal fluid by removing sodium while remaining impermeable to water. These properties are possessed by the ascending limb of the loop of Henle and the early (convoluted) part of the distal tubule. Secondly, ADH secretion must be suppressed appropriately by the low plasma osmolality so that water is not reabsorbed from the collecting duct system.

In assessing the patient with inappropriate water retention, it is thus necessary first to rule out renal failure (low GFR); second, to exclude the use of diuretic drugs acting on the thick ascending limb (e.g. furosemide; frusemide) or the early distal tubule (e.g. thiazides); and third, to determine that ADH is not being released into the circulation. With regard to the latter, it must be remembered that ADH release can be triggered not only by a rise in plasma osmolality but also by non-osmotic stimuli such as hypovolaemia, hypotension, nausea, stress, and pain. Sometimes these stimuli are present without elevation of the plasma osmolality, resulting in water retention sufficient to drive the plasma osmolality below the normal range.

Differential diagnosis of hyponatraemia

These considerations are most commonly brought to bear in assessing the clinical problem of hyponatraemia. Nearly all of the hyponatraemic states are associated with sustained action of ADH in retaining water from the collecting ducts, despite the presence of hyposmolality, which would otherwise be expected to switch off ADH release. The main exception is forced water drinking, such as that which occurs in psychogenic polydipsia: in this situation, the primary excess of ingested water and slight expansion of ECF volume both act to switch off ADH, such that maximal urine dilution occurs. Hyponatraemia only develops to the extent that water ingestion continues at a rate exceeding its maximal excretion rate through the kidney.

The other causes of hyponatraemia are summarised in Box 3.3. Relative water retention may occur in conditions where there is a sodium deficit and hypovolaemia. This is

due most commonly to sodium losses through the gastrointestinal tract (e.g. vomiting) or via the kidney (e.g. during diuretic action). As previously mentioned, in the case of loop and early distal acting diuretics, sodium loss is compounded by interference with the mechanisms for generating dilute urine in these nephron segments. Deficiency of adrenocortical hormones also results in renal sodium wasting. In all of these conditions, ADH is activated through the mechanism of hypovolaemia consequent upon ECF volume reduction. The stage is thus set for the persistence of hyponatraemia until the sodium deficit is restored.

Water retention without a major change in body sodium can occur where ADH levels are elevated with neither an osmotic nor a hypovolaemic stimulus. In the syndrome of inappropriate ADH secretion (SIADH), ADH is released into the circulation either from an ectopic site, such as a hormone-secreting tumour (e.g. lung cancer) or from the posterior pituitary, secondary to non-malignant lung disease which may stimulate intrathoracic receptors to mimic volume depletion. A variety of drugs may also stimulate central ADH release, e.g. phenothiazines, vincristine, cyclophosphamide. In SIADH, there is hyponatraemia with plasma hyposmolality but with a urine which remains inappropriately concentrated, i.e. not maximally dilute. The urine sodium concentration is relatively high, which excludes plasma volume contraction in which it would be low.

A final category of hyponatraemia is that which arises when there is salt retention but relatively greater water retention. This can occur during any of the conditions causing systemic oedema, such as congestive cardiac failure, nephrotic syndrome, and cirrhosis. The water retention in these cases is partly because of the impaired GFR and avid proximal sodium and water reabsorption, which limit delivery of solute through the diluting segments of the nephron, and partly because of ADH release into the circulation. ADH secretion in these conditions is triggered by a reduction in the 'effective' arterial blood volume related to the impaired haemodynamics prevailing in each condition (see also Chapter 6).

The management of hyponatraemia depends first on defining the cause and reversing the causative condition wherever possible. This being done, treatment for hypovolaemic states involves volume replacement with intravenous sodium chloride infusions. For hypervolaemic conditions, sodium restriction accompanied by even tighter water restriction is necessary. In SIADH and related conditions, restriction of water alone is the mainstay of treatment.

Interesting facts

In the treatment of hyponatraemia, it is critically important to relate the rate of correction to the rate of development of the disorder. Unduly slow correction of acute hyponatraemia can lead to death from cerebral oedema as water enters cerebral neurones and causes brain compression. In contrast, overly rapid correction of chronic hyponatraemia can lead to death from demyelination of cerebral neurones, which undergo osmotic shrinkage and separation from their myelin sheaths.

Again it is worth reiterating that a low plasma sodium concentration generally reflects the relative excess of water in the ECF and gives no reliable guide to the total body sodium and volume status. This must be determined from the history and by physical examination, using guidelines provided in Chapter 2.

Summary

1. Plasma osmolality is a measure of total solutes in plasma and is primarily determined by sodium and its corresponding anions.
2. Maintenance of plasma osmolality (in effect serum Na) is dependent on the regulation of water transport.
3. Urinary concentration occurs via the generation of a medullary concentration gradient by the loop of Henle, which leads to water reabsorption if aquaporins are present in the collecting duct.
4. If maximal urinary concentration cannot occur in the presence of water deprivation, hypernatraemia (and plasma hyperosmolality) will occur.
5. Urinary dilution occurs because of sodium reabsorption in the water impermeable ascending limb of the loop of Henle and the distal convoluted tubule, combined with the absence of aquaporins in the collecting duct.
6. If maximal urinary dilution cannot occur, particularly in the presence of a relative increase in water intake, hyponatraemia (and plasma hyposmolality) will occur.
7. ADH is released in response to an increase in osmolality to promote urinary concentration. It is also released in response to excessive volume loss and, in this situation, may cause hyponatraemia as increased ADH will increase water but not solute reabsorption.
8. There are several non-osmotic stimuli for ADH secretion in addition to hypovolaemia, such as pain, nausea, and stress – common features of hospital admission.

Self-assessment case study

A consultation is requested on a hospitalised patient because of hyponatraemia. The patient was admitted 72 h before following a motor vehicle accident in which injuries were sustained to the chest and head. There is no evidence of skull fracture, although two ribs are broken on the left chest wall. The patient has been rather drowsy and confused since admission, although there are no localising neurological signs. He has received some intravenous fluids since admission and there is no clinical evidence of hypervolaemia or hypovolaemia.

The plasma sodium level has fallen from 139 mmol/L on admission to 124 mmol/L, with an osmolality on the second occasion of 256 mosm/kg. A single urine sample has been obtained, and this shows a sodium concentration of 54 mmol/L and an osmolality of 460 mosm/kg.

After studying this chapter, you should be able to answer the following questions:

Q1. Does this patient show inappropriate failure to concentrate the urine or inappropriate failure to dilute the urine?

Q2. What influences might be acting to determine the plasma level of ADH in this clinical setting (A) osmolality; (B) volume status; (C) splenic rupture; or (D) pain?

Self-assessment case study answers

A1. Since the plasma osmolality is very low, and the osmotic control mechanisms should respond by diluting the urine to excrete some of the excess water retained in the extracellular fluid, the fact that the urine osmolality is relatively high suggests that a failure to dilute the urine appropriately has developed.

A2. The hyposmolality of the plasma would be expected to inhibit ADH release, and we have clinically determined that the patient is euvolaemic, which would rule out A and B.

The injuries affecting his lung and brain may act as triggers for the inappropriate release of ADH, but a splenic injury is not specifically thought to cause ADH release. However, the patient has suffered stress and is in pain, both of which act as non-osmotic stimuli to the release of ADH. This scenario is typical of the development of a syndrome of inappropriate ADH secretion (SIADH).

ACID–BASE BALANCE AND REGULATION OF pH

Chapter objectives

After studying this chapter, you should be able to:

1. Define the normal range for plasma pH.

2. Explain the role of the kidney in the steady state elimination of acid produced daily by metabolism.

3. Outline the defence mechanisms which act to prevent an abrupt change in pH in response to an acid load.

4. Describe the mechanism for acid transport in the different nephron segments.

5. Recognise the clinical and biochemical features of metabolic acidosis, list some causes and give an approach to the differential diagnosis.

6. Recognise metabolic alkalosis, list some causes, and explain the pathophysiology of this disturbance during prolonged vomiting.

Introduction

Just as the kidney is a critical organ in defending the normal set points for extracellular fluid (ECF) volume, osmolality and potassium concentration, it also plays a central role in the homeostasis of the plasma pH. Whilst chemical buffering mechanisms and respiratory elimination of carbon dioxide are important in immediate responses to disturbances in acid–base balance, it falls to the kidney to make long term adjustments in the rate of acid excretion, which allows the external balance with respect to hydrogen ion concentration to be maintained. This chapter will focus on the mechanisms whereby the kidney achieves this role and the origin of some disturbances of this system in disease. See Case 4.1: 1.

The clue in this case that there is a disturbance of acid–base metabolism is that the bicarbonate concentration,

---

Case 4.1 — Acid–base balance and regulation of pH: 1

A case of acidosis

Mrs. Mary Loy is a 48-year-old woman of Chinese background who has been sent by her family doctor to the Emergency Department because they were concerned about her clinical condition and some biochemical results.

She had been complaining for some weeks of increasing lethargy, an extensive rash and 'heavy breathing'. She had been receiving treatment for 4 years for systemic lupus erythematosus (SLE), a multiorgan autoimmune condition for which a consultant rheumatologist had prescribed prednisone. However, Mrs. Loy confessed to having discontinued this medication some 10 months earlier because she was unhappy about its side effects.

On examination, she was febrile, unwell and had an erythematous rash on her face and limbs. Her blood pressure was 110/80, pulse rate 100 beats/min and respiratory rate 20/min. Her breathing was deep and sighing. The referring doctor's letter indicated that he had obtained a urinalysis result that morning showing: pH 7, blood +++ and protein ++.

He had also obtained plasma biochemistry the previous day, the results of which are as follows:

Sodium 135 mmol/L
*Potassium 3.1 mmol/L
*Chloride 113 mmol/L
*Bicarbonate 13 mmol/L
Urea 8.0 mmol/L
Creatinine 89 μmol/L.

The family doctor is particularly concerned about the low bicarbonate, which he interprets as a sign of acid build-up, and seeks full evaluation of her clinical and metabolic problem.

*Results outside the normal range; see Appendix.

---

representing the base component of the principal physiological buffer system, is greatly reduced below the normal range. This is consistent with acid accumulation in the ECF, for which we must explore both the cause and the consequences.

The key parameter involved in acid–base regulation is the concentration of H in the ECF. The physiological set point for this parameter is 40 nmol/L, usually expressed (using the negative base 10 logarithm) as the pH, which is normally 7.40. So important is homeostasis of this parameter to the normal operation of metabolism and cellular function that pH is tightly regulated in the range 7.38 to 7.42, although a somewhat wider range is compatible with life (7.0–7.8).

Two forms of acid are generated as a result of normal metabolic processes. Oxidative metabolism produces a large amount of CO_2 daily, and this so-called 'volatile acid' is excreted through the lungs. Carbon dioxide effectively acts as an acid in body fluids because of the following reactions:

$$CO_2 + H_2O \xrightarrow{c.a.} H_2CO_3 \longleftrightarrow H^+ + HCO_3^-$$

The first reaction (formation of carbonic acid, H_2CO_3) is the rate-limiting step and is normally slow, but in the presence of the enzyme carbonic anhydrase (c.a.), the reaction is greatly accelerated. The subsequent ionisation of carbonic acid proceeds almost instantaneously. This equation can be rearranged to enhance its physiological utility in the form shown in Fig. 4.1, as the Henderson–Hasselbalch equation.

The other form of acid, the so-called 'non-volatile acid', results from the metabolism of dietary protein, resulting in the accumulation of some 70 mmol of acid per day in an average adult on a typical western meat-containing diet.

The most important mechanism preventing a change in the pH of the ECF is the carbonic acid/bicarbonate

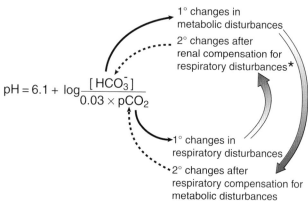

$$pH = 6.1 + \log\frac{[HCO_3^-]}{0.03 \times pCO_2}$$

Fig. 4.1 Effect of changes in HCO_3^- and pCO_2 on net pH of the plasma. This is an applied version of the Henderson–Hasselbalch equation. Normal plasma $[HCO_3^-] = 24$ mmol/L, normal $pCO_2 = 40$ mmHg, giving a normal plasma pH of 7.40. The pH will return to 7.40 as long as the ratio of $[HCO_3^-]$:$[0.03 \times pCO_2]$ is 20:1. *Note that changes in HCO_3^- concentration are also made as part of the renal correction of sustained *metabolic* acid–base disturbances as long as the kidney itself is not the cause of the primary disturbance.

buffer system outlined above. The importance of this buffer pair relates to certain key properties: bicarbonate is present in a relatively high concentration in the ECF (24 mmol/L), and the components of the buffer system are effectively under physiological control: the CO_2 by the lungs and the bicarbonate by the kidneys. These relationships are illustrated in Fig. 4.1.

It is clear from this relationship that a shift in pH can be brought about by either a primary change in the bicarbonate concentration (metabolic disturbances) or in the partial pressure of CO_2 in the blood (respiratory disturbances). However, it can also be seen that alterations in each of these parameters may represent a compensatory change whereby either the kidney or the lung can act to limit the extent of pH change which would occur because of a primary disturbance in respiratory function or in metabolism, respectively. The patterns of resulting clinical acid–base disturbances will be discussed later in this chapter.

Role of the kidney in H⁺ balance

Before we can make further progress in analysing the acid–base problem in our patient, it is necessary to consider the role the kidney plays in maintaining acid–base balance under normal conditions. Given that bicarbonate buffer is freely filtered at the glomerulus and that there is a daily load of non-volatile acid to be excreted into the urine, there must be two components to the nephron's task: reabsorption of filtered bicarbonate and addition of net acid to the tubular fluid.

Bicarbonate reabsorption

Bicarbonate is the principal physiological buffer in the plasma, and it is freely filtered at the glomerulus. If this bicarbonate were not fully reabsorbed by the tubular system, there would be ongoing losses of essential buffer into the urine, resulting in progressive acidification of the body fluids as metabolic acid production continued. In fact, bicarbonate excretion is essentially zero under normal conditions because of the extensive and efficient reabsorption of bicarbonate, principally in the proximal tubule, as shown in Fig. 4.2.

As discussed in Chapter 2, the cells in this tubular segment contain a sodium–hydrogen exchange carrier molecule known as NHE-3 in the apical cell membrane. As sodium enters the cell from the luminal fluid down its electrochemical gradient via this carrier, it effectively removes hydrogen ions from the cell cytoplasm and adds them to the luminal fluid. The hydrogen ions are generated within the cell by the action of the enzyme carbonic anhydrase, which catalyses the reaction between CO_2 and water to produce carbonic acid. This rapidly breaks down to produce the hydrogen ions that are secreted into the lumen and bicarbonate ions which are cotransported on a carrier with sodium (probably in a ratio $3HCO_3^-:1Na^+$) across the basolateral cell membrane into the plasma. (Note that this is equivalent to saying that the dissociation of cellular water yields a hydrogen ion and a hydroxyl ion, which reacts with cytoplasmic CO_2 under the influence of carbonic anhydrase to produce the bicarbonate for basolateral extrusion.) Carbonic anhydrase also exists on the brush border membrane on the luminal surface of these cells. Here it catalyses the breakdown of carbonic acid formed as the secreted hydrogen ion reacts with filtered bicarbonate, releasing water and CO_2, which passes freely across the cell membrane, allowing the cycle to repeat.

The net outcome of this process is that the filtered sodium bicarbonate passing through the proximal tubule is effectively reabsorbed, although the bicarbonate added to the plasma in a given turn of the cycle is not the same one appearing in the lumen with sodium. This process accounts for reabsorption of some 85% of filtered bicarbonate and operates at a high capacity but generates a low gradient of hydrogen ion concentration across the epithelium, with the luminal pH falling only slightly from 7.4 at the glomerulus to around 7.0 at the end of the proximal tubule. This is both because of the presence of carbonic anhydrase in the luminal compartment and because the epithelium is 'leaky' to hydrogen ions.

Net acid excretion

It is important to understand that the process described above has not done anything to remove net acid from the body since the fate of the secreted H^+ in this segment is effectively to conserve most of the filtered bicarbonate. Under circumstances requiring the removal of net acid from the body, the tubules must still carry out two more steps.

- Secrete further acid into the tubular lumen beyond that needed to reabsorb all filtered bicarbonate.
- Provide a buffer in the tubular fluid to assist in the removal of this acid (this is necessary since the maximum acidification which can be achieved in the lumen – around pH 4.5 – would not allow for excretion of the metabolic acid load needing elimination).

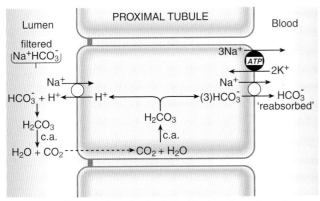

Fig. 4.2 Mechanism of proximal tubular bicarbonate reabsorption. c.a., carbonic anhydrase.

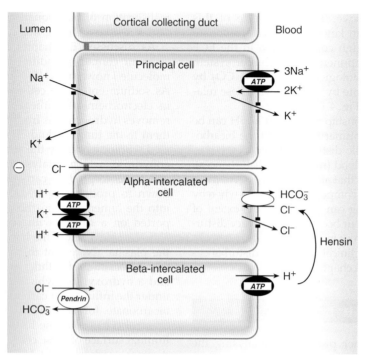

Fig. 4.3 Principal and intercalated cells in the distal nephron. The intercalated cell usually adopts a type A (alpha) phenotype but changes to a type B (beta) phenotype under alkalotic conditions.

These two requirements are fulfilled in more distal nephron segments. The collecting duct has two types of cells: principal cells and intercalated cells. The intercalated cells come in two forms – type A or alpha (which secrete acid) and type B or beta (which secrete base). Intercalated cells possess the ability to change phenotype from one to the other under the control of the extracellular matrix protein hensin. The type B cells possess an apical bicarbonate-chloride exchanger known as Pendrin (Fig. 4.3). As shown in Figs 4.4 and 4.5, acid is secreted into the lumen of the late distal tubule and collecting ducts by an H^+-ATPase located in the apical cell membrane. This pump has been found in the type A intercalated cells within the cortical collecting duct and in the apical membrane of the outer medullary collecting duct cells. The H^+ undergoing secretion in this way is generated within the tubular cells by a reaction facilitated by carbonic anhydrase, as described for the proximal tubule. Again, the bicarbonate generated within the cell by this process passes across the basolateral membrane, this time via a chloride-bicarbonate exchange carrier (anion exchanger 1), into the plasma. However, here the bicarbonate does not replace a filtered bicarbonate molecule but represents a 'new' bicarbonate, effectively counteracting the consumption of buffer, which would have occurred had the excreted acid been retained in the body.

Two types of buffer are involved in the excretion of this net acid. The glomerular filtrate contains a limited amount of non-bicarbonate buffer, which is capable of taking up some of the H^+, as shown in Fig. 4.4. The main molecule involved is monohydrogen phosphate HPO_4^{2-} which is titrated in the distal lumen to dihydrogen

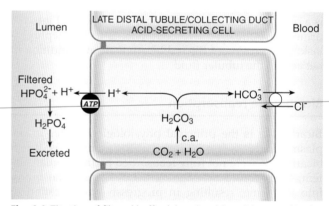

Fig. 4.4 Titration of filtered buffer (phosphate) by acid secreted in the distal nephron. Movements of filtered sodium ions are not shown. c.a., carbonic anhydrase.

phosphate (HPO_4^-), which is excreted in the urine with sodium. This reaction has limited capacity (removing up to 30 mmol of H^+/day) and tends to proceed as the urine pH falls along the distal nephron segments, typically from 7 down to 6 and below, with the pK (acid dissociation constant) of this buffer system being 6.8. This form of excreted H^+ is sometimes called 'titratable acid' as it can be quantitated by back-titrating a specimen of urine.

The other form of buffer involved in the removal of secreted acid is that manufactured by the kidney itself, namely ammonia (NH_3). Renal tubular cells, especially those of the proximal tubule, contain the enzyme glutaminase, which catalyses the production of NH_3 from the nitrogen-rich amino acid glutamine. Ammonia itself is a lipid-soluble gas, which diffuses freely through the

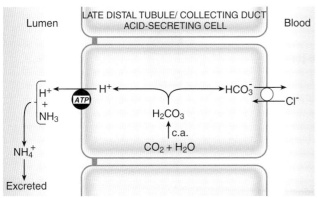

Fig. 4.5 Titration of manufactured buffer (ammonia) by acid secreted in the distal nephron. Ammonia is largely synthesised in proximal tubular cells and reaches the distal tubular lumen by gaseous diffusion from the blood. c.a., carbonic anhydrase.

kidney tissue and is converted to its protonated form ammonium (NH_4) in acidic environments (it is also concentrated in the renal medulla by recirculation in the loop of Henle). As the luminal pH falls from the proximal to the distal nephron segments, the NH_4^+ becomes increasingly 'trapped' in the luminal fluid compartment where it is washed away into the urine, associated with chloride ions. Again, this constitutes removal of an unwanted H^+ from the body, with the restoration of a 'new' bicarbonate molecule to the ECF. The importance of this mechanism for acid excretion is that it is linked to an abundant and regulated source of buffer production (NH_3) of essentially unlimited capacity. Thus, under conditions of acid build-up (especially chronic acidosis), NH_3 synthesis is stimulated, and acid excretion (as ammonium) is greatly increased, allowing systemic acid–base balance to be maintained (Fig. 4.5).

Note that despite the action of NH_3 to buffer the build-up of free acid in the late segments of the nephron, the pH of the tubular fluid does fall along the collecting duct system, resulting in final urinary pH as low as 4.5. This occurs both because the distal nephron is relatively impermeable to H^+ and because there is no carbonic anhydrase in the luminal compartment in these tubular segments. This means that the dehydration of carbonic acid formed in the lumen is slow, allowing H^+ to accumulate.

In summary, under conditions of normal dietary protein consumption, a slightly alkaline plasma pH of 7.40 is maintained despite the generation of about 70 mmol of hydrogen ion (as non-volatile acid) per day. The kidney's role in maintaining this pH homeostasis is achieved by generating acidic urine in which the net daily excess of acid can be removed. It does this in the following ways.

- Reabsorbing all bicarbonate buffer filtered into the urine.
- Secreting H^+ for excretion with filtered buffers such as phosphate.
- Secreting H^+ for excretion with the manufactured buffer ammonia.

Disturbances of acid–base balancedosis

Following on from the above principles, we can now examine how the kidney is involved in the response to acid–base disturbances and will first consider the situation of excess acid accumulation or acidosis. This may arise as a result of either of two primary disturbances.

Respiratory acidosis

Respiratory acidosis results from the accumulation of CO_2 in the body because of the failure of pulmonary ventilation. This itself may occur after lesions either in the central nervous system (e.g. depression of cerebral function, spinal cord injury) or in peripheral nervous pathways involved in ventilating the lungs (peripheral nerve and muscle disorders), or in some forms of lung disease involving impaired gas diffusion (also refer to *Systems of the Body: The Respiratory System*).

The decrease in body fluid pH resulting from carbonic acid generation is initially buffered to a limited extent by the reaction of carbonic acid with intracellular buffers such as haemoglobin, leading to the release of small amounts of bicarbonate into the plasma. However, long term restoration of body fluid pH balance requires the excretion by the kidney of the net acid retained during the period of hypoventilation.

This is achieved by the three steps described above, namely total reabsorption of filtered bicarbonate, titration of all available filtered buffers, and increased generation of ammonia within the kidney to allow for a higher-than-baseline level of net acid excretion as ammonium ion. This latter step is stimulated both by intracellular acidosis and by the elevated pCO_2, which is associated with respiratory acidosis. Over a few days, a new steady state is achieved in which renal excretion of net acid matches that being retained by the lungs, the urine pH being low, and the plasma bicarbonate being raised above baseline values (Fig. 4.6).

Metabolic acidosis

Metabolic acidosis (or, more correctly, non-respiratory acidosis), in contrast, is associated with the accumulation of non-volatile acid within the body. There are essentially three components to the protective response which limits the fall in pH which would otherwise occur.

Physicochemical buffering

The first defence against a fall in the pH of the body fluids after the addition of an acid load is the buffering of H^+ by available bases, particularly bicarbonate which is abundant in the ECF. This results in a fall in the plasma bicarbonate, and hence a lesser fall in the plasma pH than would otherwise have occurred. A variety of extracellular and intracellular proteins provide a further reserve of H^+ binding sites,

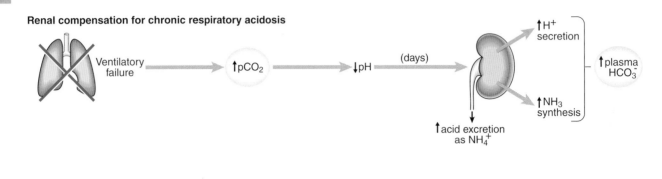

Renal compensation for chronic respiratory acidosis

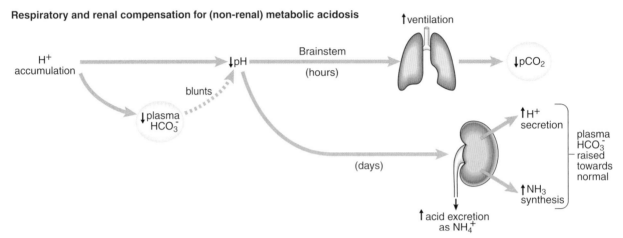

Respiratory and renal compensation for (non-renal) metabolic acidosis

Fig. 4.6 Mechanisms of renal and respiratory compensation for acid–base disturbances. The immediate action of physicochemical buffers is omitted for clarity.

and a limited amount of tissue phosphate also contributes some buffer capacity. These reactions are essentially complete within a few minutes of the addition of acid to the body fluids, though further buffering occurs in bone and other tissues over the ensuing hours and days.

Respiratory response

Despite initial buffering, the pH of the plasma will still fall somewhat during acidosis, and this acts as a potent stimulus to increase the ventilation rate via the activation of chemoreceptors within the brainstem (ventral medulla), which respond to a fall in pH of the cerebrospinal fluid. Clinically, this manifests as a deep, rapid breathing pattern (Kussmaul respiration). Over a matter of minutes to hours, this response drives the CO_2 below normal and thus serves to blunt the fall in ECF pH by shifting the carbonic acid equilibrium reaction (Fig. 4.1). This respiratory response provides a medium-term compensation for the acidosis produced by the metabolic disturbance. Note that whilst the resulting plasma pH is brought up towards 7.40, it is not fully normalised and never 'overshoots' because of respiratory compensation alone.

Renal response

Steady state correction of the acid–base disturbance requires the development over several days of an increased capacity by the kidney to excrete the metabolic acid load.

This involves reabsorption of all filtered bicarbonate, maximum titration of filtered buffers with secreted H^+, and increased intrarenal synthesis of ammonia, which combines with secreted hydrogen ions in the luminal compartment and appears in the urine as large quantities of ammonium. The urine pH falls to minimum levels (around 4.5), and the plasma bicarbonate, lowered initially by the reaction with added acid and subsequently by the hyperventilation response, is elevated back up into the normal range. The net result is a restoration of plasma pH to normal.

Before leaving the subject of renal acid secretion, several factors which have been identified as regulators of this process should be listed. The principal factors causing an increase in H^+ secretion by the nephron include:

- Increase in the filtered load of bicarbonate

- Decrease in ECF volume

- Decrease in plasma pH

- Increase in blood pCO_2

- Hypokalaemia

- Aldosterone.

Note that the first two factors listed result in increased proximal bicarbonate reabsorption, whilst the latter factors act in distal nephron segments to enhance net acid

Case 4.1 Acid–base balance and regulation of pH: 2

The arterial blood gases

Returning to the case of Mrs. Loy, crucial early data needed to clarify her acid–base status are the pH and pCO_2 of the arterial blood. These are obtained immediately after her admission to hospital and give the following results:

pH 7.37
*pCO_2 22 mmHg
*HCO_3^- 13 mmol/L
pO_2 103 mmHg.

These data confirm that her problem is primarily an acidosis (pH < 7.40) of metabolic origin (low HCO_3^-) which has undergone a considerable degree of respiratory compensation (low pCO_2). However, the presence of the low bicarbonate concentration implies that the kidney has not achieved long term correction of the underlying acid accumulation.

The question now arises: what is the source of the metabolic acid load that is playing a major part in this presentation?

Before completing an analysis of her acid–base problem, we might take note of one clue present in the data available already. Whatever the cause of metabolic acid build-up, there is some problem with kidney function in this case since urinalysis showed a pH of 7. According to the description above of an expected renal response to acidosis involving excretion of a maximally acidic urine (pH < 5), the urine pH in this case is quite inappropriate and would appear to point to a primary problem located within the kidney itself. As will be seen, this was indeed the case.

excretion. The common mediator in the case of the last four factors is probably a decrease in the intracellular pH of the tubular cells, which not only activates the hydrogen ion secretory mechanism but also enhances tubular ammonia synthesis. See Case 4.1: 2.

Patterns of metabolic acidosis

Two basic types of metabolic acidosis can be distinguished on the basis of the effect they have on readily measurable plasma parameters. In one type, acid might be added as hydrochloric (mineral) acid, or there might be a primary loss of bicarbonate buffer from the ECF. In this pattern, there is no addition to the plasma of a new acid anion. In the second type, the accumulating acid might be in the form of an organic acid, where the acid anion accumulates in the plasma to replace the falling bicarbonate.

These concepts are shown in diagrammatic form in Fig. 4.7. When the concentrations of the commonly measured cations in the blood (sodium and potas-

sium) are added, there is in normal plasma an apparent discrepancy of some 15 mmol/L over and above the sum of the two commonly measured anions (chloride and bicarbonate). This 'anion gap' is largely explained by the multiple negative charges on plasma protein molecules. It can be seen that where mineral acid is added, or bicarbonate is lost (pattern A), the fall in plasma bicarbonate is compensated by a rise in chloride, resulting in no change in the apparent anion gap. In pattern B, however, the bicarbonate may fall to the same extent, but this is accounted for by the addition of the organic acid anion, which, being itself unmeasured, adds to the apparent anion gap, and the plasma chloride does not change from normal. This simple analysis provides an initial tool for the diagnosis of the cause of metabolic acidosis, where this is not obvious.

Some causes of normal anion gap metabolic acidosis are given in Table 4.1. Rarely, the cause is the addition of hydrochloric acid or ammonium chloride, usually in a setting of medical investigation or treatment. More commonly, there is a problem either in the gastrointestinal tract involving loss of bicarbonate from the lower bowel or in the kidney. In the latter case, the normal mechanisms for H^+ secretion into the lumen of the nephron may be impaired, either in the proximal tubule (such as by the carbonic anhydrase inhibitor acetazolamide) or in the distal nephron (where the processes involved in urinary acidification are defective). As a group, these disorders of renal acid excretion are called renal tubular acidoses and will be discussed further later in this chapter.

Causes of the increased anion gap pattern of metabolic acidosis are given in Table 4.2. The organic acid load in these conditions may be classified as to whether it is of endogenous or exogenous origin. In some cases, when specifically suspected, such as lactate in lactic acidosis, the organic acid anion can be measured in the blood. In other cases, however, the clinical history provides a strong clue as to the cause, for example, the accumulation of ketoacids in diabetic ketoacidosis or of salicylate following aspirin intoxication (this latter disorder being complicated by respiratory alkalosis because of ventilatory stimulation). Of note is the predisposition of alcoholic patients to several forms of increased anion gap metabolic acidosis. These include starvation ketosis, lactic acidosis and intoxication by methanol or ethylene glycol (when consumed as alternatives to alcohol). Where metabolic acidosis is associated with advanced renal failure, the cause is usually the accumulation of complex organic acids normally excreted by filtration and proximal tubular secretion, and the result is an increased anion gap. See Case 4.1: 3.

Renal tubular acidosis

Metabolic acidosis can arise as a result of the failure of renal tubular segments to secrete hydrogen ions in the absence of any major impairment of the glomerular

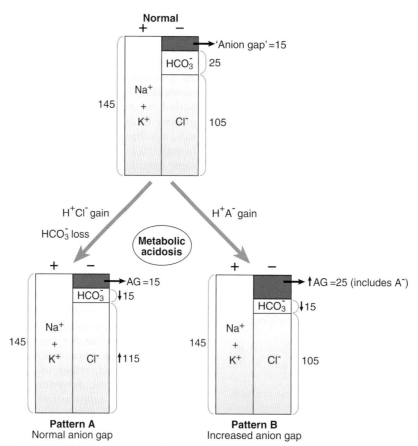

Fig. 4.7 Patterns of metabolic acidosis. All figures are in mmol/L. AG, anion gap.

Table 4.1 Causes of normal anion gap metabolic acidosis

Disorder	Mechanism
Inorganic acid addition:	
Infusion/ingestion of HCl, NH₄Cl	Exogenous acid load
Gastrointestinal base loss:	
*Diarrhoea	Loss of bicarbonate from gut
Small bowel fistula/drainage	Loss of bicarbonate from gut
Surgical diversion of urine into gut loops	Secretion of $KHCO_3$ by bowel mucosa
Renal base loss/acid retention:	
Proximal renal tubular acidosis	Renal tubular bicarbonate wasting
Distal renal tubular acidosis	Impaired renal tubular acid secretion

*Diarrhoea alone is rarely associated with marked acidosis unless it is severe and prolonged.

Table 4.2 Causes of increased anion gap metabolic acidosis

Disorder	Anion(s)	Clues to diagnosis
Endogenous acid load		
Diabetic ketoacidosis	Acetoacetate, beta-OH butyrate	Hyperglycaemia, ketonuria
Starvation ketosis	Acetoacetate, beta-OH butyrate	Hypoglycaemia
Lactic acidosis	Lactate	Shock, hypoxia, liver disease
Renal failure	Organic acids	Reduced glomerular filtration rate
Exogenous acid load		
Salicylate poisoning	Salicylate	Associated with respiratory alkalosis
Methanol poisoning	Formate	Visual complaints, often alcoholic
Ethylene glycol poisoning	Glycolate, oxalate	Oxalate crystalluria, often alcoholic

filtration rate. This acidosis of renal tubular origin is not associated with accumulation of any organic acid anion, and so the anion gap remains normal. Two basic variants of the condition, which can be either congenital or acquired, are described.

- In **proximal renal tubular acidosis** (RTA), the defect lies in the mechanism normally present within the proximal tubular epithelium for reabsorbing bicarbonate (refer to Fig. 4.2). Thus, either because of a specific defect in one of the components of the

Acid–base balance and regulation of pH: 3

The diagnosis

Mrs. Loy's electrolyte profile was examined, and an anion gap of 12 mmol/L was calculated (see original biochemistry data). There was no history of gastrointestinal disturbance, and the urine pH was noted to be inappropriately high at 7. An interim diagnosis of renal tubular acidosis was made.

Further investigation, directed towards defining the immunological activity of her underlying connective tissue disease, revealed that the levels of antinuclear antibodies (including antibodies to double-stranded DNA) were elevated, and serum complement levels were low, consistent with activated SLE. In addition, the urine contained many red cells and red cell casts (see Chapter 7), and a large amount of protein. Renal biopsy confirmed severe diffuse inflammation affecting the glomeruli as well as the tubulointerstitium.

A diagnosis of reactivated SLE was made, with the complications of diffuse lupus nephritis (see Chapter 7) and renal tubular acidosis. The distal tubular dysfunction in this setting reflects a disruptive effect of the interstitial inflammatory changes on the transport properties of the tubules.

cellular acid secretory mechanism in this segment or because of non-specific damage to, or malfunction of, the proximal tubular epithelium as a whole, filtered bicarbonate is incompletely reabsorbed. This results in a large flow of bicarbonate, together with sodium, through later nephron segments. Plasma bicarbonate falls, blood pH falls, and bicarbonate appears in the urine.

- In **distal RTA,** the defect is in the late distal tubule and collecting duct segments, where acid secretion is mediated by an H$^+$-ATPase. In inherited ('classical') forms of this disorder, the defect is either in the hydrogen pump itself or the anion exchanger in the basolateral membrane (Fig. 4.8). In other forms, such as that induced by amphotericin (an antifungal antibiotic), the impairment of net acid secretion results from the back-leak of hydrogen ions across an epithelium which is made abnormally permeable to these ions.

Some causes of proximal and distal RTA are given in Box 4.1. Both proximal and distal RTA may be inherited as a primary defect, but several other conditions may produce secondary RTA in either segment. Notably, an alteration in proximal tubular function can be induced by high paraprotein levels as in myeloma or by the carbonic anhydrase inhibitor acetazolamide. Distal RTA, in contrast, can be caused by conditions associated with polyclonal hyperglobulinaemia, including systemic lupus erythematosus (SLE), as in the patient studied in this chapter (see also *Systems of the Body: The Musculoskeletal System*). Other forms of structural tubu-

lointerstitial disease can produce the same defect, and several drugs and toxins are also prone to damage this segment selectively.

Apart from the differences in clinical setting and cause between the proximal and distal types of RTA, several physiological differences exist. In the distal form, the impaired operation of the collecting duct H$^+$ pump means that, no matter how severe the systemic acidosis, the urine pH can never be lowered appropriately and generally remains above 5.5. Bicarbonate loss is not prominent since proximal reabsorption is generally intact. However, in early or mild forms of proximal RTA, there is a considerable leak of bicarbonate into the urine, which again has an inappropriately high pH since the distal segments are unable to acidify the urine as long as large amounts of bicarbonate are flooding through the lumen from the proximal segments. However, when acidosis is more severe in proximal RTA, the plasma bicarbonate falls because of buffering of the accumulated acid. Therefore, a point may be reached where the reduced filtered amount of bicarbonate can be largely reabsorbed by the defective proximal tubular reabsorptive mechanism. The intact distal segments can then reabsorb a small distal leak of bicarbonate, as normally occurs. In this situation, the distal tubular secretory pump can operate normally and generate a transtubular H$^+$ concentration gradient, resulting in a lowering of the final urine pH. When this occurs, bicarbonate loss ceases, and ammonium excretion rises so that a new steady state arises in which acid retention stabilises, albeit at a reduced plasma bicarbonate concentration.

There are also differences in some of the associated features of proximal *versus* distal RTA. The proximal type may be associated with the loss of other molecules normally reabsorbed in the proximal tubule, giving rise to aminoaciduria, glycosuria, and phosphaturia. A different problem occurs in distal RTA as a result of progressive accumulation of acid over many years. As a consequence of buffering of H$^+$ in bone, calcium is released from the skeleton and may be deposited in the tissues, including the kidney (nephrocalcinosis). Furthermore, the high urinary excretion of calcium may result in stone formation (see Chapter 12), often associated with urinary tract infection. Impairment of skeletal growth can occur in this condition and also in proximal RTA when the disorder is congenital or starts in early childhood.

Much of the symptomatology of both kinds of RTA relates to electrolyte depletion. Urinary losses of sodium are abnormally high in both forms, resulting in a degree of hypovolaemia. Both forms are typically associated with hypokalaemia because of stimulated potassium secretion in the late distal and cortical collecting ducts. This is caused by a high luminal flow of sodium and bicarbonate in proximal RTA and by electrically-driven potassium secretion to replace faulty H$^+$ secretion in distal RTA.

An important and common variant of distal RTA is hyperkalaemic distal RTA (sometimes called type 4

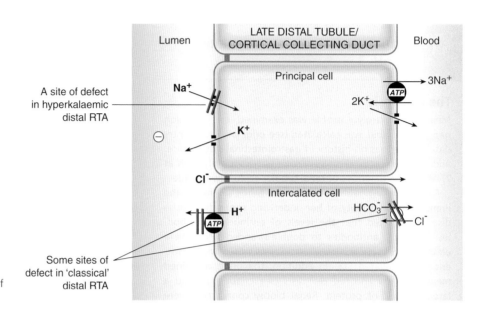

Fig. 4.8 Sites of defect in two variants of distal renal tubular acidosis (RTA).

Box 4.1 Some causes of renal tubular acidosis (RTA)

Proximal RTA (Type II)

Congenital (Fanconi syndrome, cystinosis, Wilson's disease)
Paraproteinaemia (e.g. myeloma)
Drugs (carbonic anhydrase inhibitors, Tenofovir)

Distal RTA (Type I)

Congenital
Hyperglobulinaemia
Autoimmune connective tissue diseases (e.g. systemic lupus erythematosus)
Toxins and drugs (toluene, lithium, amphotericin)

Hyperkalaemic distal RTA (Type IV)

Hypoaldosteronism
Obstructive nephropathy
Renal transplant rejection
Drugs (amiloride, spironolactone)

Case 4.1 Acid–base balance and regulation of pH: 4

Treatment and outcome

Mrs. Loy's treatment focused on the control of her underlying connective tissue disease. Immunosuppression using prednisone and cyclophosphamide was initiated with a view to reducing the activity of her SLE. The metabolic acidosis and hypokalaemia were corrected initially with infusions and later with oral supplements of alkaline salts of sodium and potassium.

Over the ensuing weeks, her condition improved dramatically, with the fevers and rash subsiding, urinary protein and red cell excretion reduced, and plasma electrolyte profile reverted towards normal. Within several weeks it was possible to discontinue her electrolyte and buffer therapy, and ongoing management was directed towards long term stabilisation of the connective tissue disease.

RTA). In this case, the normal anion gap metabolic acidosis is associated with hyperkalaemia, which points to a different site of the defect in the acid-secreting segment of the nephron. As shown in Fig. 4.8, if a disruption occurs in the normal operation of the principal cell type in this tubular segment, sodium reabsorption will be impaired, resulting in a loss of the normal lumen negativity (see Chapter 2). This electrical change impairs the rate of secretion of both potassium and hydrogen ions into the lumen, resulting in systemic acidosis with hyperkalaemia. This lesion has been described in a variety of conditions causing distal tubulointerstitial damage (such as urinary tract obstruction with infection) and also during treatment with drugs interfering with principal cell sodium transport (such as amiloride). A similar defect results from deficiencies in aldosterone secretion or action, including diseases of the adrenal cortex and of the renin secretory mechanism in the kidney. Hyporeninaemic hypoaldosteronism is commonly found in the elderly and those with diabetes.

The management of all forms of RTA is directed in the first instance towards reversing the underlying condition affecting tubular function, if possible. The next principle is that sufficient bicarbonate buffer must be provided to replace that consumed by the acid being accumulated. Provision of some of this bicarbonate as potassium salt will help replete potassium lost in classic forms of the disorder, whilst in the hyperkalaemic variant of distal RTA, measures to assist in the excretion of potassium (e.g. loop or thiazide diuretics, or corticosteroids, as appropriate) may be necessary. Treatment may also be required for specific complications in the various forms of the condition, such as removal of stones and treatment of infections which sometimes complicate classic distal RTA.

Disturbances of acid–base balance: alkalosis

To complete our survey of acid–base disturbances, we can consider the two primary perturbations which might result in alkalosis.

Respiratory alkalosis

Any form of sustained hyperventilation will produce a reduction in the blood pCO_2 with a resulting increase in plasma pH. The respiratory stimulus most commonly arises from anxiety states, but it may also be because of drugs stimulating the respiratory centre, other brain disorders and chronic liver disease.

The homeostatic response to respiratory alkalosis involves an initial phase of physicochemical buffering by intracellular proteins, which give up H^+, resulting in a small decrease in the plasma bicarbonate. More sustained compensation occurs over the ensuing days, during which renal tubular H^+ secretion is inhibited by the high extracellular pH and the reduced pCO_2. Bicarbonate reabsorption is inhibited, as is ammonium excretion, and the result is a reduction in net acid excretion and a fall in the plasma bicarbonate. In many cases, the respiratory disturbance is not unduly prolonged, and the renal compensation subsides as ventilation is normalised.

Metabolic alkalosis

In this disorder, there is a primary increase in the plasma bicarbonate concentration and the plasma pH. The causes fall into two groups according to whether there is an associated contraction of the ECF volume or not.

Hypovolaemic metabolic alkalosis is the most common pattern and includes disorders such as vomiting and gastric suction, in which acid-rich gastric juices are lost from the body. Metabolic alkalosis associated with volume contraction also occurs during treatment with most diuretics (other than carbonic anhydrase inhibitors and potassium-sparing drugs). Here there is increased acid loss into the urine related to the diuretic action on the tubules. The alkalosis associated with volume contraction is perpetuated by secondary renal responses, described in more detail below.

Normovolaemic (or hypervolaemic) metabolic alkalosis occurs when the primary disturbance provokes both bicarbonate retention and a degree of volume expansion. This most commonly occurs in corticosteroid excess states such as primary hyperaldosteronism (Conn's syndrome),

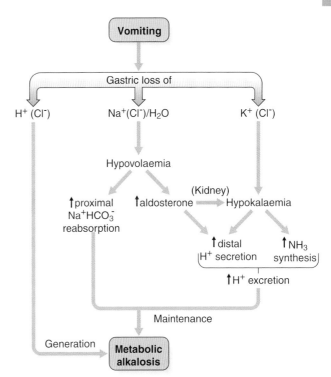

Fig. 4.9 Vomiting: generation and maintenance of metabolic alkalosis. Note that the gastric loss of H^+ is primarily responsible for generating the systemic alkalosis, whilst the other mechanisms shown act through the kidney to maintain the alkalosis as long as sodium and potassium losses are uncorrected. Chloride is the deficient anion accompanying all cations shown.

Cushing's syndrome, and related disorders. Potassium loss in these conditions also contributes to systemic alkalosis as H^+ ions move into cells in exchange for K^+ ions moving into the ECF. Occasionally, overuse of antacid salts can produce a similar pattern though without external potassium imbalance.

The homeostatic response to metabolic alkalosis involves initial buffering of the rise in plasma bicarbonate by titration of extracellular and intracellular buffers, including plasma proteins. Soon afterwards, the increased pH acts to inhibit ventilation through the medullary chemoreceptors, such that the pCO_2 starts to rise. Since, however, this is ultimately associated with an unacceptable degree of hypoxia, the extent to which this form of compensation occurs is limited, such that the maximum pCO_2 attained is rarely more than 55 mmHg.

In the absence of counterbalancing stimuli, the expected renal response to sustained metabolic alkalosis would be to decrease tubular acid secretion, inhibit bicarbonate reabsorption, and excrete the excess bicarbonate into the urine. However, in the most common form of metabolic alkalosis, that caused by sustained vomiting, this response is distorted by other changes associated with the loss of gastric fluid. As shown in Fig. 4.9, the loss of H^+ initiates the alkalosis ('generation' phase), which is actually worsened by the losses of sodium, water, and potassium ('maintenance' phase). The sodium

Table 4.3   Summary of 'simple' acid–base disturbances

Disorder	pH	Primary change	Compensatory response	Rule of thumb in predicting compensatory response
Metabolic acidosis	Decreased	Decreased HCO_3^-	Decreased pCO_2	Drop in pCO_2 = 1–1.5 × drop in HCO_3^- pCO_2 = (pH - 7.00) × 100 pCO_2 = 15 + HCO_3^-
Metabolic alkalosis	Increased	Increased HCO_3^-	Increased pCO_2	Rise in pCO_2 = 0.25-1 x rise in HCO_3^- < 55 mmHg pCO_2 = 0.7 $[HCO_3^-]$ + 20 mmHg (range: ± 5)
Respiratory acidosis	Decreased	Increased pCO_2	Increased HCO_3^-	Acute: 1 mmol/L rise in HCO_3^- for every 10 mmHg rise in pCO_2 Chronic: 3.5–5 mmol/L rise in HCO_3^- for every 10 mmHg rise in pCO_2
Respiratory alkalosis	Increased	Decreased pCO_2	Decreased HCO_3^-	Acute: 2 mmol/L fall in HCO_3^- for every 10 mmHg fall in pCO_2 Chronic: 4–5 mmol/L fall in HCO_3^- for every 10 mmHg fall in pCO_2

losses are associated with hypovolaemia, which triggers both proximal bicarbonate reabsorption and aldosterone release, which stimulates distal acid secretion, thereby aggravating the systemic alkalosis. Furthermore, the hypokalaemia resulting from potassium loss (more through the kidney than from gastric fluid) also stimulates distal acid secretion and tubular ammonia synthesis (see earlier), both of which enhance acid excretion and maintain the alkalosis. The net result is an inappropriately acid urine and a failure of the kidney to effect long term correction of the systemic pH disturbance.

The cornerstone of management in hypovolaemic metabolic alkalosis states, exemplified by vomiting, is to provide adequate volume replacement as sodium chloride (isotonic saline infusions), which switches off the volume-conserving mechanisms mentioned above and allows the kidney to excrete the excess alkali in the urine. Replacement of potassium helps correct hypokalaemia and its consequences in the kidney.

The non-hypovolaemic forms of metabolic alkalosis, by way of contrast, are resistant to treatment with sodium chloride but can usually be managed by cessation of alkali therapy or correction of mineralocorticoid excess. The latter may involve either adrenal gland surgery or blockade of mineralocorticoid effect in the kidney by treatment with spironolactone.

Summary of findings in principal acid–base disturbances

Table 4.3 provides an overview of the changes in pH, bicarbonate concentration and pCO_2 in the four major simple acid–base disorders. Taken in conjunction with clinical information, the results of these analyses are usually sufficient to enable a diagnosis to be made of the nature and cause of the disturbance. Rules of thumb are shown

to indicate the predicted compensatory change in pCO_2 or bicarbonate levels expected in each of the simple (uncomplicated) acid–base disorders. When the available data for a given patient is not consistent with these changes, a complex or 'mixed' acid–base disorder can be inferred, and the elements of the disturbance are usually deduced in conjunction with a thorough clinical evaluation.

Summary

1. The normal range for plasma pH is 7.38 to 7.42 and is tightly regulated because it affects the normal operation of metabolism and cellular function.
2. The kidney is involved in the steady state elimination of acid produced daily by metabolism, both by bicarbonate reabsorption and acid secretion within the renal tubule.
3. The defence mechanisms which act to prevent an abrupt change in pH in response to an acid load include physico-chemical buffering, respiratory compensation, and renal compensation.
4. Acid transport in the different nephron segments occurs directly, through bicarbonate absorption, net hydrogen ion excretion, or indirectly regulated through changes in urinary flow regulated by changes in sodium transport.
5. In metabolic acidosis, there is a primary decrease in plasma bicarbonate concentration and the plasma pH. Metabolic acidosis is associated with the accumulation of non-volatile acid within the body. Acid might be added as hydrochloric (mineral) acid, or there might be a primary loss of bicarbonate buffer from the ECF. In this pattern, there is no addition to the plasma of a new acid anion – RTA is the most common cause. In the second type, the accumulating acid might be in the form of an organic acid, where the acid anion accumulates in the plasma to replace the falling bicarbonate. A new production of lactate, keto-anions

or uraemic acids (e.g. phosphoric acid), or toxic agents such as ethylene glycol are commonly responsible.

6. In metabolic alkalosis, there is a primary increase in plasma bicarbonate concentration and the plasma pH. The causes fall into two groups according to whether there is an associated contraction of the ECF volume

or not. Common causes where ECF volume is reduced include prolonged vomiting and diuretic therapy. The most common cause where ECF volume is preserved is mineralocorticoid excess, such as is found in Conn's syndrome.

Self-assessment case study

A consultation is requested on an 81-year-old man who has been admitted to the hospital with an acute myocardial infarction. There has been significant damage to the left ventricle such that cardiac output is markedly reduced. Furthermore, on day 5 after admission, his course is complicated by the development of acute ischaemia in the left leg, attributed to occlusion of a major leg artery following embolisation of a thrombus from the left ventricular cavity.

The patient's plasma electrolyte results are as follows:

Sodium 135 mmol/L

*Potassium 5.2 mmol/L

Chloride 97 mmol/L

*Bicarbonate 14 mmol/L

*Urea 14.0 mmol/L

*Creatinine 140 umol/L.

(*Values outside normal range; see Appendix.)

Arterial blood gas analysis reveals the following: pH 7.33, pCO_2 29 mmHg, pO_2 (breathing room air) 58 mmHg.

After studying this chapter, you should be able to answer the following questions:

Q1. What is the overall pattern of acid–base disturbance in this patient?

Q2. What is the anion gap in this patient?

Q3. What is the likely cause of the disturbance in this case?

Q4. What would you expect the urine pH to be?

Q5. What are the principles of treatment?

Q6. What would the effect of a bicarbonate infusion be on his plasma potassium concentration?

Self-assessment case study answers

A1. Metabolic acidosis (has low plasma pH and bicarbonate), with incomplete respiratory compensation (pCO2 is low indicating hyperventilation, but the pH has not normalised).

A2. The anion gap is (135 + 5.2) − (97 + 14) = 29.2 mmol/L. This is higher than the normal range (12–18 mmol/L), suggesting that the acidosis can be attributed to the appearance of a `new' acid anion.

A3. Given the patient's poor cardiac output, poor peripheral perfusion, and ischaemic leg, it is likely that considerable anaerobic metabolism is occurring in the tissues, with a generation of lactic acid as the endpoint. Thus, lactate is likely to be the unmeasured anion expanding the anion gap.

A4. Given that renal function is not greatly impaired and that there is a significant systemic acidosis, over a period of days, the kidney would increase its capacity for acid excretion, including the generation of increased amounts of ammonia

with which acid is excreted as ammonium ions. The urine pH would be expected to fall below 6.0.

A5. Reversing the cause of the poor tissue perfusion would be a primary goal, and this would involve optimum management of his heart failure, as well as removal or dissolution of his femoral artery embolus, which would hopefully reverse the hypoxic conditions in his tissues. The provision of adequate oxygen supplementation in his inspired air would assist in this. Treatment of the acidosis itself is generally recommended only where the pH remains below 7.25 because of inadequate compensation. This may involve oral or intravenous supplementation with sodium bicarbonate.

A6. The plasma potassium would fall if bicarbonate is infused to correct the acidosis since extracellular acidosis promotes potassium movement out of cells, and this is reversed by raising the extracellular pH.

Self-assessment questions and answers

Q1. What would the effect on systemic acid–base balance be if a patient were given long term treatment with a carbonic anhydrase inhibitor such as acetazolamide?

A1. Acetazolamide interferes with the ability of the proximal tubule to reabsorb bicarbonate ions, which depends on the enzyme carbonic anhydrase acting both within proximal tubular cells and in the proximal tubular lumen. Blockade of

this enzyme by acetazolamide leads to bicarbonate wasting and a degree of systemic metabolic acidosis of the normal anion gap type.

Q2. Where in the nephron is the steepest gradient of pH between the plasma and the luminal fluid?

A2. Acidification of the luminal fluid against a steep hydrogen ion concentration gradient occurs chiefly in the most distal nephron segments, particularly the outer medullary collecting duct where acid-secreting pumps are abundant in the apical cell membrane of the tubular epithelial cells, and the epithelium has a low hydrogen ion permeability, allowing maintenance of the steep transtubular pH gradient.

Q3. Name three changes in the plasma which stimulate an increase in hydrogen ion secretion by the nephron.

A3. A decreased plasma pH, an increased blood pCO_2 and hypokalaemia all stimulate tubular acid secretion. Note that increased circulating levels of aldosterone also enhance hydrogen ion secretion in the distal nephron.

Q4. Give three causes of metabolic acidosis with a normal anion gap.

A4. Infusion or ingestion of hydrochloric acid, diarrhoea or equivalent lower gastrointestinal loss, and failure of renal tubular mechanisms to reabsorb bicarbonate or secrete hydrogen ions (renal tubular acidosis) all cause metabolic acidosis with a normal anion gap.

Q5. Name three factors which perpetuate the systemic alkalosis which follows prolonged vomiting.

A5. In addition to the initiation of alkalosis because of loss of gastric acid, there is stimulation of proximal bicarbonate reabsorption because of the hypovolaemia, which follows gastric losses of sodium and water. This hypovolaemia also triggers aldosterone release, which enhances distal acid secretion and perpetuates systemic alkalosis. Finally, potassium is also lost in the vomitus and is excreted by the kidney because of high circulating aldosterone levels. Hypokalaemia promotes tubular acid secretion and renal ammonia synthesis, again amplifying the systemic alkalosis.

GLOMERULAR FILTRATION AND ACUTE KIDNEY INJURY

5

Chapter objectives

After studying this chapter, you should be able to:

1. Define the determinants of renal blood flow and glomerular filtration.

2. Describe the mechanism of glomerular filtration.

3. Understand the factors that govern autoregulation within the kidney.

4. Understand the concept of clearance and be familiar with the different methods of assessment of renal function.

5. Determine whether oliguria is physiological or because of established renal failure.

6. Recognise the clinical circumstances in which acute kidney injury (AKI) is likely to occur.

7. Describe the cellular and biochemical mechanisms which underlie AKI caused by acute tubular necrosis.

8. Outline a logical clinical, laboratory, and radiological approach to the assessment of a patient presenting with renal failure.

9. Define the acute clinical complications and the biochemical and haematological abnormalities in AKI.

10. Effectively anticipate, prevent, and treat the complications occurring in AKI.

Introduction

As described in previous chapters, the primary functions of the kidney are to maintain body fluid, electrolyte, and acid-base homeostasis and to excrete nitrogenous wastes. These functions rely on a normal anatomical outflow pathway, normal renal circulation, and normal intrarenal mechanisms for regulating the process of urine formation. Abnormalities in any of these structures or processes can underlie the development of acute kidney injury (AKI), characterised by an abrupt fall in the glomerular filtration rate (GFR). After studying this chapter, you should be able to describe the mechanism of glomerular filtration, the factors normally involved in its regulation, and the causes, consequences, and treatment of AKI. See Case 5.1: 1.

Renal blood flow

Renal blood flow is between 1.0 and 1.2 L/min/1.73 m^2 of body surface area. The majority of blood flow to the kidney is directed to the cortex, with only a small proportion delivered to the medulla, where sodium transport by the thick ascending limb of the loop of Henle accounts for high oxygen consumption. Thus the renal medulla is sensitive to reductions in renal blood flow and oxygen delivery that may induce hypoxia and result in tubular damage, causing AKI.

The main determinant of the overall renal blood flow is the state of vasoconstriction of the renal arterial tree. Changes in the intrarenal vascular resistance mediate significant alterations in renal blood flow under pathophysiological conditions, whilst over a wide range of physiological mean arterial pressure levels, renal vasoregulation contributes to the maintenance of a stable renal blood flow and hence GFR (see below, under autoregulation).

Glomerular filtration

As described in Chapter 2, the key process involved in the kidney's excretory function is the formation of an ultrafiltrate of plasma in the glomeruli, where capillary tufts arising from the arterial circulation meet the blind ends of the tubular system in which urine is modified and conducted into the urine drainage system.

The structure of the glomerulus will be discussed in detail in Chapter 6. In brief, the process of filtration occurs across a complex barrier consisting of the thin fenestrated endothelial lining of the glomerular capillary, the glomerular basement membrane, and the foot processes of the epithelial cells (derived from the end of the tubular system) apposed to the external wall of the capillary. This filtration barrier allows free passage of solutes (up to a molecular weight of around 60,000 D) but retains cells and protein within the circulation. The selec-

---

Case 5.1   Glomerular filtration and acute kidney injury: 1

A presentation with anuria

Joan Wood is a 60-year-old woman who presented to the emergency department with a 4-day history of abdominal pain and vomiting, during which she had been unable to tolerate any food or fluids orally. She had passed no urine in the last 24 h.

Her past history included poorly controlled hypertension, with current treatment being an angiotensin-converting enzyme inhibitor (ramipril 10 mg/day), a loop diuretic (furosemide; frusemide 40 mg/day), and a dihydropyridine calcium channel blocker (amlodipine 5 mg/day).

Clinically she was febrile at 38.6 °C. Her blood pressure was 100/60 mmHg with a postural drop of 10 mmHg. She was tachycardic, with a pulse rate of 100 beats/min. Her jugular venous pressure was only just visible lying flat, and her mucous membranes were dry. Her abdomen was distended, with tenderness in the left iliac fossa and an ill-defined mass was present. Bowel sounds were absent, consistent with bowel obstruction.

Bladder catheterisation yielded 50 mL of urine, and urinalysis showed protein trace and blood trace.

Clinical evaluation and computed tomography (CT) scanning suggested that the likely diagnosis was diverticular disease complicated by an abscess, resulting in systemic sepsis.

This patient is clearly critically unwell, with sepsis and dehydration arising from a surgical disorder of the bowel. The failure to pass urine in this setting (anuria) is a crucial element of the presentation, suggesting the development of impaired renal excretory function and a reduced GFR.

This scenario gives rise to the questions:

1. What is the mechanism of glomerular filtration, and how is it normally regulated?
2. How can the cause of an abnormally low rate of urine production be determined?

---

tive properties of this barrier, and the consequences of its disruption, will be discussed further in the next two chapters.

The filtration process itself is based on purely passive forces, of which the hydrostatic pressure generated by the heart is the principal driving force. However, as shown in Fig. 5.1, this outward filtration pressure is partially opposed by two pressures acting to restrain filtration, namely the hydrostatic pressure within the lumen of the tubular system itself and by the oncotic pressure because of plasma proteins which are retained within the capillary. Thus the net ultrafiltration pressure (P_{uf}) comprises the hydrostatic pressure in the glomerular capillaries (P_{gc}) minus the hydrostatic pressure in the tubules (P_t) minus the oncotic pressure generated by plasma proteins (π_{gc}).

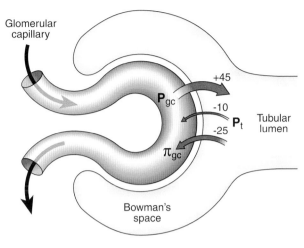

$$\mathbf{P}_{uf} = P_{gc} - P_t - \pi_{gc}$$

Fig. 5.1 Diagram of glomerulus showing the forces involved in glomerular filtration. P_{gc}, hydrostatic pressure in glomerular capillary; P_t, hydrostatic pressure in tubular lumen; P_{uf}, net ultrafiltration pressure; π_{gc}, oncotic pressure (osmotic pressure because of plasma proteins) in the glomerular capillary. Representative pressures are shown in mmHg.

An overall expression for GFR which indicates all of its determinants is as follows:

$$GFR = K_f \times P_{uf}$$

where K_f is the ultrafiltration coefficient, which is made up of the product of the hydraulic permeability of the filtration membrane times the surface area available for filtration.

Typical mean values for the pressure terms (obtained from micropuncture studies in experimental animals) indicate that: P_{gc} = 45 mmHg, P_t = 10 mmHg, π_{gc} = 25 mmHg, giving rise to a P_{uf} of 10 mmHg.

Factors that interfere with any of these determinants of glomerular filtration may lead to an abrupt fall in GFR and thus AKI unless adequate compensatory responses occur. The most important physiological determinant is the capillary hydrostatic pressure, which may be reduced either by a reduction in perfusion pressure reaching the afferent arteriole, by an increase in afferent arteriolar tone, or by a decrease in efferent arteriolar tone (see below). The pressure in the tubular system may rise significantly during ureteric obstruction, thus reducing the GFR. Changes in the plasma oncotic pressure are less important in altering GFR under physiological or pathological conditions. Pathological change involving the glomeruli may lead to alterations in the ultrafiltration coefficient by decreasing the hydraulic permeability and/or by obliterating the total capillary surface area available for filtration. Conditions such as glomerulonephritis (see Chapter 7) and diabetes mellitus (see Chapter 8) impair glomerular filtration by these mechanisms.

Under physiological conditions, the regulation of the filtration rate in individual glomeruli is determined by the balance between the resistance in the afferent and efferent arterioles. As shown in Fig. 5.2, the hydrostatic pressure across the wall of the glomerular capillaries will be increased by factors either dilating the afferent arteriole or constricting the efferent arteriole, increasing the single nephron GFR in either case. Conversely, factors leading to afferent arteriolar constriction or efferent arteriolar dilatation will reduce the filtration rate of the affected glomerulus. Some circulating substances known to have these effects are shown in Fig. 5.2. It should be noted, however, that in the normal kidney, minor perturbations in levels of individual substances do not have significant net effects on GFR because of compensatory changes in other factors which tend to maintain a haemodynamic steady state. However, if renal function is impaired, particularly because of a low renal perfusion pressure (e.g. renal artery stenosis or cardiac failure), maintenance of GFR is highly dependent on intrinsic compensatory mechanisms such as afferent arteriolar vasodilatation (predominantly because of prostaglandins) and efferent arteriolar vasoconstriction (predominantly because of angiotensin II). Thus, factors which interfere with these compensatory mechanisms, such as non-steroidal anti-inflammatory drugs (which inhibit prostaglandin synthesis) and angiotensin-converting enzyme inhibitors or angiotensin II receptor blockers (which interfere with angiotensin II action), blunt these compensatory responses and may precipitate AKI (see Chapter 14).

It should be noted that angiotensin II has a particularly important but complex role in the regulation of glomerular filtration. Whilst local production of this peptide acts predominantly on the efferent arteriole to maintain single nephron GFR, higher circulating levels are capable of producing afferent arteriolar vasoconstriction, which tends to reduce glomerular filtration. Furthermore, angiotensin II causes contraction of the mesangial cells, which support the glomerular capillary network, leading to a reduction in surface area available for filtration and so further acting to reduce filtration. The net effect in a particular physiological or pathophysiological circumstance depends on the balance between these actions and other haemodynamic compensations which occur.

Autoregulation of renal blood flow and GFR

Renal blood flow is generally kept constant over a wide range of blood pressures. This phenomenon, called autoregulation, ensures constancy of glomerular filtration and thus solute excretion despite changes in systemic haemodynamics within certain limits (Fig. 5.3). Whilst a variety of neural and vasoactive pathways may be involved in stabilising the renal blood flow under these conditions, two particular mechanisms have been invoked to explain the autoregulation of GFR.

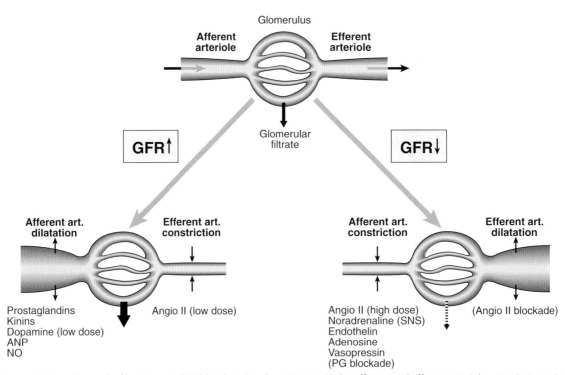

Fig. 5.2 Factors altering glomerular filtration rate (GFR) by changing the resistance in the afferent and efferent arterioles. Angio II, angiotensin II; ANP, atrial natriuretic peptide; NO, nitric oxide; PG, prostaglandin; SNS, sympathetic nervous system.

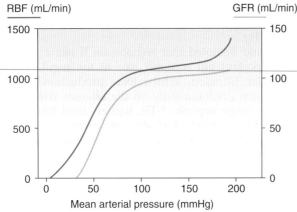

Fig. 5.3 Autoregulation of renal blood flow and glomerular filtration rate (GFR).

First, the **myogenic mechanism** refers to the intrinsic capacity of afferent arteriolar smooth muscle cells to increase their state of contraction in response to an increase in renal perfusion pressure. This response, probably mediated by vasoactive agents produced by endothelial cells acting on smooth muscle cells in the afferent arteriole, serves to blunt the transmission of changed arteriolar pressure into the glomerular capillary bed.

The second mechanism is **tubuloglomerular feedback** (TGF). This describes the process whereby the GFR in individual nephrons is regulated according to the rate of solute flow through that nephron. As described in Chapter 2, the juxtaglomerular apparatus consists of a structure at which the distal tubule of a given nephron comes into close proximity with the afferent and efferent arterioles of the same nephron. The tubular wall contains specialised cells known as the macula densa (Fig. 5.4; see also Fig. 2.10). Hence, the ionic composition (and indirectly, the flow rate) of the tubular fluid can be sensed by the macula densa, which signals directly to the vascular structures of the glomerulus to influence GFR. In brief, during conditions of avid tubular sodium chloride reabsorption, the sodium chloride concentration of the luminal fluid is reduced at the macula densa. Filtration in the corresponding glomerulus is increased, primarily by dilatation of the afferent arteriole. Conversely, when sodium chloride concentration and fluid delivery are high at the macula densa, afferent arteriolar tone is increased, and single nephron GFR falls. This feedback mechanism, probably designed to limit the loss of fluid and electrolytes from damaged nephrons, also contributes to the process of autoregulation. This is because increases in renal perfusion pressure would otherwise tend to lead to increased filtration and solute loss, which TGF effectively blunts. The mediator of the vasoconstrictor response involved in TGF appears to be locally produced adenosine, acting via the adenosine 1 receptor on the afferent arteriole. It is possible that other vasoactive mechanisms also play a part.

Renal excretion and the clearance formula

The rate at which a solute (s) is excreted by the kidney (E_s) is given simply by the product of the concentration of the solute in the urine (U_s) and the urine flow rate (V), which is the urine volume over a defined period. That is:

$$E_s = U_s \times V$$

where the units of E are mmol/min (or equivalent). This expression is useful in assessing absolute removal rates of solute by the kidney and hence evaluating total body mass balance.

The renal clearance (C_s) of solute (s) in contrast, is defined as the apparent volume of plasma from which the substance is completely removed per unit time during passage through the kidneys. It is equivalent mathematically

to the ratio of the excretion rate to the simultaneous plasma concentration for that substance (P_s):

$$C_s = (U_s \times V) / P_s$$

The units of clearance are mL/min (or equivalent). The clearance calculation provides a measure of the relative efficiency of the kidney in removing a given solute from the plasma and a means of comparison between substances which are handled differently by the nephron. The range of possible clearance rates is from zero (for a substance which is either not filtered at all or is filtered and then completely reabsorbed by the tubular system) up to a maximum equivalent to the renal plasma flow rate (for a substance which is filtered and totally secreted by the tubular system). Interpretation of clearance calculations depends on knowing whether the substance is freely filtered at the glomerulus. The procedure requires the presence of a steady state in the plasma concentration throughout the time frame of the period under study.

Measuring the GFR

The utility of the clearance concept in renal physiology is illustrated best by its application to the determination of GFR. As shown in Fig. 5.5, the renal handling of the plant polysaccharide inulin is such that it is freely filtered at the glomerulus and undergoes no reabsorption or secretion during its passage through the tubular system. It follows from a simple mass balance that the amount being filtered into the early part of the tubular system equals the amount being excreted at the end of that system. As shown in Fig. 5.5, this gives rise to the inference that the GFR can be measured by determining the clearance of inulin, which is possible experimentally simply by measuring its concentration in the plasma and urine, as well as the urine flow rate, during a steady state infusion.

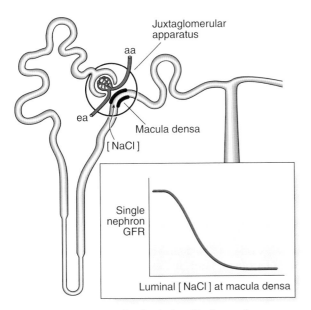

Fig. 5.4 Tubuloglomerular feedback. [NaCl] refers to the concentration of NaCl in the luminal fluid at the macula densa (top of the ascending limb of the loop of Henle). The inset shows the shape of the relationship between the [NaCl] at the macula densa and the glomerular filtration rate (GFR) in the same nephron.

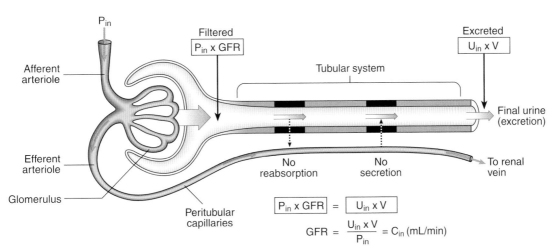

Fig. 5.5 Schematic illustration of the application of the clearance concept to the determination of the glomerular filtration rate (GFR). C_{in}, clearance of inulin; P_{in}, inulin concentration in plasma brought to the glomerulus; U_{in}, inulin concentration in final urine; V, urine flow rate.

Unfortunately, there are logistical difficulties involved in determining inulin clearance since it needs to be infused and is difficult to assay. Whilst a variety of other substances behave in a way similar to inulin and can be used clinically (e.g. iothalamate), in practice a great advantage is gained by using the clearance of an endogenous molecule whose behaviour approximates that of inulin for clinical determination of GFR. Such a substance is creatinine, derived from the metabolic breakdown of creatine, a component of skeletal muscle. For a given individual, the amount of creatinine entering the circulation per day is dependent almost exclusively on skeletal muscle mass. As long as kidney function is stable, this same daily amount will be excreted in the urine, given by the product of U_{cr} and V. Creatinine, like inulin, is freely filtered at the glomerulus and undergoes no tubular reabsorption, although there is a small degree of secretion by the tubules when renal function is impaired. Nonetheless, under most conditions, the clearance of endogenous creatinine provides a measure of GFR which is sufficiently robust for clinical use. Moreover, because $U_{cr} \times V$ is a constant (k) for a given individual under steady state conditions, there is a fixed relationship between the GFR and plasma creatinine, in the form of a rectangular hyperbola as shown in Fig. 5.6.

Several important deductions can be made from the inspection of this relationship. First, plasma creatinine only starts to increase substantially when approximately 50% of renal function (GFR) is lost. Thus, a significant reduction in GFR can be present before the plasma creatinine is recorded outside the 'normal' reference range for a laboratory. Second, each such relationship is specific to a given individual with a particular muscle mass, making a comparison of plasma creatinine between patients of different morphology difficult. For example, in patients with a low muscle mass, particularly elderly females, plasma creatinine can lie within the normal range in the presence of marked reductions in renal function. This is equivalent to saying that patients with increasing muscle masses have different GFR *versus* plasma creatinine graphs, displaced to the right in Fig. 5.6 for increasing muscle mass.

To obviate some of these difficulties in interpretation of plasma creatinine, several nomograms have been devised which give a reasonably accurate estimate of GFR from the plasma creatinine in an individual of a certain age, weight, and gender. One such formula is that of Cockcroft and Gault, namely:

Estimated GFR (mL/min)

$$= \frac{(140 - \text{age}) \times \text{weight (kg)}}{814 \times \text{plasma creatinine (mmol/L)}}$$

The result should be multiplied by 0.85 for women to allow for the relatively lower proportion of body weight which is muscle. This formula has proved useful in the modification of drug doses in the context of reduced GFR.

However, the formula most widely used at present to estimate GFR is the CKD-EPI creatinine equation, which

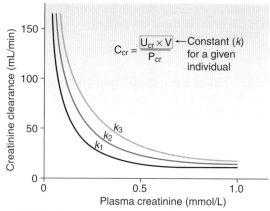

Fig. 5.6 Relationship between creatinine clearance (an estimate of glomerular filtration rate) and plasma creatinine concentration. C_{cr}, creatinine clearance; P_{cr}, plasma creatinine concentration; U_{cr}, urine creatinine concentration; V, urine flow rate. k_1 represents the curve for a small–average patient, while k_2 and k_3 show the position of the curve for progressively heavier patients.

estimates GFR (eGFR) from serum creatinine, age, sex, and race. The equation is complex, using a two slope spline to model the relationship between eGFR and creatinine whilst also modelling a relationship for age, sex, and race. This allows for a relatively accurate prediction of eGFR, even in patients with higher levels of kidney function, a group that was less reliably represented by older models such as the modification of diet in renal disease formula.

Urea is one of the main metabolic products of protein metabolism, and its excretion into the urine is one of the key functions of the kidney. Urea ($NH_2.CO.NH_2$) is synthesised in the liver from ammonium ions, derived from amino acid catabolism, plus carbon dioxide. It is freely filtered at the glomerulus but undergoes approximately 50% reabsorption during passage through the nephron. Thus, the clearance of urea is approximately half the GFR, and plasma urea varies inversely with the GFR. However, the fraction of filtered urea which is reabsorbed is not constant, being greater during conditions of dehydration and low urine flow rate because of vasopressin induced urea reabsorption in the medullary duct. This makes urea less valuable as a direct measure of GFR than creatinine since it is influenced not only by the GFR but also by the state of hydration. Furthermore, urea production is related to the amount of protein absorbed from the gut and the protein catabolic rate (Box 5.2). Consideration of the factors in this box allows for an informed interpretation of the results of plasma creatinine and urea levels. This will be of value later in our consideration of Mrs. Campbell.

Pathophysiology of oliguria

We turn now to a consideration of the origin and significance of the greatly reduced urine volume in the present

Box 5.1 Factors causing an increase in plasma creatinine and urea concentrations

Creatinine	Urea
Decreased GFR	Decreased GFR
Increased skeletal muscle mass (long-term)	Decreased urine flow rate
	Increased protein intake:
	Diet
	Gastrointestinal bleeding
	Increased protein catabolic rate:
	Sepsis
	Steroid therapy
	Some tetracycline antibiotics

GFR, glomerular filtration rate.

Box 5.2 Changes in plasma biochemistry in acute kidney injury

Hyperkalaemia
Decreased bicarbonate
Elevated urea
Elevated creatinine
Elevated uric acid
Hypocalcaemia
Hyperphosphataemia

patient. The urinary volume varies widely on a daily basis in normal individuals because of regulatory mechanisms aimed at maintaining a normal and constant body fluid volume. As described in Chapter 2, the main factors that are regulated to control body fluid volume and osmolality are the rates of reabsorption of sodium and water during their passage through the nephron. During states of sodium depletion and extracellular fluid (ECF) volume contraction, sodium reabsorptive mechanisms are activated, resulting in the excretion of urine with a low-sodium content. Similarly, during water deprivation, the kidney can concentrate urine sufficiently to maintain water balance at an intake of less than 500 mL/day. This capacity is largely related to the anatomical and physiological integrity of the tubular structures within the renal medulla and their responsiveness to antidiuretic hormone, which is released during states of dehydration.

Thus, a low urine flow rate itself may be a normal response to hypovolaemia, often accompanied by systemic and renal haemodynamic changes ('pre-renal' oliguria). By definition, AKI is only present when there is evidence for a reduced GFR; indeed, this diagnosis can be made in the presence of a normal or even increased urine volume under certain circumstances. However, when there is sustained oliguria, defined as a urine volume of less than 400 mL/24 h in adults, the likelihood

of a low GFR is increased, but it is necessary to establish whether this is essentially 'physiological' and reversible, or pathological and indicative of structural renal damage.

The clinical history and examination are often helpful in suggesting which of these patterns of oliguria is present in a particular patient. Thus, sustained hypovolaemia or shock, or the presence of toxins known to cause tubular necrosis (see below), suggests that widespread damage to the parenchyma is likely, whilst shorter lived or lesser insults make 'physiological' oliguria more likely. The fractional excretion of sodium ($FeNa_+$) is thought to be useful in making the distinction between pre-renal causes of AKI, where FeNa is low because of appropriate sodium reabsorption to restore fluid balance, and established acute tubular necrosis, where FeNa is high because of tubular dysfunction. However, the evidence behind this diagnostic technique is limited, and several factors (diuretic use, CKD, cirrhosis) render this calculation unreliable. In broad terms, the functional oliguria associated with physiological responses to hypovolaemia is reversible with appropriate fluid replacement therapy, whilst that associated with structural damage is less likely to be so. Making this clinical differentiation has important therapeutic implications, as will be illustrated later in the present patient. See Case 5.1: 3.

Causes of acute kidney injury

AKI is a clinical term that encompasses many causes of abrupt renal impairment; that is, a fall in GFR occurring over a period of hours or days, which results in impaired fluid and electrolyte homeostasis and the accumulation of nitrogenous wastes. AKI occurs in response to a wide variety of insults, the most common causes being haemodynamic, immunological, toxic, and obstructive. Classically, the causes of AKI are divided into pre-renal, renal, and post-renal causes depending on the site of the initiating insult (Table 5.1).

The commonest causes of AKI acquired out of hospital are prolonged ischaemic injury in some 50% of cases and nephrotoxic injury in 35%. In hospital-acquired kidney injury, the cause is usually multifactorial. The major predisposing factors include volume depletion (often caused by vomiting, diarrhoea, or diuretics) and treatment with drugs (such as angiotensin-converting enzyme inhibitors, angiotensin II receptor blockers or non-steroidal anti-inflammatory drugs), and radiocontrast agents. Elderly, diabetic and chronically hypertensive patients are at particular risk because of their predisposition to underlying vascular disease and poor renal autoregulatory responses. In the hospital population, hypotension, heart failure, sepsis, and aminoglycoside use are common additional factors involved in the genesis of AKI. Sustained circulatory impairment leading to ischaemia induced acute tubular necrosis (ATN) accounts for the majority of cases of AKI overall.

Glomerular filtration and acute kidney injury: 2

Investigations

Initial blood tests in Mrs. Wood showed an elevation in the white cell count, with a neutrophilia consistent with infection.

The plasma urea concentration was elevated at *26 mmol/L, and creatinine was elevated at *350 µmol/L. The plasma sodium was 145 mmol/L, and the potassium was elevated at *6.1 mmol/L.

Acidosis was present, indicated by the reduced bicarbonate at *18 mmol/L. The serum albumin was 48 g/L, calcium was 2.20 mmol/L, and phosphate was *1.8 mmol/L.

From this data, we can conclude that Mrs. Wood's oliguria is associated with acute kidney injury, given the marked elevation of plasma creatinine which implies a reduced GFR.

The questions now arise:

1. What has caused the acute kidney injury in this case?
2. What are the pathologic conditions and natural history of ATN?
3. How have the plasma biochemistry abnormalities come about?
4. What complications of acute kidney injury can be anticipated and treated?

*Results outside the normal range; see Appendix.

Acute tubular necrosis

When the kidney sustains a severe hypoxic insult, injury and death of tubular cells occur, and the resulting clinico-pathological syndrome is referred to as ATN. This most commonly occurs because of prolonged renal ischaemia during a period of hypotension. Other causes include direct toxic injury to the tubules by endogenous chemicals such as myoglobin (released from damaged muscle cells – rhabdomyolysis) or haemoglobin (released from red blood cells during acute episodes of haemolysis). Less commonly, ATN results from exposure to nephrotoxic drugs (see Chapter 11) and heavy metals.

Several biochemical processes have been implicated in the development of injury to tubular cells, particularly following the onset of renal ischaemia. These include depletion of cellular adenosine triphosphate (ATP), increase in intracellular calcium, disruption of cytoskeletal structures, loss of epithelial polarity, activation of apoptosis (programmed cell death), and increased oxygen free radical production. The latter mechanism may be particularly important as a cause of tissue injury during the reperfusion phase after a period of ischaemia.

Table 5.1 Causes of acute kidney injury

Pre-renal	Renal	Post-renal
Hypovolaemia	Acute tubular necrosis (ischaemic or toxic)	Bilateral ureteric obstruction
Decreased effective blood volume	Interstitial nephritis (e.g. drugs – see Chapter 14)	Ureteric obstruction in a single kidney
Decreased cardiac output	Glomerular disease (e.g. acute glomerulonephritis)	
Renovascular obstruction	Small vessel disease (e.g. microvasculitis)	Bladder outflow obstruction
	Intrarenal vasoconstriction (e.g. in sepsis)	
	Tubular obstruction (e.g. urate crystals)	

Pathology of ATN

Histologically, the changes in ATN are most prominent in the cells of the proximal tubule, particularly in its latter third (S3 segment). Blebs appear in the apical brush border, with sloughing of the brush border membrane into the lumen or involution into the cytoplasm. The integrity of the tight junctions is disrupted, and loss of epithelial cell polarity occurs. Integrins, which normally contribute to cell–cell adhesion, are redistributed to the apical membrane, resulting in the shedding of both live and dead cells into the lumen, which contributes to cast formation and tubular obstruction. Interstitial oedema is prominent because of leakage of tubular fluid across damaged tubular walls (Fig. 5.7). The glomeruli are generally relatively well preserved.

Pathophysiology of ATN

A variety of mechanisms have been proposed to explain the persistence of reduced glomerular filtration in the context of ATN, even after the instigating stimulus has been corrected or removed. These include sustained renal vasoconstriction, probably mediated by intrarenal humoral factors, reduced glomerular permeability, mechanical obstruction by sloughed cells and proteinaceous casts, and back-leak of filtrate from the tubular lumen. It is likely that a different pattern of mechanisms is involved depending on the exact cause or contributing factors in a given case of ATN.

Course of ATN

Impaired kidney function and oligoanuria during ATN typically persist for 1 week or more, after which complete cellular recovery can occur, accompanied by a return of GFR towards normal and a marked increase in urine output. This recovery is because of epithelial cell

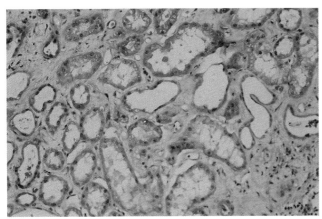

Fig. 5.7 Micrograph (stained with haematoxylin and eosin) showing acute tubular necrosis. Note the atrophy of the tubular epithelium, the dilatation of tubules and interstitial oedema (wide separation between adjacent tubules).

Case 5.1 Glomerular filtration and acute kidney injury: 3

Progress

Mrs. Wood's acute kidney injury was attributed to ATN based on prolonged renal ischaemia caused by dehydration, hypotension, and sepsis, on a background of treatment with a diuretic and an angiotensin-converting enzyme (ACE) inhibitor.

Initial treatment consisted of ceasing her antihypertensives, rehydration with normal saline, and commencement of intravenous antibiotics. A surgical opinion was sought, and a conservative approach to the management of her diverticular abscess was recommended in the first instance.

Over the following 2 days, Mrs. Wood's general condition improved considerably, with loss of fever and improvement of tissue hydration, with her blood pressure rising to 150/85. However, her urine output remained very poor, and the plasma creatinine concentration increased further to *600 µmol/L. Mild hyperkalaemia and acidosis persisted.

Given these developments, consistent with a sustained reduction in GFR because of tubular necrosis, Mrs. Wood was seen by the consultant nephrologist who arranged for her to commence intermittent haemodialysis via a temporary catheter inserted into her jugular vein. She tolerated these treatments well, and there was further improvement in her clinical condition and electrolytes over the following week. She received parenteral nutrition over this period.

Ten days after admission, an increase in urine output was noted, and over the next few days, her plasma urea and creatinine concentrations started to fall towards normal, and her dialysis was discontinued. She was now eating and drinking and was recommenced on an antihypertensive drug regime to control her blood pressure. On surgical review, the decision was made to defer surgery on her bowel until further settling of her inflammatory mass had occurred. She was discharged from the hospital 2 weeks after admission.

regeneration, probably under the control of locally produced peptide growth factors such as insulin-like growth factor 1 and epidermal growth factor.

As long as kidney function can be temporarily replaced with a form of dialysis during the period of suppressed GFR, if required, with correction of electrolyte disturbances and maintenance of adequate nutrition, the patient can recover and reattain normal renal function. Close attention to the replacement of fluid and electrolytes is important during the early recovery phase, as a period of polyuria and uncontrolled electrolyte loss is common as tubular regeneration proceeds. See Case 5.1: 3.

Overview: assessment and management of a patient with AKI

A logical approach to the evaluation of a patient with AKI is presented in Table 5.2. All patients presenting with AKI require a careful history and examination, urinalysis and urine microscopy, plasma biochemistry analysis, and full blood count. In general, urinary tract obstruction should be excluded early on with a renal ultrasound. Subsequent investigations depend on whether the cause of AKI is considered to be pre-renal, renal, or post-renal in nature. Clues should also be sought to determine whether there is a background of chronic kidney disease, which is suggested by anaemia, hyperphosphataemia, hypocalcaemia, and small kidney size. Previously documented serum creatinine levels are also very useful, if available, to assess the acuity of kidney injury.

Biochemical changes in AKI

When the kidneys fail over a short time period, the metabolic disturbances which occur reflect the failure of their normal homeostatic role in maintaining body fluid volume and composition within a narrow normal range. Changes in plasma biochemistry usually seen in this situation are shown in Box 5.2. It is important to note that this box does not include any direct indication of altered body fluid volume in AKI. As a result of an impaired capacity to excrete fluid, this is usually manifested as hypervolaemia and, in extreme cases, pulmonary oedema, which must be assessed clinically and radiologically.

Hyperkalaemia results in part from potassium retention because of a failure of filtration and tubular secretion of potassium by the damaged kidney. There is, in addition, an increased endogenous potassium load associated with some causes of AKI, such as muscle crush injury. This electrolyte disturbance is particularly serious because of its potential to produce life-threatening cardiac asystole through its effect on the excitability of

Table 5.2 Assessment of a patient with acute kidney injury

Procedure	Information sought
Clinical history and examination	Clues to the cause of acute kidney injury (see Table 5.1) Indicators of the severity of metabolic disturbance Estimate of volume status (hydration) (see Table 2.1 and Clinical Skills box in Chapter 2)
Urinalysis and urine microscopy	Markers of glomerular or tubulointerstitial inflammation, urinary tract infection, or crystal uropathy
Plasma biochemistry	To assess the extent of GFR reduction and metabolic consequences
Full blood count	To determine the presence of anaemia, leucocytosis, and platelet consumption
Renal ultrasound	To determine kidney size, presence of obstruction, abnormal renal parenchymal texture
Plus, where appropriate:	
Abdominal CT scan*	To define structural abnormalities of the kidneys or urinary tract
Radionuclide scan	To assess abnormal renal perfusion
Cystoscopy ± retrograde pyelograms	To evaluate/relieve urinary tract obstruction
Renal biopsy	To define the pathologic conditions of renal parenchymal disease

*CT, computed tomography; note that this should ideally be performed without the use of contrast agent in the context of impaired GFR.
GFR, glomerular filtration rate.

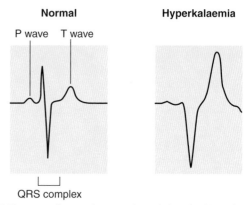

Fig. 5.8 Electrocardiogram in severe hyperkalaemia. Note the widening of the QRS complex and the high peaked T waves compared to the normal tracing. The plasma potassium in this patient was 7.6 mmol/L.

cardiac conducting tissue. It can also lead to profound skeletal muscle weakness.

Other factors which may contribute to hyperkalaemia include conditions or drugs which directly influence the capacity of the distal tubule to secrete potassium, as is sometimes seen in cases where the urinary tract is infected and obstructed, or in low aldosterone states, or when potassium-sparing diuretics or angiotensin-converting enzyme (ACE) inhibitors are being used. Metabolic acidosis, itself a consequence of AKI and associated conditions, also frequently contributes to hyperkalaemia by promoting the transcellular exchange of potassium ions for hydrogen ions.

ECG abnormalities are often the first indication that severe hyperkalaemia is present (Fig. 5.8). Such changes, usually associated with a serum potassium greater than 6.5 mmol/L, require emergency treatment with an infusion of calcium gluconate to stabilise the membrane potential in the cardiac conducting tissue, followed by agents to shift potassium into cells (nebulised beta-agonists, intravenous sodium bicarbonate, intravenous glucose, and insulin). These measures must be accompanied by interventions to remove potassium from the body (ion exchange resins or dialysis).

Metabolic acidosis (reflected by a low bicarbonate) occurs in kidney disease because of the retention of organic acids and failure of the kidney to secrete and excrete the net hydrogen ion load (see Chapter 4). An additional acid load may be generated in some settings of AKI, such as with lactate production in the presence of poor tissue perfusion.

Elevated urea and creatinine are manifestations of the retention of nitrogenous products of metabolism because of reduced filtration. Both substances have additional significance as markers of the GFR, with creatinine being more useful for this purpose (see above). The likelihood of uraemic symptoms correlates best with urea level, although urea is not the only toxin responsible for the development of the symptoms. Uraemia is characterised by impaired mental function (drowsiness and confusion), anorexia, nausea and vomiting and, in severe cases, asterixis and pericarditis.

Hyperphosphataemia also results from failure of filtration but is aggravated in situations in which a high phosphate load is generated (such as tissue breakdown in rhabdomyolysis or tumour lysis syndrome). The total plasma calcium is generally low at the onset of AKI, although this often normalises or overcorrects as recovery proceeds.

Complications of AKI

Complications may arise because of the kidney injury itself or the illnesses associated with the development of kidney failure.

The most important factors in contributing to morbidity and mortality rates are cardiovascular complications arising from fluid overload, arrhythmias, acute myocardial ischaemia, and hypertension. Systemic infection is another major cause of adverse outcomes in AKI. This is probably because of the effect of the abnormal metabolic environment on immunological functions, although it often relates directly to the cause of the AKI, such as Gram-negative septicaemia or burns.

Neurological disturbances often parallel the rate of the rise of blood urea, sometimes resulting in a depressed level of consciousness or seizures.

Gastrointestinal haemorrhage occurs frequently in these patients, often based on an impaired coagulation mechanism. This may be caused by a platelet function defect induced by uraemia, reduced tissue integrity predisposing to bleeding, and sometimes systemic coagulopathy related to the primary cause of kidney injury.

Another factor contributing to high morbidity and mortality rates in AKI is impaired nutritional status. Factors contributing to this may include anorexia in the period before the development of kidney injury; a catabolic state commonly associated with kidney injury; uncontrolled acidosis, which accelerates protein breakdown; and inadequate provision of nutrients in the early phase of management.

Management of AKI

The principles of management of AKI can be summarised as shown in Table 5.3. Note that the table does not include the measures required to correct the underlying cause of AKI, e.g. relieving urinary tract obstruction when present.

It should be clear from the above that the availability of renal replacement therapy in the form of acute dialysis is of critical importance in saving lives from this medical emergency. This can be a particularly cost-effective form of intervention, where appropriate, given that the kidney has the capacity for complete recovery in many of the conditions underlying this presentation.

Table 5.3 Principles of management of acute kidney injury

Problem	Management
Fluid volume disturbance	Rehydrate if hypovolaemic; withhold fluid and give high-dose diuretic if hypervolaemic; dialysis for resistant pulmonary oedema
Metabolic disturbances:	
Hyperkalaemia	Intravenous calcium, bicarbonate, glucose plus insulin; oral/rectal ion exchange resin; dialysis
Acidosis	Bicarbonate supplements; dialysis
Uraemic syndrome	Dialysis
Infection	Antibiotics and surgery if appropriate
Nutritional deficiencies	Enteral or parenteral feeding in conjunction with dialysis

Summary

1. Understanding the physiology of glomerular filtration will improve your understanding of the measurement of GFR.
2. GFR is rarely directly measured but rather estimated using various equations.
3. The estimation of GFR relies on serum creatinine being in the steady state.
4. Oliguria may be an appropriate response to hypovolaemia or may be related to structural kidney damage.
5. AKI can be thought of as being pre-renal, renal, or post-renal, and it is important to understand how to differentiate these causes.
6. Metabolic disturbances occur in AKI, including hyperkalaemia and metabolic acidosis.
7. The management of AKI involves ensuring euvolaemia, correcting electrolyte disturbances, and monitoring for complications.
8. If AKI is unable to be reversed with correcting the cause and rehydration, short-term dialysis may be required.

Self-assessment case study

A previously well 32-year-old man is brought to the emergency department having been involved in a motor vehicle accident. The circumstances of the accident are initially unclear. However, the ambulance officers who attended the accident noted that he was trapped in the vehicle for 3 h before being freed. At this time, he was hypotensive with a systolic blood pressure of 80 mmHg and had significant injuries to his lower limbs with probable fracture of both femora. He was treated with fluid resuscitation, and his systolic blood pressure stabilised at 100 mmHg. At the time of admission to the emergency department, abdominal, thoracic, and cerebral injuries were excluded, and his injuries were assessed as being confined to his lower limbs. He was tachycardic, and his blood pressure was 100/60 mmHg, and his jugular venous pressure was not visible even though he was lying flat. In preparation for surgical stabilisation of his lower limbs, he had a urinary catheter inserted, and 50 mL of dark urine, which tested strongly positive for blood on

Continued

Self-assessment case study – cont'd

urinalysis, was drained, after which minimal urine output was documented.

Initial laboratory investigations revealed the following results:

*Haemoglobin 79 g/L

Sodium 140 mmol/L

*Potassium 7.8 mmol/L

Chloride 98 mmol/L

*Bicarbonate 11 mmol/L

*Urea 13 mmol/L

*Creatinine 190 μmol/L.

(*Results outside normal range; see Appendix.)

After studying this chapter, you should be able to answer the following questions:

Q1. What is the urine microscopy finding most likely to confirm this patient's diagnosis?

A. Presence of red cells

B. Absence of red cells

C. Presence of white cells

D. Absence of white cells

Q2. This man has acute tubular necrosis. What is the most likely cause?

A. Prolonged hypoxic insult to the kidneys

B. Direct toxic injury to the tubules by endogenous substance

C. Direct toxic injury to the tubules by nephrotoxic drugs

D. Tubular injury related to interstitial nephritis

Self-assessment case study answers

A1. B, Absence of red cells. This presentation strongly suggests rhabdomyolysis as a cause for this patient's AKI. Myoglobinuria occurs, and myoglobin is detected on the dipstick measure as blood. However, when the urine is examined for the presence of red cells, they will not be present

A2. B, Direct toxic injury to the tubules by endogenous substance. Myoglobin is directly toxic to the tubules.

PROTEINURIA AND THE NEPHROTIC SYNDROME

6

Chapter objectives

After studying this chapter, you should be able to:

1. Describe the anatomy of the normal glomerulus, including its three cell types and their arrangement and the structure of the glomerular capillary wall and glomerular basement membrane (GBM).

2. Discuss the components of normal and abnormal proteinuria and differentiate tubular and glomerular proteinuria.

3. Understand the role of the glomerulus and its components (cells and GBM) in preventing proteinuria.

4. Discuss the pathophysiology and differential diagnosis of oedema.

5. Understand the features and pathophysiology of nephrotic syndrome and its complications.

6. List the main diseases that cause nephrotic syndrome in children and adults.

7. Describe the renal histopathological features of minimal change disease.

8. Discuss the natural history of minimal change disease and the other major causes of nephrotic syndrome.

9. Discuss the response to treatment of the major causes of nephrotic syndrome.

Introduction

In producing an ultrafiltrate of plasma as the first stage in urine production, the glomerulus must retain plasma proteins within the lumen of its capillary network. This ability to retain plasma proteins by preventing their filtration into the tubular lumen is determined by the size- and charge-selective properties of the glomerular filtration barrier (GFB). When diseases damage the integrity of this barrier, plasma proteins may escape across it into the tubular lumen.

The proximal segments of the nephron have the capacity to reabsorb and metabolise very efficiently any proteins that appear in the tubular lumen. Under normal circumstances, small plasma proteins which are able to pass across the GFB are taken up (endocytosed) by proximal tubular cells via luminal membrane receptors such as megalin-cubilin on their brush-border membrane, to be broken down in lysosomes. However, protein may appear in the final urine (proteinuria) if the amount filtered by the glomerulus overwhelms tubular reabsorptive mechanisms or if tubular cells are damaged.

Severe proteinuria may damage the kidney or have systemic consequences because of the loss of albumin and other proteins from the blood.

In this chapter, the causes and consequences of proteinuria will be considered and illustrated by a case of severe proteinuria occurring in a child (see Case 6.1: 1).

Pathophysiology of oedema formation

Oedema literally means 'swelling' and refers to the accumulation of fluid within the tissues. This fluid is located outside the vascular system in the interstitial space (see Chapter 2).

Under normal circumstances, the balance between hydrostatic and osmotic pressure gradients (Starling's forces) across capillary walls prevents oedema formation (Fig. 6.1A). The hydrostatic pressure of the column of blood within systemic capillaries is determined by the pumping action of the heart and resistance to flow within the arterial tree and capacitance of the venous system. Capillary hydrostatic pressure varies in different tissues but is on average about 25 mmHg. This favours the movement of plasma filtrate into the surrounding interstitial compartment, which has a lower hydrostatic pressure. This hydrostatic pressure gradient is opposed by osmotic forces, which favour the movement of fluid from the interstitium (which has a colloid osmotic pressure, or oncotic pressure, of about 1 mmHg) into the capillary lumen (where plasma proteins exert an oncotic pressure of about 25 mmHg). Capillary hydrostatic pressure falls along the length of the capillary, whereas capillary oncotic pressure rises as water moves into the interstitial space. Thus these forces favour net water movement into the interstitium at the arterial end of the capillary (hydrostatic > oncotic pressure), balanced under normal conditions by an equivalent

---

Case 6.1 — Proteinuria and the nephrotic syndrome: 1

Generalised oedema

Kylie Major presented to her general practitioner (GP) with facial swelling of 3 days duration. Kylie was a 6-year-old girl who had been completely healthy in the past and had had no antecedent illnesses before the presentation. Her GP found obvious pitting oedema (swelling which can be indented by digital compression) in her face and around her ankles. Her blood pressure was 95/60. Her jugular venous pressure was normal, her chest was clear to auscultation, and there was no shifting dullness on percussion of her abdomen, indicating that there were no clinically obvious ascites (free peritoneal fluid). Dipstick analysis of a fresh urine sample was strongly positive for protein but negative for blood. Her GP thought her generalised oedema was most likely caused by proteinuria.

Consideration of the presenting features of this patient leads to the following questions:

1. What are the forces which prevent the development of oedema normally?
2. What are the major diseases that cause oedema? How are the forces opposing oedema formation disrupted in these conditions?
3. How does proteinuria cause oedema?

These questions will be addressed in the first section of this chapter.

---

movement of water in the other direction at the venous end (oncotic > hydrostatic pressure). Oedema fluid within the interstitial space is limited also by drainage via lymphatic vessels.

The above principles apply to other capillary beds, but the details of the forces involved vary (see, e.g. Chapter 5 for a discussion of forces in the glomerulus, a capillary bed designed to achieve net movement of fluid out of the lumen).

Oedema arises because of a localised or generalised disruption of Starling's forces within capillaries or because of a failure of lymphatic drainage of the interstitial space (Fig. 6.1B). Thus, factors that favour oedema formation include a loss of integrity of the capillary wall, an increase in hydrostatic pressure within the capillary lumen (e.g. caused by high venous pressures within the systemic or pulmonary circulation as occurs in congestive cardiac failure, and within portal veins in **cirrhosis**), reduction in plasma oncotic pressure because of hypoalbuminaemia, or obstruction of lymphatic flow. The main causes of oedema are listed in Table 6.1.

If oedema formation were determined only by Starling's forces in capillaries, then bodyweight should not increase. However, in most conditions causing generalised oedema (see Table 6.1), the kidneys actively

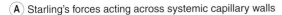

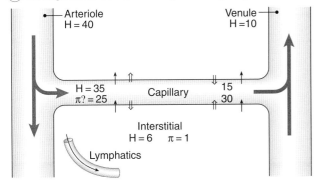

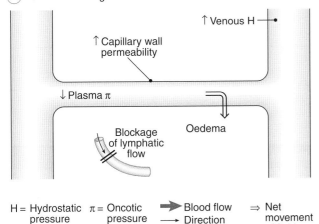

H = Hydrostatic   π = Oncotic   ➡ Blood flow   ⇒ Net
    pressure   pressure   → Direction   movement
    in mmHg   in mmHg   of force   of fluid

Fig. 6.1 (A) Starling's forces acting across systemic capillary walls. The net movement of fluid depends on the balance between capillary and interstitial hydrostatic (H) and oncotic (π) pressures. Representative values (in mmHg) are shown. (B) Factors favouring oedema formation. Reduction in plasma oncotic pressure, increase in capillary wall permeability or venous hydrostatic pressure, or lymphatic blockage will increase oedema formation.

retain salt and water, causing weight gain and aggravating the build-up of oedema fluid. Salt and water retention in these circumstances may arise as a response to a reduction in 'effective' arterial blood volume because of impaired cardiac output or loss of fluid from the circulation into the tissues, leading to several responses designed to protect against hypovolaemia (see Chapter 2). These responses include systemic haemodynamic changes, which occur quickly, and intrarenal changes, which lead to salt and water retention over days to weeks. The intrarenal factors include:

- reflex activation of the sympathetic nervous system
- activation of the renin–angiotensin–aldosterone system and vasopressin (antidiuretic hormone, ADH) release
- resistance to the action of natriuretic peptides
- altered glomerular haemodynamics
- peritubular forces in the proximal tubule.

These neuronal, hormonal, and intrarenal mechanisms, which together augment sodium reabsorption at multiple sites along the nephron, are discussed in more detail in Chapter 2. It is important to recognise that evidence also exists to suggest that renal salt and water retention may actually precede the development of circulatory changes in these conditions. In the case of the nephrotic syndrome, this may arise because of a fall in glomerular filtration rate (GFR) as glomerular damage progresses or from poorly understood mechanisms promoting distal tubular sodium reabsorption early in the course of the disease process.

The predominant site of oedema can give a clue to the cause. Thus, with right-sided heart failure, peripheral oedema (affecting the extremities) should be accompanied by a raised jugular venous pressure and hepatic congestion. With left-sided heart failure, pulmonary congestion alone is expected. With cirrhosis, ascites (fluid accumulation in the peritoneal cavity) is seen earlier than in other causes of generalised oedema because of portal venous hypertension. Peripheral oedema also occurs with cirrhosis owing to hypoalbuminaemia.

When there is marked proteinuria, peripheral and/or facial oedema develops because of hypoalbuminaemia. This combination of findings is called the nephrotic syndrome (or nephrosis), which will be discussed further below. The site of oedema is also influenced by the effect of gravity. Thus, in ambulant patients, mild oedema is frequently seen first around the ankles (where venous hydrostatic pressure is highest in the erect posture), whereas in bedridden patients, it may be over the sacrum as this is the most dependent position. With severe nephrotic syndrome, oedema can be more widespread and may involve the lungs and pleural and peritoneal cavities. If renal salt and water retention is a predominant pathophysiological event, as occurs in some forms of nephrosis (particularly where the GFR is reduced), the blood volume may be increased, and jugular venous pressure raised.

The three main generalised oedema states are congestive cardiac failure, cirrhosis, and nephrotic syndrome. These may be differentiated by finding signs of cardiac disease in the case of congestive cardiac failure, liver failure in the case of cirrhosis, and heavy proteinuria in cases of nephrotic syndrome. The latter is clearly the problem in the present patient and will be the subject of the rest of this chapter.

Glomerular anatomy and the filtration barrier

Each human kidney contains about one million glomeruli, each of which is a specialised capillary network fed by a single afferent arteriole and drained by a single efferent arteriole. The glomerulus is populated by three intrinsic cells: the capillary endothelial cell, the epithelial cell, which lies over it with the GBM in between, and the

Table 6.1 Main causes of oedema

	Pathophysiological factors	Predominant site
Local		
Infection, trauma	Capillary leak	Local
Venous obstruction (e.g. thrombosis)	Increased venous hydrostatic pressure	Local
Lymphatic obstruction	Lymphatic obstruction	Local
Generalised		
Congestive cardiac failure	Increased venous hydrostatic pressure, renal salt and water retention	Jugular veins (intravascular, not 'oedema'), lower limb, pulmonary
Cirrhosis	Decreased plasma oncotic pressure, renal salt and water retention, increased venous hydrostatic pressure	Ascites, lower limb
Nephrotic syndrome	Decreased plasma oncotic pressure, renal salt and water retention	Facial, lower limb
Septicaemia	Capillary leak	Lower limb, pulmonary
Allergic reactions (angio-oedema)	Capillary leak	Facial
Cyclical ('idiopathic')	?	Lower limb
Drugs	Increased venous hydrostatic pressure, renal salt and water retention	Lower limb

mesangial cell. Under normal circumstances, protein is largely excluded from the glomerular filtrate by an intact GFB. As shown in Fig. 6.2, the GFB comprises three layers: the endothelial cell, the GBM, and the visceral glomerular epithelial cell (also known as 'podocyte'). Each layer appears to provide a barrier to the filtration of protein, but this function is subserved predominantly by the GBM and by the slit pore between cytoplasmic extensions ('foot processes') of the podocyte. The podocyte can be visualised as a small-headed octopus with its many discrete feet ('foot processes') draped over and covering the outer surface of each glomerular loop. Between the podocytes are slit pores, across which are spread thin diaphragms consisting of newly recognised proteins such as nephrin. Mutations of various podocyte proteins, including nephrin, have been identified as causing familial nephrotic syndrome, and their identification has brought an understanding of the molecular structure of the slit diaphragm and podocyte–GBM interactions.

The GBM also consists of specialised structural proteins, including certain collagens and charged heparin-like molecules. These molecules are arranged so that discrete pores prevent the movement of large molecules (size selectivity) and charged ions (charge selectivity) across the GBM. Thus albumin, which is negatively charged and has a molecular weight of 67 kDa, does not pass across the normal GBM. Haemoglobin has a similar molecular weight to albumin but is not charged; therefore, when released from red blood cells (haemolysis), it can pass across the GBM and is excreted in the urine (haemoglobinuria). Smaller proteins such as myoglobin (17 kDa) and monomeric light chains (22 kDa) pass across freely, whereas larger molecules such as ferritin (480 kDa) may only pass across severely disrupted GBMs.

Although the mesangial cell is not anatomically part of the GFB, it can alter the filtration of proteins because of its contractile properties (which alter the surface area of GFB available for filtration) and its ability to absorb, metabolise and discharge macromolecules into renal lymphatic channels.

Normal and abnormal proteinuria

Normal urine contains a small amount of protein, less than 150 mg/day in adults. Normal urinary protein consists of proteins of small molecular weight which have been filtered across the GFB and not reabsorbed by tubular cells, and proteins such as Tamm–Horsfall protein (also known as Uromodulin) which are secreted by tubular cells. Heavy exercise, fever, and prolonged standing ('orthostasis') may increase proteinuria in otherwise normal individuals. As explained above, larger proteins such as albumin are found in only small amounts in normal urine.

Abnormal proteinuria most commonly arises because of failure of the GFB filtration barrier ('glomerular proteinuria'), but it can also result from decreased protein reabsorption into or increased protein release from tubular epithelial cells ('tubular proteinuria'; see Fig. 6.3). Tubular proteinuria consists of low molecular weight proteins (generally less than 40 kDa) and usually amounts to less than 1 g/day. Glomerular proteinuria consists of proteins of greater molecular size and may be up to many grams per day. In some glomerular diseases in which the injury is of a limited nature, such as minimal change disease, protein loss into the urine is largely restricted to molecules the size of albumin or less ('selective proteinuria'), whereas with more extensive damage, immunoglobulins and even larger proteins may be found in the urine ('nonselective proteinuria'). Note that even with glomerular proteinuria, the tubules do have some capacity to reabsorb a fraction of the filtered protein. When glomerular proteinuria is severe, nephrotic syndrome may develop, as occurred with the current patient.

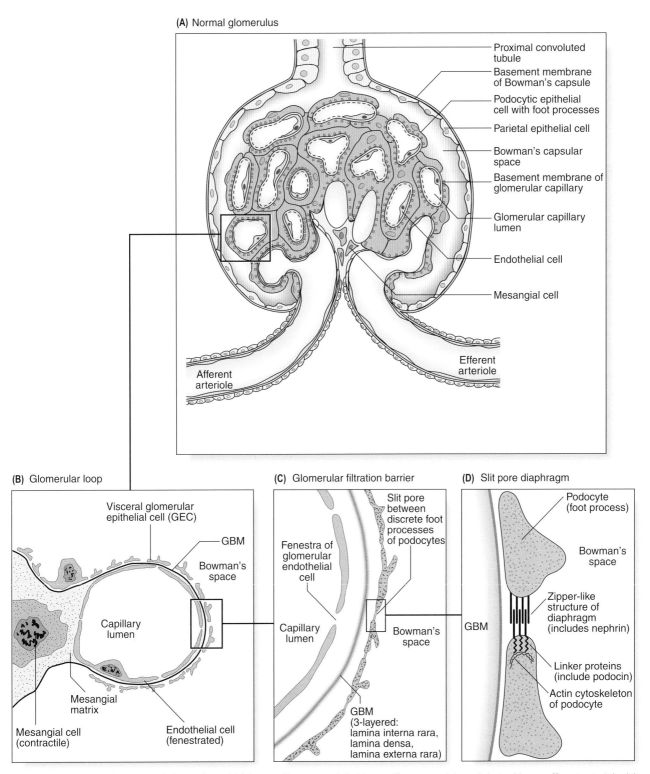

(A) Normal glomerulus

Proximal convoluted tubule
Basement membrane of Bowman's capsule
Podocytic epithelial cell with foot processes
Parietal epithelial cell
Bowman's capsular space
Basement membrane of glomerular capillary
Glomerular capillary lumen
Endothelial cell
Mesangial cell

Efferent arteriole
Afferent arteriole

(B) Glomerular loop

Visceral glomerular epithelial cell (GEC)
GBM
Bowman's space
Capillary lumen
Mesangial matrix
Mesangial cell (contractile)
Endothelial cell (fenestrated)

(C) Glomerular filtration barrier

Slit pore between discrete foot processes of podocytes
Fenestra of glomerular endothelial cell
Capillary lumen
Bowman's space
GBM (3-layered: lamina interna rara, lamina densa, lamina externa rara)

(D) Slit pore diaphragm

Podocyte (foot process)
Bowman's space
GBM
Zipper-like structure of diaphragm (includes nephrin)
Linker proteins (include podocin)
Actin cytoskeleton of podocyte

Fig. 6.2 (A) Structure of the normal glomerulus, which is a capillary network fed by an afferent arteriole and drained by an efferent arteriole; (B) glomerular loop, consisting of a capillary lumen lying beneath podocytes) and adjacent to mesangium; (C) glomerular filtration barrier comprising glomerular endothelial cells surrounded by the glomerular basement membrane (GBM) and podocytes; (D) slit diaphragm of podocyte with newly recognised structural and signalling proteins.

The principal causes of proteinuria are listed in Box 6.1. The most important of these in clinical terms are those conditions that cause damage to the glomerulus. Glomerular disease may be primary (glomerulonephritis) or secondary to systemic diseases such as diabetes mellitus. In addition, glomerular disease may occur as a component or consequence of widespread renal scarring, which occurs late in the course of any chronic renal disease. In the latter situation, the glomerular scarring is called 'glomerulosclerosis'.

See Case 6.1: 2.

Interesting facts

Urinary dipsticks are used in screening for proteinuria and vary in their specificity and sensitivity for albumin. Some are highly specific and able to detect albumin in low concentration ('microalbuminuria'). To quantitate protein excretion, the urine sample needs to be collected over a specified period of time or a factor introduced to take account of how concentrated the urinary sample is. Urinary creatinine concentration is a useful correction factor because, in an individual patient, the daily excretion of creatinine tends to remain constant. Thus it is common practice to express urinary protein as a ratio to urinary creatinine.

Nephrotic syndrome

Clinical features

Nephrotic syndrome (or nephrosis) consists of a diagnostic triad of heavy proteinuria, which leads to

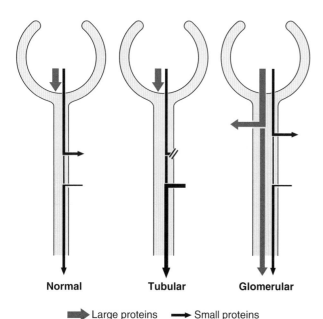

Fig. 6.3 Proteinuria, occurring in normal kidneys or because of tubular or glomerular disease.

hypoalbuminaemia, which in turn causes oedema in a range of anatomical locations (Table 6.2 and Fig. 6.4).

Complications of nephrotic syndrome are relatively common, and their frequency increases with the severity

Box 6.1 Principal causes of proteinuria

Normal kidneys
Normal (<150 mg/24 h)
Exercise
Fever
Orthostasis

Abnormal kidneys
Tubular diseases (≤1 g/24 h)
Glomerular disease (>1 g/24 h)
  Primary glomerulonephritis
  Secondary glomerular disease in:
    systemic diseases such as diabetes mellitus, **amyloidosis**
    generalised renal scarring

Case 6.1 Proteinuria and the nephrotic syndrome: 2

Investigations

Kylie's GP organised some blood and urine tests. Her serum creatinine was normal, and serum albumin was very low at *13 g/L. Microscopic examination of spun urinary sediment was normal except for the presence of many hyaline (proteinaceous) casts. Urinary protein excretion was *6 g/day and consisted mainly of albumin. Serum cholesterol was *9.6 mmol/L, and serum triglycerides were normal.

When Kylie returned to be reviewed by her GP 2 days later, she had gained an extra 3 kg in weight, and her oedema was worse. In addition, she was complaining of pain in her right calf, which appeared to be more swollen than the left. Her GP suspected a deep vein thrombosis in her right calf and treated her with anticoagulants.

In summary, the results of Kylie's tests indicated that her generalised oedema was caused by hypoalbuminaemia, which in turn was because of heavy proteinuria. As the proteinuria was predominantly albuminuria, it can be considered as 'selective,' suggesting a restricted injury to the glomerular filtration barrier.

Her subsequent clinical course raises the following questions:

1. Why did the oedema progress?
2. Was the hypercholesterolaemia related to her renal disease?
3. What was the relationship between her renal disease and the deep venous thrombosis?

*Values outside normal range; see Appendix.

Table 6.2 Nephrotic syndrome

Pathophysiology	
Diagnostic triad	
Proteinuria >3.5 g/day	Disease of the glomerular capillary wall
Serum albumin <30–35 g/L	Urinary protein loss
Oedema	Low plasma oncotic pressure
	Salt and water retention by kidneys
Complications	
Hypercholesterolaemia	Increased hepatic synthesis and reduced metabolism of lipoproteins
Thrombosis	Venous obstruction caused by oedema
	Increased hepatic synthesis of clotting factors
	Urinary loss of antithrombotic proteins
Infection	Urinary loss of immunoglobulins and other defence proteins
Kidney failure	Intravascular volume depletion (acute)
	Intrarenal oedema (acute)
	Primary renal disease causing glomerular damage
	Proteinuria causing interstitial inflammation and fibrosis
Malnutrition	Severe protein loss

of the proteinuria. Some of the complications arise because of loss of 'protective' factors in the urine, and others are caused by increased hepatic production of 'damaging' factors, apparently as part of a generalised compensatory hepatic synthetic response primarily involving albumin. The major complications of nephrosis and their pathogenesis are described in Table 6.2. These complications are clinically relevant and, in untreated nephrotic syndrome, have an important bearing on what happens to the patient. Chronic kidney disease may develop because of progression of the primary disease or because of toxic effects of filtered protein which in large amounts may injure tubular cells or cause them to produce proinflammatory and profibrotic cytokines, leading to interstitial inflammation and fibrosis.

It has been established that this patient has severe nephrotic syndrome with complications. The next questions to be asked include the following.

- What type of kidney disease caused the nephrosis?
- Can and should the disease be treated?

These questions will be answered below.
See Case 6.1: 3.

NEPHROTIC SYNDROME

Diagnostic features	Complications

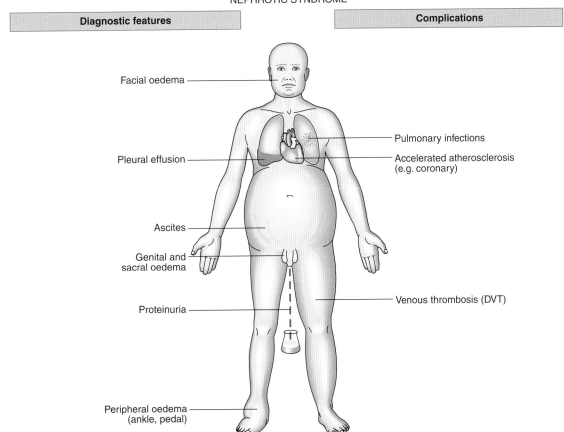

Fig. 6.4 Diagnostic clinical features and complications of nephrotic syndrome (representative site of complication shown but may occur at multiple sites).

Interesting facts

Many patients with severe proteinuria develop hypoalbuminaemia and nephrosis, whereas others with similar degrees of proteinuria do not. The difference may depend on the relative capacity of the liver to synthesise albumin, and to some extent, on the cause of proteinuria.

Renal biopsy

Percutaneous renal biopsy, in which a small specimen of kidney tissue is obtained under local anaesthesia using a specialised needle, can be used to establish diagnosis and prognosis in patients with suspected renal parenchymal disease, including those with nephrotic syndrome. Although it is a safe procedure, it can be complicated by bleeding and so is used selectively. It may not be used when the diagnosis is in little doubt, when it is unlikely to lead to a change in therapy, or when the chance of complication is greater than usual.

Renal biopsy specimens are examined by light microscopy with standard and special stains, by electron micros-copy and by immunofluorescence microscopy. The main parameters examined are listed in Table 6.3. Abnormalities may be segmental (involving part of a glomerulus only) or global (the whole glomerulus), and focal (involving a few glomeruli only) or diffuse (most glomeruli).

The classification of glomerular disease depends largely on histopathological features of renal biopsy specimens. There are many types of glomerular disease, and the classification system is somewhat complicated and is revised every few years or so. Therefore, the student should not aim to become an expert. A basic understanding of how renal biopsies are examined and of a few important varieties of glomerular disease (described below and in Chapters 7 and 8) is sufficient for most non-nephrologists.

With minimal change disease, light and immunofluorescence microscopy are normal. The only abnormality is diffuse fusion or effacement of foot processes of the podocyte seen on electron microscopy (Fig. 6.5). This occurs because of disruption of the actin cytoskeletal network of podocytes.

Causes of nephrotic syndrome

The main causes of nephrotic syndrome are listed in Table 6.4. The condition may arise as an isolated (primary) pathologic condition or as a component of a systemic disease.

In a child with new onset nephrotic syndrome and normal blood pressure, benign (or inactive) urinary sediment (see Chapter 7) and normal serum creatinine, minimal change disease is by far the most likely diagnosis. The patient's age and associated clinical features are very useful in predicting the diagnosis in other cases, though a renal biopsy would usually be performed. Membranous glomerulonephritis is the principal cause of nephrotic syndrome in adults. It usually occurs in isolation ('primary' or 'idiopathic') but sometimes develops as a complication of diseases such as **systemic lupus erythematosus** or cancer. Focal sclerosing glomerulonephritis can occur in any age group.

Case 6.1 — Proteinuria and the nephrotic syndrome: 3

Diagnosis

Kylie was referred to a nephrologist to have a renal biopsy. However, the nephrologist informed Kylie's GP that in this particular instance, there was no need to perform a renal biopsy as the clinical features and (subsequent) response to treatment predicted both diagnosis and prognosis with high sensitivity and specificity.

This portion of the patient's history raises the following questions:

1. How can glomerular disease be diagnosed?
2. Is a kidney biopsy always necessary to make the diagnosis?

Table 6.3   Renal biopsy: parameters

Light microscopy	
Glomerulus	Glomerular capillary wall thickness, cellularity, matrix, sclerosis
	Focal *versus* diffuse, segmental *versus* global
Blood vessels	Wall thickness, inflammation, occlusion
Tubule cells	Hypertrophy, atrophy, luminal casts
Interstitium	Inflammation, fibrosis
Special stains	Silver, Congo red, immune cell markers, complement (e.g. C4d)
Electron microscopy	
Glomerular epithelial cell podocytes	Discrete *versus* fused
Glomerular basement membrane	Thickness, regularity
Site of electron-dense deposits	Mesangial, subendothelial, subepithelial
Immunofluorescence microscopy	
Glomerular pattern	Capillary wall *versus* mesangial, linear *versus* granular
Ligand of fluorescent antibody	Immunoglobulins, complement component, light chain, fibrinogen

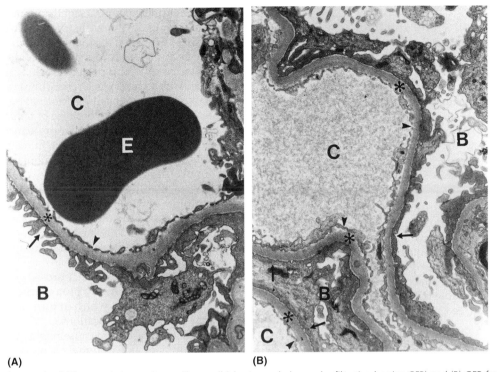

(A)   **(B)**

Fig 6.5 Electron micrograph of (A) normal glomerular capillary wall (also termed glomerular filtration barrier, GFB) and (B) GFB from a patient with minimal change disease showing extensive fusion of the foot processes (podocytes) of glomerular epithelial cells. C, capillary lumen; B, Bowman's space; *, basement membrane; arrowhead, fenestrated glomerular endothelial cell; arrow, podocytes (which are normally discrete but fused in minimal change disease); E, red blood cell.

Table 6.4 Major causes of nephrotic syndrome

	Usual age	Response to treatment	Risk of chronic kidney disease
Primary			
Minimal change disease	Child or adolescent	Yes	No
Focal sclerosing GN	Child or adolescent, adult, elderly	(Yes)	Yes
Membranous GN	Adult, elderly	(Yes)	Yes
Mesangiocapillary GN	Adult	Yes	Yes
Secondary			
Diabetic nephropathy	Adult, elderly	(No)	Yes
Amyloidosis	(Adult)*, elderly	(No)	Yes
Systemic lupus erythematosus	Adult, elderly	Yes	Yes

*Less frequent. Other parentheses indicate that this is sometimes the case.
GN, glomerulonephritis.

Interesting facts

In most cases of primary nephrotic syndrome (e.g. minimal change disease, focal segmental glomerulonephritis), the underlying factor that causes the disease is unknown. Membranous glomerulonephritis has recently been found to be caused in the majority of cases by antibodies against the phospholipase A2 receptor (PLA2R), which is found on podocytes, less commonly by antibodies against thrombospondin type-1 domain-containing 7A, and rarely by antibodies to other proteins. PLA2R antibody titres in serum are useful in both the diagnosis and monitoring of disease activity in PLA2R positive membranous nephropathy.

Natural history and response to treatment

Treatment of nephrotic syndrome depends on the exact pathological diagnosis. In general, primary forms of glomerulonephritis causing nephrotic syndrome are treated with corticosteroids. These have an anti-inflammatory action involving depletion of T lymphocytes and impairment of polymorphonuclear leucocyte function. In some cases, immunosuppressive drugs such as cyclophosphamide, rituximab, or calcineurin inhibitors are used. With secondary glomerulonephritis, treatment is directed towards the underlying disease, though this may be modified considerably with renal involvement.

Case 6.1 Proteinuria and the nephrotic syndrome: 4

Treatment

Kylie was treated with corticosteroids, and her nephrotic syndrome resolved completely within a few weeks. Two years later, her disease relapsed, and once again, she responded rapidly to corticosteroids. She has remained completely well since.

The response to treatment varies considerably depending on the diagnosis, as summarised in Table 6.4. The response is excellent with minimal change disease, but relapses are not infrequent. The response is much less predictable with other diagnoses. In the face of continuing nephrosis, the patient is at risk of developing complications (see Table 6.2), some of which can be prevented or treated (see Case 6.1: 4).

Interesting facts

Although the severity of proteinuria tends to predict the risk of complications of nephrosis, this is not always the case. For example, minimal change disease is unique because chronic kidney disease does not develop, even when proteinuria is massive and unremitting. Thus kidney scarring in proteinuria is determined not only by the amount of filtered protein but also by intrinsic properties of the particular protein and other proinflammatory and profibrotic events.

2. Normal urine contains a small amount of protein, less than 150 mg/day in adults. Normal urinary protein consists of proteins of small molecular weight which have been filtered across the GFB and not reabsorbed by tubular cells, and proteins such as Tamm–Horsfall protein (also known as Uromodulin) which are secreted by tubular cells. Abnormal proteinuria most commonly arises because of failure of the GFB filtration barrier ('glomerular proteinuria'), but it can also result from decreased protein reabsorption into or increased protein release from tubular epithelial cells ('tubular proteinuria').

3. Oedema arises because of a localised or generalised disruption of Starling's forces within capillaries or because of a failure of lymphatic drainage of the interstitial space. The three main generalised oedema states are congestive cardiac failure, cirrhosis, and nephrotic syndrome.

5. Nephrotic syndrome (or nephrosis) consists of a diagnostic triad of heavy proteinuria, which leads to hypoalbuminaemia, which in turn causes oedema in a range of anatomical locations.

6. The main diseases that cause nephrotic syndrome in children include minimal change disease, whilst in adults, causes include membranous glomerulonephritis and focal segmental glomerulosclerosis.

7. Treatment for the major causes of nephrotic syndrome varies by disease – minimal change disease is exquisitely sensitive to corticosteroid therapy, whilst other causes such as amyloidosis often requires more intense immunosuppression such as cytotoxic agents.

Summary

1. The glomerulus is populated by three intrinsic cells: the capillary endothelial cell, the epithelial cell which lies over it with the GBM in between (termed GFB), and the mesangial cell.

Self-assessment case study

Eric Daniels, a 65-year-old man who had been in good health previously, presented with a 4-month history of progressive swelling of his ankles. He had no previous history of cardiac or hepatic disease, and on examination, there was no evidence of cardiac or hepatic failure. Urinalysis was positive for protein (+++) but was otherwise normal.

After studying this chapter, you should be able to answer the following questions:

Q1. What is the most likely clinical diagnosis?

Q2. Name two other features required to make this clinical diagnosis.

Q3. Why has the patient developed oedema?

Q4. List at least three possible complications of this condition and the pathophysiological factors involved.

Q5. In a patient of this age, what is the most likely renal histopathological diagnosis?

Q6. Describe the likely renal histopathological features.

Self-assessment case study answers

A1. In the absence of hepatic and cardiac disease, the most likely diagnosis is nephrotic syndrome.

A2. Proteinuria and hypoalbuminaemia.

A3. Urinary protein loss leads to hypoalbuminaemia. Peripheral oedema develops, partially because of hypoalbuminaemia and therefore low plasma oncotic pressure (so that excess oedema fluid leaks from the capillaries), and also because of renal sodium and water retention.

A4. Deep venous thrombosis owing to hypercoagulability caused by increased hepatic synthesis of thrombotic factors and urinary loss of antithrombotic factors; hyperlipi-

daemia caused by increased hepatic synthesis of lipoproteins; increased risk of infection because of urinary loss of immunoglobulins and other defence proteins; chronic kidney disease owing to the natural progression of the disease.

A5. Membranous glomerulonephritis. There are several other possible diagnoses, including focal segmental glomerulosclerosis and amyloidosis.

A6. Thickening of capillary loops on light microscopy; electron-dense deposits between the GBM and visceral glomerular epithelial cell on electron microscopy; IgG and C3 in a capillary wall distribution on immunofluorescence microscopy.

Self-assessment questions and answers

Q1. List four factors that will favour the formation of oedema at the level of a capillary.

A1. Increase in hydrostatic pressure within the capillary lumen, reduced concentration of plasma proteins causing reduced plasma oncotic pressure, increased leakiness of the capillary wall, and reduced lymphatic flow.

Q2. Which three structures comprise the glomerular capillary wall?

A2. Glomerular endothelial cell, GBM, and visceral glomerular epithelial cell.

Q3. What is the definition of nephrotic syndrome?

A3. Heavy proteinuria causing hypoalbuminaemia and oedema.

Q4. List the principal complications of nephrotic syndrome and their pathophysiology.

A4. Hypercholesterolaemia, thrombosis, infection, renal failure, malnutrition. See Table 6.3 for pathophysiology.

Q5. What pathological features are expected in the renal biopsy of a patient with minimal change disease?

A5. Normal light and immunofluorescence microscopy, diffuse fusion of podocytes on electron microscopy.

GLOMERULONEPHRITIS AND THE ACUTE NEPHRITIC SYNDROME

7

Chapter objectives

After studying this chapter, you should be able to:

1. Describe the components of acute nephritic syndrome and its variations.

2. Describe other forms of presentation of glomerulonephritis (GN) and their classification by clinical presentation, renal biopsy appearance and cause.

3. Understand the pathogenesis of post-streptococcal GN.

4. Differentiate acute nephritis occurring with post-streptococcal GN, IgA disease and systemic diseases.

5. Discuss the consequences of glomerular disease.

6. Describe the parameters of urinary sediment examination.

7. Discuss the natural history of post-streptococcal GN.

Introduction

Acute glomerulonephritis (GN) refers generally to inflammatory renal diseases affecting the glomeruli of some or all of the million nephrons of each kidney. Although this classification is based largely on the pathological appearance of glomeruli, other components of the nephron, blood vessels and renal interstitium are involved to a variable extent. Many of the acute glomerulonephritides are primary or idiopathic, whereas, with others, a secondary cause is identified. The pathogenesis of GN varies with the diagnosis and may involve multiple factors. With many forms, it is only partially understood. In this chapter, the pathogenesis of GN will be explained by a discussion of the presentation and diagnosis of a case of acute nephritic syndrome.

There are a bewildering number of types of primary and secondary GN, and the systems of classification are overlapping and confusing. For this reason, the student is urged to concentrate on the common or classic forms of disease which are discussed in this chapter (see Case 7.1: 1).

Urinary sediment examination

To confirm the presence of renal inflammation, a sediment examination should be performed on a centrifuged sample of fresh urine. Although these techniques are now routinely performed by experienced pathology laboratories, microscopic examination of spun urine sediment is still manually performed by nephrologists and their trainees. To allow quantification of the urinary abnormalities, this should be done in a standardised fashion. Ten mL of urine is centrifuged for 5 min, 9.5 mL of the urine is then discarded, the sediment is resuspended in the remaining 0.5 mL of urine by gentle tapping of the test tube, and this resuspended sediment is examined under a microscope. Normal urine may contain up to ten red blood cells, ten white blood cells and one to two hyaline (but not granular or cellular) casts per high power field.

The finding of an excess number of red or white cells may be explained by abnormalities anywhere in the urinary tract. It should be noted that a positive dipstick test for blood indicates the presence of haem pigment, whereas microscopy is required to confirm the presence of red blood cells (this is discussed in more detail in Chapter 12). When cells or cellular debris aggregate in the tubular lumen, they may form casts of the tubule. Granular or cellular (epithelial, red, or white cell) casts indicate the presence of renal parenchymal disease, whereas hyaline casts are formed from Tamm-Horsfall protein and tend to be a non-specific finding. An 'active' sediment contains elements consistent with renal inflammation and/or cell necrosis, whereas a 'benign' sediment may contain a few cells and only hyaline casts. Urine should be examined as a fresh sample because casts may break down within 1 to 2 h. Fig. 7.1 shows examples of urinary casts. See Case 7.1: 2.

Interesting facts

Healthy individuals pass on average up to two million erythrocytes in their urine per day, with the actual number in an individual varying from four-fold less to more than this. These cells generally come from the kidney and are thus 'dysmorphic' in appearance. As urinary dipsticks for haem pigment can detect as few as 5–20 erythrocytes/μL, normal urinary blood should usually not be detectable by dipstick testing.

Case 7.1 — Glomerulonephritis and the acute nephritic syndrome: 1

Nephritic syndrome

Michael is a 22-year-old man who presented to the local hospital of a small country town complaining of headache and dark urine. He had also noticed a reduction in urine output (oliguria) even though he had a normal fluid intake. In the past, Michael has had frequent sore throats and skin infections. Approximately 2 weeks before the presentation, he had another sore throat which resolved spontaneously after 8 days. The resident doctor noted that he had facial swelling and blood pressure of 165/105 mmHg. His jugular venous pressure was raised 2 cm, and rales (sounds produced by the passage of air through fluid in the lower respiratory tract) were heard on auscultation at the bases of both lungs. There was a creamy exudate on his tonsils and mild pharyngeal erythema. Dipstick analysis of urine revealed blood +++ and protein +. The doctor suspected that Michael had acute GN.

The important clinical features in this patient include the occurrence of oliguria, dark urine, hypertension, and fluid overload 2 weeks after a sore throat. The questions that arise from this clinical history include the following:

1. What is the pathophysiology of each of the clinical features?
2. Are the clinical features interrelated?
3. What is the relationship of the sore throat to the acute illness which followed 2 weeks later?
4. What made the doctor suspect a diagnosis of GN?

The answers to these questions will be revealed in the initial sections of this chapter. Before this, however, we must discuss the examination of urinary sediment, the first and one of the most important tests in a suspected case of renal disease, which provides a non-invasive glimpse of the inflammatory processes which occur within the kidney.

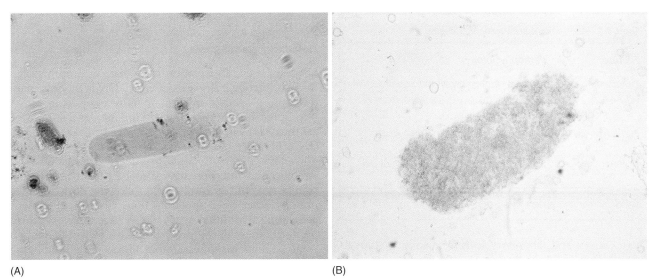

Fig. 7.1 Urinary casts: (A) hyaline, (B) red cell. Casts form within the tubular lumen and therefore take on the shape of the lumen with parallel sides. (Photographs courtesy of Prof. J. Lawrence.)

Case 7.1 Glomerulonephritis and the acute nephritic syndrome: 2

Initial investigations

Urinary sediment examination showed more than *100 red cells/μL and a moderate number of white cell and red cell casts. Serum creatinine was elevated at *160 μmol/L. Based on this, the doctor told Michael he had 'nephritis'.

The obvious question to be asked at this stage is: which of the clinical and laboratory features of the patient are diagnostic, characteristic, or consistent with the nephritic syndrome (or nephritis)?

*Values outside the normal range; see Appendix.

Box 7.1 Presentation of glomerular disease

Nephritic syndrome*
Nephrotic syndrome†
Asymptomatic proteinuria and/or microscopic haematuria
Macroscopic haematuria
Acute kidney injury (acute renal failure)
Progressive chronic kidney disease
Hypertension

*Haematuria, hypertension, renal functional impairment, and oliguria.
†Heavy proteinuria, hypoalbuminaemia, and oedema.

Presentation and consequences of glomerular disease

Patients with glomerular disease may present in several different ways; these are listed in Box 7.1. The spectrum of the presentation includes asymptomatic microscopic haematuria and/or proteinuria discovered on a routine medical check, acute or chronic kidney disease (CKD), hypertension, or full-blown (or a limited form of) nephrotic or nephritic syndromes. The nephrotic syndrome is described in Chapter 6. It is important to be able to recognise these different presentations and to predict the pathologic condition associated with each one and possible underlying causes.

The nephritic syndrome consists of haematuria, hypertension, and renal functional impairment (reduced glomerular filtration rate (GFR), reflected by the raised serum creatinine), as was found in the present case. The haematuria and active urinary sediment are indicative of renal inflammation; oliguria and renal functional impairment are a consequence of glomerular infiltration with inflammatory cells and release of vasoactive hormones and cytokines, and hypertension is the result of salt and water retention and vasoactive hormone release.

The consequences of glomerular disease and the underlying pathophysiology of each feature are described in Table 7.1. Renal functional impairment in glomerular disease is multifactorial and arises because of the acute inflammatory process (proliferation of intrinsic glomerular cells, glomerular infiltration with leucocytes, and haemodynamic changes induced by vasoactive hormones and cytokines) and chronic renal scarring (caused by continuing inflammation, hypertension, proteinuria, and other factors). Hypertension occurs in acute nephritis because of salt and water retention (a consequence of the reduction of GFR), glomerular capillary and arteriolar scarring, and neurohumoral changes, in particular activation of the renin–angiotensin system.

The diagnosis of glomerular disease and, specifically, nephritic syndrome can almost always be established by a combination of clinical features, serological tests, and renal biopsy. This was the case with the current patient.

Table 7.1 Consequences of glomerular disease

Feature	Pathophysiology
Proteinuria	Impaired filtration barrier function of GCW
Haematuria	Leak into Bowman's space across GCW or into the tubular lumen
Renal impairment	Structural and/or functional damage to glomeruli and tubulointerstitium
Hypertension	Salt and water retention, activation of the renin–angiotensin system

GCW, glomerular capillary wall.

These clinical and laboratory features also give clues to the pathogenesis of the disease and its complications. See Case 7.1: 3.

Investigation of glomerulonephritis

Several serological tests are useful for establishing, confirming, or supporting a specific diagnosis in patients with GN (Table 7.2). A positive test result suggests the primary diagnosis but does not prove that it is the cause of renal disease. Some of these serological abnormalities are actually involved in the pathogenesis of the renal lesion and will be discussed in more detail later in this chapter.

A renal biopsy usually establishes the diagnosis definitively. The components of renal biopsy examination are discussed in Chapter 6 (Table 6.3). In the current patient, the history, positive ASOT, low serum C3, and renal biopsy appearances were all consistent with a diagnosis of post-streptococcal GN.

Differential diagnosis of acute glomerulonephritis

GN may occur in isolation or as part of a multisystem disease. Amongst diseases in which GN is the sole manifestation, a specific precipitant is recognised in only a few. In the current case, the precipitant was a streptococcal throat infection occurring 2 weeks before the onset of GN. This once-common disease is seen less frequently nowadays, except in underprivileged populations. The streptococcal infection may also be a skin infection. A similar type of GN can be seen following bacterial infections of other types (postinfectious GN). Many patients presenting with other types of GN give a history of respiratory illness in the preceding days to weeks. Only in some patients is the respiratory illness of definite pathogenetic significance. A common form of GN that needs to be distinguished from post-streptococcal GN is IgA disease (or mesangial IgA nephropathy). IgA disease is a common type of GN, characterised by acute nephritis and, in particular, macroscopic haematuria occurring at the time or within a few days of a viral sore throat. The shorter prodrome and its frequently recurrent nature help to distinguish it at the presentation from post-streptococcal GN (Table 7.3 and Fig. 7.3).

Acute nephritic syndrome can occur in several conditions that are either restricted to the kidney or involve multiple organs (systemic diseases). Some of the important examples are listed in Box 7.2. Amongst these, IgA disease is the only common disease. Nevertheless, it is important to consider the other conditions because, without rapid treatment, irreversible renal failure may develop. Rapidly progressive GN, in which renal failure develops over a period of days to weeks, is characteristic of several of these conditions, including primary crescentic GN, microscopic polyangiitis, and Goodpasture's syndrome.

Case 7.1 | **Glomerulonephritis and the acute nephritic syndrome: 3**

Diagnostic investigations

The history of a sore throat 14 days before the onset of acute nephritis was consistent with a diagnosis of post-streptococcal GN. Serum antistreptococcal O titre (ASOT) was elevated, and serum concentration of the third complement component (C3) was low, indicating complement activation, and was consistent with the presumed diagnosis. In this disease, the renal lesion represents an immunological reaction to nephritogenic antigens in the microorganism responsible for the sore throat.

The patient was referred to a nephrologist who arranged a renal biopsy (Fig. 7.2). On light microscopy, all glomeruli were infiltrated with neutrophil leucocytes, and there was a proliferation of mesangial and endothelial cells. Electron microscopy showed large electron-dense deposits lying between the podocytes of the visceral glomerular epithelial cells and the glomerular basement membrane. Immunofluorescence microscopy was positive for IgM, IgA, and C3 in a granular capillary wall pattern. (A renal biopsy is frequently unnecessary in this situation because the clinical and other laboratory features can be highly suggestive of the diagnosis and the long term prognosis is usually good.)

The results of these diagnostic investigations lead to several questions which will be answered in the following sections of this chapter:

1. Which serological tests are necessary to establish the diagnosis and classification of GN?
2. Which renal biopsy features are useful or necessary to classify GN?
3. What insights do these features give to the pathogenesis of the renal lesion?

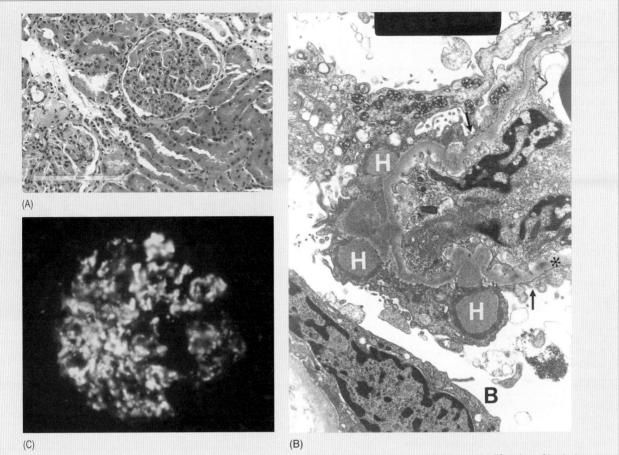

Fig. 7.2 Renal biopsy of the patient with post-streptococcal glomerulonephritis. (A) Light microscopy showing proliferation of intrinsic glomerular cells and infiltrating neutrophil leucocytes. (B) Electron microscopy showing large immune deposits ('humps' H) projecting into the Bowman's space (B) between the glomerular basement membrane (*) and glomerular epithelial cell (arrows). (C) Immunofluorescence microscopy showing a coarse granular pattern for IgG along the glomerular capillary wall.

Interesting facts

IgA disease is the most common form of GN worldwide. Its presentation is very variable, ranging from isolated microscopic haematuria to (rarely) a rapidly progressive GN. Although the clinical course is benign in the majority of patients, IgA disease is so common that it is (after diabetes) the second most frequent condition causing end-stage kidney disease.

Pathogenesis of acute glomerulonephritis

Current classification systems for GN are confusing, which is not surprising given the incomplete knowledge of the pathogenesis and the overlapping morphological characteristics of many types of GN. Important concepts regarding classification will be outlined below.

GN may be initiated by an immune response to an exogenous antigen such as a microbial product (including streptococcal products as in the current case) or an endogenous antigen (such as DNA with systemic lupus erythematosus; SLE). Less commonly, it may be initiated by an autoimmune response to a renal antigen, such as a component of the glomerular basement membrane in Goodpasture's syndrome (Figs 7.4A and 7.5). The antibodies involved in these responses may form the basis for diagnostic serological tests for these diseases (see Table 7.2). Several other effector mechanisms involving leucocytes, platelets, complement, coagulation factors, and humoral products of intrinsic and infiltrating cells act in concert with these immune mechanisms to cause glomerular injury.

When the antigen forms part of a circulating immune complex or is deposited in the kidney (e.g. on the glomerular capillary wall) to form an immune complex *in situ*, the immunofluorescence pattern is discontinuous or granular (Fig. 7.4B). In this case, corresponding electron-dense deposits are seen with electron microscopy. This pattern is seen, for example, in membranous GN, post-streptococcal GN and SLE. In most cases, it is unclear whether the immune complex forms primarily in the circulation or in the kidney.

Table 7.2 Important diagnostic serological tests for glomerulonephritis

Test	Diagnosis
Serum complement	
Low C3	Post-streptococcal GN, mesangiocapillary GN
Low C3 and C4	Systemic lupus erythematosus
Others	
ANA, anti-double-stranded DNA antibody, ENA	Systemic lupus erythematosus
ANCA	Microscopic polyangiitis or granulomatosis with polyangiitis
Anti-GBM antibody	Goodpasture's syndrome
ASOT	Post-streptococcal GN
HBsAg	Hepatitis B
Anti-HCV	Hepatitis C
HIV	HIV associated kidney disease and AIDS
VDRL	Syphilis
Anti-phospholipase A2 receptor	Primary membranous GN

ANA, antinuclear antibody; ANCA, antineutrophil cytoplasmic antibody; ASOT, antistreptococcal O titre; GBM, glomerular basement membrane; HBsAg, hepatitis B surface antigen; HCV, hepatitis C virus; VDRL, Venereal Disease Research Laboratory (serological test for syphilis); ENA, extractable nuclear antigens.

Table 7.3 Clinical and pathological differences between post-streptococcal glomerulonephritis (GN) and IgA disease

	Post-streptococcal GN	IgA disease
Antecedent pharyngitis	Yes, 10–14 days	Yes, 0–4 days
Acute nephritis	Yes	Yes
Other presentations	No	Yes*
Recurrence	No	Yes
Long term prognosis	Excellent	Variable
Diagnostic tests		
Serological	Low C3, positive ASOT	–
Renal biopsy	Glomerular neutrophil infiltration (LM)	Mesangial IgA (IF)†
	Subepithelial electron-dense deposits (EM)	Mesangial electron-dense deposits (EM)

*Other presentations of IgA disease include macroscopic haematuria, nephrosis (uncommon), hypertension, chronic kidney disease.
†See Fig. 7.3.
ASOT, antistreptococcal O titre; LM, light microscopy; EM, electron microscopy; IF, immunofluorescence microscopy.

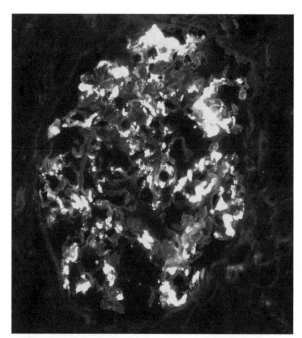

Fig. 7.3 Immunofluorescence of renal biopsy from a patient with IgA disease, showing positive immunofluorescence for IgA in a mesangial distribution. Contrast this with the 'capillary wall' distribution in Figs 7.2C and 7.4.

Box 7.2 Important causes of acute nephritic syndrome

Primary
Post-streptococcal glomerulonephritis
Post-infectious glomerulonephritis
IgA disease*
Mesangiocapillary (membranoproliferative) glomerulonephritis
Crescentic glomerulonephritis

Secondary to systemic disease
Systemic lupus erythematosus
Microscopic polyangiitis and granulomatosis with polyangiitis

*Can present less commonly as a systemic vasculitis with skin, joint, gastrointestinal, and renal involvement (Henoch–Schönlein purpura).

In contrast, when the antibody is directed against an intrinsic renal antigen, the immunofluorescence pattern is continuous or linear, as seen in Goodpasture's syndrome (Fig. 7.4A). In the latter situation, there should be no electron-dense deposits seen with electron microscopy.

Whether or not immune complex formation leads to the development of GN depends on numerous factors, including the nature of the antigen, the size of the complex, the antibody, the clearance of complexes by phagocytic cells, and other glomerular haemodynamic, cellular, and humoral influences (Fig. 7.5).

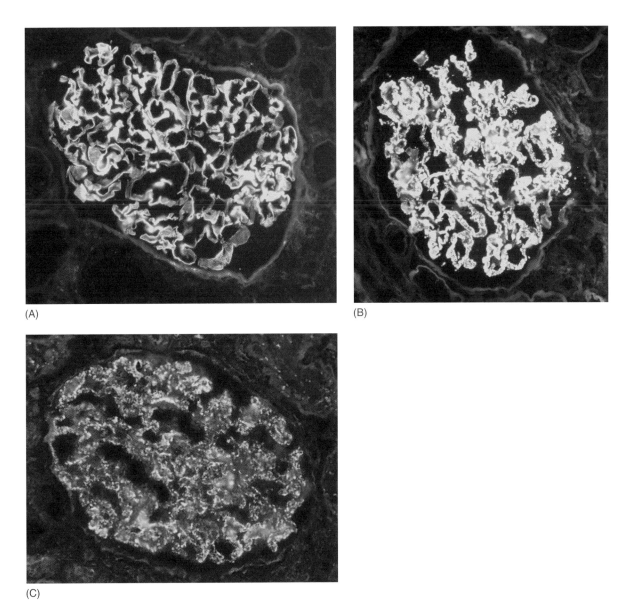

(A)

(B)

(C)

Fig. 7.4 Immunofluorescence pattern of a renal biopsy specimen of glomerulonephritis initiated by: (A) autoimmune response to glomerular antigen (linear), and (B) immune response to circulating or planted extrarenal antigen (granular) and (C) staining for phospholipase A2 receptor, the antigen in most cases of membranous glomerulonephritis. Half of the glomerulus in (A) is replaced by a glomerular crescent which is not immunofluorescent. In both (A) and (B), the immunofluorescence is in a glomerular capillary wall distribution.

Pathology of acute glomerulonephritis

The glomerulus may be altered in multiple ways in GN. Intrinsic cells (endothelial, mesangial, and epithelial) may proliferate; circulating leucocytes may infiltrate; platelets may accumulate; mesangial matrix may expand; the glomerular basement membrane may change; and scarring may develop.

A hallmark of severe disease is the development of a glomerular crescent, which is a cellular, fibrinous and, later, fibrous lesion in Bowman's space, arising from the proliferation of extracapillary cells including glomerular epithelial cells and macrophages (Fig. 7.6). The greater the size and the number of crescents, the more severe the disease. Crescents may be seen in many forms of GN and, when large and numerous (in more than 50% of glomeruli), they are associated with a rapidly progressive clinical course in certain forms of vasculitis and in primary crescentic GN (Table 7.4). The presence of crescents is associated with reduced glomerular filtration by virtue of its association with more severe glomerular damage and mechanical blockage of filtration through Bowman's space.

The glomerulus contains a capillary network and can thus be regarded as an 'extension' of the circulatory system, so it is not surprising that processes that cause systemic immune injury to blood vessels ('vasculitis') commonly cause GN. An example of this is antineutrophilic cytoplasmic antibody (ANCA) positive GN which can cause injury in the kidneys, lungs, or less often other tissues.

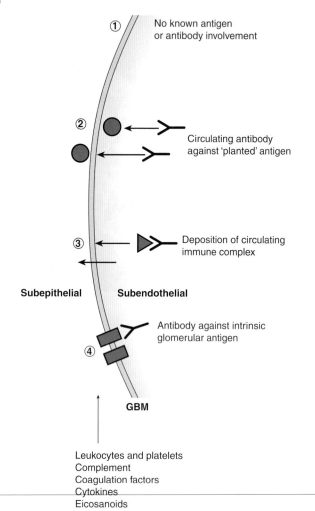

Fig. 7.5 Schematic representation of immunopathogenetic mechanisms of acute glomerulonephritis and the influence of other cellular and humoral mediators. Antigens may be deposited on the glomerular basement membrane before antibody deposition or as part of circulating antigen–antibody complexes or may be self-antigens (usually modified) in the glomerular basement membrane.

Table 7.4 Important types of glomerulonephritis (GN) and their usual clinical picture

Presentation	Primary	Secondary
Nephrotic syndrome	Minimal change disease	Diabetes mellitus*
	Membranous nephropathy	Amyloidosis*
	Focal segmental glomerulosclerosis (also known as focal sclerosing GN)	Systemic lupus erythematosus
	Mesangiocapillary GN	
Acute nephritic syndrome	Postinfectious GN	Systemic lupus erythematosus
	Post-streptococcal GN	
	IgA disease	
	Mesangiocapillary GN	
Rapidly progressive GN	Crescentic GN	Microscopic polyangiitis
		Granulomatosis with polyangiitis (formally known as Wegener's granulomatosis)
		Goodpasture's syndrome

Asymptomatic haematuria/proteinuria can occur with almost all listed conditions.
*These conditions are associated with non-inflammatory glomerulopathy rather than true glomerulonephritis.

Outcome of glomerulonephritis

Given that glomerulonephritides presenting with an acute nephritic picture may have a guarded prognosis, it is logical to ask about the natural history of this particular patient and whether treatment could alter the clinical course. See Case 7.1: 4.

The outcome of acute GN varies greatly with the type of disease. In diseases in which the inciting antigen or event disappears spontaneously (as in the current case) or with treatment, the renal disease may resolve. In some circumstances, such as IgA disease and SLE, the disease may smoulder on or recur. When the disease remains active, smoulders on, or recurs, the tendency is for progressive kidney scarring and kidney failure to occur over a variable period of time.

Clinicopathological correlations in glomerulonephritis

No current system of classification lends itself ideally to the study of GN and so understanding the condition can be a daunting task.

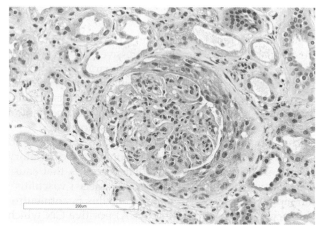

Fig. 7.6 Cellular crescent (*) occupying three-quarters of the circumference of a glomerulus and compressing the glomerular tuft.

| Case 7.1 | Glomerulonephritis and the acute nephritic syndrome: 4 |

Outcome

The patient received antihypertensive therapy and a loop diuretic to control fluid accumulation. Within weeks his serum creatinine returned to normal, and his oedema and hypertension resolved. After 6 months, his urinary sediment was inactive.

Thus, the patient's acute nephritis settled without specific treatment of the renal inflammation. But does this apply to other forms of acute nephritis?

Some primary and secondary glomerulonephritides are usually associated with nephrotic syndrome, as discussed in Chapter 6. Other forms of GN, such as postinfectious GN and IgA disease, may present with an acute nephritic syndrome, whilst others, such as SLE and mesangiocapillary GN, may present with either acute nephritis or nephrosis. In the context of an acute nephritic presentation, clinical clues should be sought to the presence of an underlying systemic condition (Fig. 7.7). As mentioned above, it is important to recognise the rare cases of rapidly progressive GN as they require emergency treatment.

GN can therefore be described as a combination of findings distilled from clinical presentation (acute kidney injury (AKI) vs chronic kidney disease, nephrotic vs nephritic), renal biopsy appearance (e.g. mesangial hypercellularity) and cause. Some diseases fit neatly into this paradigm (e.g. nephritic syndrome associated with mesangiocapillary GN because of antibodies against streptococcal antigen) whilst others do not (e.g. lupus nephritis can present as AKI or CKD, nephritic or nephrotic syndrome, mesangiocapillary, membranous or focal segmental glomerulosclerosis (FSGS) pattern on renal biopsy). The significant overlap in these aspects of diagnosis of GN make its study especially difficult. Use of the worksheet in the accompanying e-book will assist in understanding the classification of GN.

Thus, medical students should limit their studies to the most common and/or clinically important diseases. These are listed in Table 7.4.

Some important diagnostic features of the glomerular pathology in these diseases are listed in Table 7.5. These characteristic morphological and immunological features are sufficient to allow a definitive histological diagnosis to be made in the majority of cases. Further discussion of each condition included in Table 7.5 is beyond the scope of this text.

Interesting facts

Granulomatosis with polyangiitis was formally known as Wegener's granulomatosis, named after the physician who described the condition in 1936. However, the use of the term 'Wegener's granulomatosis' has fallen out of favour because of the discovery that Dr. Friedrich Wegener was a member of the Nazi party before and during World War II.

Clinical skills box: Urinalysis

The examination of urine is a key aspect of the assessment of kidney health. The diagnosis of kidney disease can be quickly made by examining its colour, turbidity, and odour. In addition, the urine dipstick provides a rapid assessment of urinary characteristics. The dipstick comprises a series of colorimetric pads on a stick which is dipped into a jar of urine, ideally midstream, and then left for up to 1 min to enable testing, either visually or using an automated detection system.

Key characteristics include:

- Colour – urine should be a clear to somewhat yellow colour. Red urine suggests haematuria but can also be because of myoglobinuria or colourings from ingested beetroot or medications such as rifampicin (in which case the microscopy shows no significant red blood cells). Urine may also be pink (because of Propofol), green (methylene blue), black (haemoglobinuria), or purple (significant bacteriuria).
- Turbidity – because of infection, crystalluria or chyluria.
- Odour – pungent (because of infection) or other unusual smells with aminoaciduria.
- Specific gravity (SG) – usually between 1.005 to 1.030, with higher SG corresponding to higher concentrations of solutes. Dehydration is a common cause, but glycosuria may also cause a high SG.
- pH – usual range is 4.5 to 8. This is most useful when diagnosing renal tubular acidosis, where an

inappropriately high urinary pH (>5.5) is usually found. A high urinary pH may be found in patients with urinary tract infection (UTI) because of urease-producing organisms.

- Heme (blood) – is positive in the presence of heme pigment, usually because of Hb in red blood cells, but also where there is free Hb (haemoglobinuria) or myoglobin (as in rhabdomyolysis).
- Leukocyte esterase ('leukocytes') – is positive in the presence of neutrophils or macrophages but may be falsely negative if proteinuria or glycosuria is present.
- Nitrite – is detected in the presence of organisms that produce the enzyme nitrate reductase (e.g. Enterobacteriaceae). Therefore, the presence of nitrites is relatively specific but not that sensitive to UTIs.
- Protein – is present when there is significant proteinuria. However, kidney disease may present early with albuminuria, in which case the total protein content in urine may not reach the threshold for protein detection by dipstick. It is usually reported as trace, 1+, 2+, 3+.
- Glucose – is present in glycosuria. In patients with normal kidney function, glycosuria does not usually appear until the plasma glucose exceeds 10 mmol/L, but patients with tubular dysfunction may have urinary loss of glucose because of lack of glucose reabsorption.

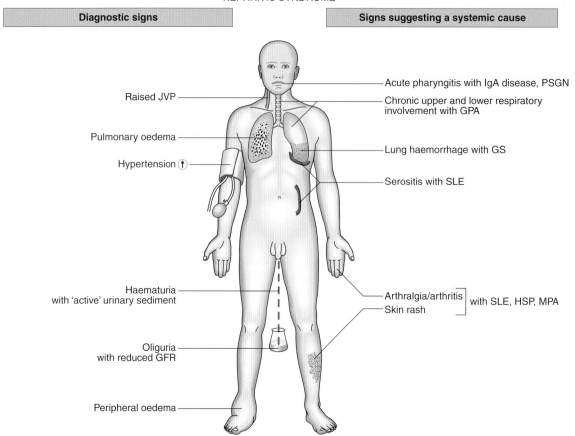

Fig. 7.7 Signs diagnostic of nephritic syndrome or suggestive of an underlying systemic condition. JVP, jugular venous pressure; PSGN, post-streptococcal glomerulonephritis; GPA, granulomatosis with polyangiitis; GS, Goodpasture's syndrome; SLE, systemic lupus erythematosus; HSP, Henoch–Schönlein purpura; MPA, microscopic polyarteritis.

Table 7.5   Principal diagnostic glomerular appearances of important types of glomerulonephritis (GN)

	Light microscopy	*Electron microscopy*	*Immunofluorescence*
Minimal change disease	Normal	Diffuse foot process fusion	Negative
Membranous nephropathy	Thick GCW without glomerular hypercellularity	Subepithelial EDD ('lumps')	Finely granular, CW
Focal sclerosing GN	Focal segmental GS	Diffuse foot process fusion	IgM (segmental)
Mesangiocapillary GN	Thick GCW with glomerular hypercellularity	Subendothelial EDD, mesangial interposition	CW Ig and C
Postinfectious/post-streptococcal GN	Hypercellular glomerulus	Subepithelial EDD ('humps')	CW Ig and C3
IgA disease	Mesangial proliferation	Mesangial EDD	Mesangial IgA
Diabetes mellitus	GS	Thick GBM, mesangial expansion	CW pseudolinear
Amyloidosis	Variable Negative birefringence with Congo Red stain	Amyloid fibrils	–
Systemic lupus erythematosus	Various patterns	EDD – multiple sites	CW and mesangial, Ig, C3, C1q
Rapidly progressive GN	Crescents	Variable	CW negative or granular or linear

C, complement; CW, capillary wall; EDD, electron-dense deposits; GBM, glomerular basement membrane; GCW, glomerular capillary wall; GS, glomerular sclerosis.

Interesting facts

Goodpastures syndrome is named after Ernest Good-pasture, a pathologist who described two cases of GN complicated by severe idiopathic pulmonary haemor-rhage at the height of the 1918–19 influenza pandemic. Forty years later, two Australian physicians described a series of nine similar cases and recalled Goodpastures classic description, naming the disease after him.

Rapidly progressive GN is a rare medical emer-gency. It can occur as primary kidney disease or as part of a systemic illness such as granulomatosis with poly-angiitis (GPA), microscopic polyangiitis, Goodpasture's syndrome, and, rarely, Henoch–Schönlein purpura (a multisystem variant of IgA disease) or SLE. It is charac-terised clinically by a nephritic picture with rising serum creatinine and histologically by the presence of glomeru-lar crescents. With appropriate early treatment, the dis-ease may be halted or even cured; without treatment, end-stage kidney failure occurs quickly.

Summary

1. Acute nephritic syndrome comprises a constellation of proteinuria, haematuria, mild oedema, and hypertension. It may present as AKI or CKD.
2. GN is a condition that can be described by clinical presentation (nephritic vs nephrotic, AKI vs CKD), renal biopsy appearance (e.g. mesangioproliferative, membranous, glomerulosclerosis) and cause (e.g. post-streptococcal infection, abnormally structured IgA deposits).
3. Management of GN comprises supportive therapy (e.g. blood pressure control, management of electrolyte disturbances) and targeting of the underlying abnormality (e.g. targeting B-lymphocytes to reduce aberrant antibody production).

Self-assessment case study

Joe Shapiro, an 18-year-old man, presented to his local prac-titioner with macroscopic haematuria. Three days before his presentation, he had had a sore throat. At 15 and 16 years old, he had a similar episode of macroscopic haematuria.

After studying this chapter, you should be able to answer the following questions:

Q1. Explain how urinary examination would help narrow the differential diagnosis in this case.

Q2. Based on the other clinical features, what is the most likely diagnosis?

Q3. What other clinical features are required to make a diagnosis of 'the nephritic syndrome'? What is the pathogen-esis of each feature?

Q4. What are the main renal histopathological features of this disease?

Self-assessment case study answers

A1. The presence of red blood cells (especially dysmor-phic), casts and protein in the urine would all point to an upper urinary tract (i.e. renal parenchymal) origin for the bleeding; red blood cells without the other urinary abnormalities would point to a lower tract origin; posi-tive dipstick for blood without red cells on microscopy would point to pigmenturia (i.e. haemoglobinuria or myoglobinuria).

A2. The recurrent nature of the haematuria and sore throat occurring only a few days before presentation points to a diagnosis of mesangial IgA disease rather than post-strepto-coccal or postinfectious glomerulonephritis.

A3. The nephritic syndrome consists of macroscopic haematu-ria, elevated serum creatinine and hypertension. The haematu-ria is caused by the leakage of the red cells from the glomerulus into the tubular lumen. Hypertension is because of renal salt and water retention and, in part to the release of vasoactive hormones. Reduced renal function is caused by structural dam-age (e.g. proliferation within the glomerulus and tubulointer-stitial inflammation and scarring) and intrarenal haemodynamic changes because of vasoactive hormone release.

A4. Mesangial proliferation on light microscopy; mesan-gial electron-dense deposits on electron microscopy; IgA in mesangial distribution on immunofluorescence microscopy.

Self-assessment questions and answers

Q1. What are the diagnostic clinical features of acute nephritic syndrome? Describe their pathogenesis.

A1. Haematuria (because of leakage of blood cells across the glomerular capillary wall), hypertension (caused by salt and water retention and activation of the renin–angiotensin system), renal functional impairment (because of vasoactive hormone release and structural injury). See Table 6.2.

Q2. List three conditions causing acute glomerulonephritis (GN) in which the serum concentration of complement components C3 and/or C4 may be reduced.

A2. Post-streptococcal GN, mesangiocapillary GN, systemic lupus erythematosus (SLE).

Q3. Which diagnostic serological tests are also involved in the immunopathogenesis of SLE, granulomatosis with polyangiitis, Goodpasture's syndrome, hepatitis B and C, respectively?

A3. Anti-dsDNA antibody, ANCA, anti-GBM antibody, HBsAg, anti-HCV antibody, respectively.

Q4. Describe five clinical features that may distinguish post-streptococcal GN from IgA disease.

A4. See Table 6.4.

Q5. List three ways in which antibodies may be associated with the glomerular basement membrane in acute GN.

A5. In situ immune complex formation, deposition of circulating immune complex, reaction with intrinsic glomerular antigen.

DIABETIC NEPHROPATHY AND CHRONIC KIDNEY DISEASE

8

Chapter objectives

After studying this chapter, you should be able to:

1. Understand the natural history of diabetic nephropathy.

2. Discuss the common causes of chronic kidney disease (CKD).

3. Describe the presentation and natural history of CKD.

4. Appreciate the progressive nature of CKD.

5. Discuss the main consequences of CKD and their pathogenesis.

6. Understand the principles of treatment of patients with CKD.

Introduction

Diabetes mellitus, both type I and type II, is the commonest cause of chronic kidney disease (CKD). For example, in Australia, which has very reliable national statistics on end-stage kidney disease (ESKD), it now accounts for almost 40% of patients commencing dialysis or receiving a kidney transplant. The incidence of diabetic nephropathy as a cause of ESKD is similar in Europe and even higher in New Zealand and the United States.

Whatever the cause of CKD, once a certain level of kidney dysfunction has been reached, kidney disease tends to progress towards end-stage. We understand some, but not all, of the reasons for this progression. Kidney failure affects almost all organ systems of the body and, as kidney dysfunction progresses, increasingly, these effects take on more clinical significance.

In this chapter, we will discuss CKD and its consequences using an illustrative case of progressive kidney failure because of diabetic nephropathy. See Case 8.1: 1.

Presentation of CKD

The development of diabetic kidney disease in this patient was not surprising, as she already manifested other evidence of diabetic microvascular complications in the form of diabetic retinopathy requiring laser photocoagulation. Microvascular complications tend to affect multiple organs concomitantly. By the time her serum creatinine was measured, she already had moderate renal impairment. However, a diagnosis of CKD may be made at any time during the course of the disease. In diabetic nephropathy, this may range from early in an asymptomatic patient following the detection of albuminuria to very late in a patient with few symptoms but marked biochemical abnormalities. The range of presentations of CKD is shown in Box 8.1.

Note that in this patient, several clinical features suggested that salt and water were being retained because of a low glomerular filtration rate (GFR). Thus, hypertension raised jugular venous pressure, pulmonary crepitations, and oedema were manifestations of expanded extracellular fluid and plasma volume. Another factor contributing to her oedema was hypoalbuminaemia resulting from heavy proteinuria (see Chapter 6).

The natural history of CKD tends to vary according to the cause. For example, the typical clinical course for a patient with type 1 diabetes who develops CKD (as some 40% do) is illustrated in Fig. 8.1. After about 5 years of type I DM, microalbuminuria develops (albumin excretion below the range usually detected by dipstick urinalysis). Overt proteinuria then develops over the next few years, followed by progressive kidney impairment, which leads, after another 5 years or so, to ESKD. The course tends not to be quite as predictable in patients with type 2 diabetes.

Case 8.1 Diabetic nephropathy and chronic kidney disease: 1

Diabetes mellitus and kidney impairment

Raylene Tomlein is a 35-year-old woman who has had type 1 diabetes mellitus since she was 23 years old. At 30 years old, she was first diagnosed with diabetic retinopathy and has received regular laser photocoagulation. She first noticed mild ankle swelling when she was 32 years old, and this has slowly increased in severity. For 2 years before the current presentation, she had been on antihypertensives. Her blood pressure is currently 155/90. She has mild peripheral oedema, and her jugular venous pressure wave is visible 3 cm above the clavicle at 45 degrees. There are bibasal pulmonary crepitations. Otherwise, her physical examination is normal.

Urinalysis is positive for protein (+++) and blood (trace). Urinary protein excretion was *4.5 g/24 h. Serum creatinine was elevated at *290 µmol/L. Ultrasound examination shows echogenic kidneys of symmetrically reduced bipolar length.

This patient has clinical features (oedema, hypertension), which suggest that her kidney disease may have been present for at least 2 years. This raises the following important questions:

1. How can we differentiate acute kidney injury from chronic kidney disease?
2. How does CKD present?
3. What is the significance of her other clinical features, namely diabetic retinopathy, hypertension, and proteinuria?

These issues will be discussed below.
*Values outside normal range; see Appendix.

Box 8.1 Presentations of CKD

Asymptomatic serum biochemical abnormality
Asymptomatic proteinuria/haematuria
Hypertension
Symptomatic primary disease
Symptomatic uraemia
Complications of CKD

Differentiating AKI and CKD

Kidney failure is defined as a reduced GFR, which causes the kidneys to lose the ability to excrete nitrogenous wastes such as urea and creatinine; this increases their concentration in the serum (uraemia). Certain clues help to differentiate an acute reversible increase in serum creatinine concentration (acute kidney injury) from a chronic irreversible rise (CKD) (see Chapter 5

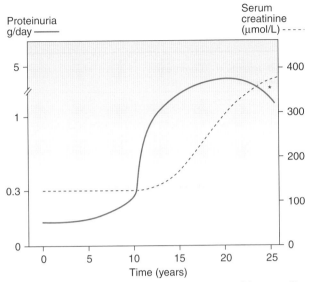

Fig. 8.1 Typical clinical course of a patient with type 1 diabetes mellitus who develops nephropathy, from the onset of diabetes. *Proteinuria often falls late in CKD as GFR becomes severely impaired.

Table 8.1	Differentiation of acute and chronic kidney disease	
	Acute	*Chronic*
History	Short (days–weeks)	Long (months–years)
Haemoglobin concentration	Normal	Low
Renal size	Normal	Reduced
Renal osteodystrophy*	Absent	Present
Peripheral neuropathy†	Absent	Present

*Osteodystrophy is a bone disease.
†Peripheral neuropathy is a disease or dysfunction of nerves supplying the limbs and peripheral tissues.

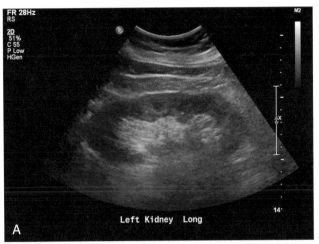

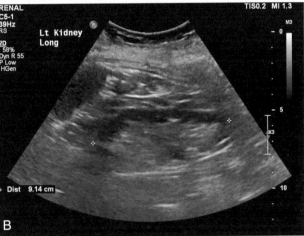

Fig. 8.2 Renal ultrasonography is useful in differentiating acute and chronic kidney disease. (A) Normal-sized kidney of acute kidney injury. Note that the normal kidney appears darker (less echogenic) than the adjacent liver. The kidney is 11.5 cm in bipolar length. (B) Small, echogenic kidney of severe CKD. Note that a scarred kidney is brighter (more echogenic) than normal and therefore less easy to distinguish from surrounding structures. The kidney is 9.14 cm in bipolar length.

and Table 8.1). In the current patient, the long history and the reduction in kidney size on ultrasonography (Fig. 8.2) indicate a chronic process. Similarly, a low haemoglobin concentration is typical of chronic rather than acute kidney disease. Additionally, it is useful to compare current levels of serum creatinine to previous ones if available.

Stages of CKD

CKD may be divided into different stages depending on the GFR and degree of proteinuria (Table 8.2). The functional changes need to be present for at least 3 months to indicate that the disease is chronic. Such a division is useful because it summarises the probable degree of kidney damage present and predicts the likelihood of progression to ESKD.

A patient may present at any stage of the disease. A term such as mild kidney impairment may be used when the GFR is only mildly reduced (e.g. greater than 60 mL/min) and the disease is not clearly progressive. ESKD, in contrast, may be defined by the need for dialysis therapy or renal transplantation to sustain life (see Chapter 9). You will notice from Table 8.2 that there may be very marked kidney dysfunction in the presence of minimal symptoms.

Because of the lack of symptoms in early disease, screening patients at high risk for CKD development is important to identify patients that may benefit from early treatment. High risk patients, such as those with

Table 8.2 Stages of chronic kidney disease (CKD)

Stage of CKD	GFR* (mL/min)	Symptoms of uraemia or its complications	Serum biochemical derangements	Comment
1. Normal GFR†	≥90	None	None	Not clearly progressive
2. Mild	60–89	None	Subtle	Early bone disease commences; increased risk of vascular disease
3. Moderate	30–59	Mild	Mild	Anaemia develops
4. Severe	15–29	Moderate	Moderate	Salt and water retention and uraemic symptoms may be evident
5. End-stage	<15	Severe	Severe	Dialysis or renal transplantation necessary

*See Chapter 5 for a discussion of normal glomerular filtration rate (GFR) (approximately 100 mL/min) and how it is affected by age, sex, and body weight. The change in GFR needs to be present for at least 3 months.
†But, with abnormal proteinuria, urine sediment and/or blood pressure.
Current CKD nomenclature used by KDIGO: CKD is defined as abnormalities of kidney structure or function, present for >3 months, with health implications. CKD is classified based on cause, GFR category (G1–G5), and albuminuria category (A1–A3), abbreviated as CGA.

Table 8.3 Common causes of ESKD

	*Percentage incidence
Diabetes mellitus	40
Glomerulonephritis	25
Hypertension	10
Polycystic kidney disease	5
Vesicoureteric reflux	5
Unknown	5
Other	10

*Approximate incidence in Australia and New Zealand (source ANZDATA Registry, 2015–18): these are representative of data for other developed countries.
ESKD, end-stage kidney disease.

Interesting facts

Currently, there are more than two million people worldwide suffering from ESKD, and this number is predicted to more than double over the next decade.

The increase in patients with ESKD is being driven largely by the increased incidence of diabetes. In 2019 there were over 450 million people worldwide with diabetes, and this number is predicted to rise to 700 million by 2045, with the burden of disease weighted towards low-middle income countries. There are already many people in these countries who cannot access renal replacement therapy, and this number is likely to increase with the increasing incidence of ESKD.

Interesting facts

Thirty years ago, analgesic nephropathy was the second most common cause of ESKD in Australia (after glomerulonephritis), accounting for one-quarter of cases. Because of legislation outlawing the sale of compound analgesics since 1980, it is now a rare cause of ESKD. The use of phenacetin in these analgesics was similarly associated with high rates of ESKD in some parts of Europe and the United States.

diabetes, hypertension, cardiovascular disease, or a family history of kidney disease, should be screened regularly to identify a reduction in eGFR, albuminuria, or new onset of hypertension.

Causes of CKD

The major causes of ESKD are listed in Table 8.3. Diabetes mellitus (as in the current patient) is the most common cause. Glomerulonephritis forms the second largest group, and, amongst these, IgA disease is the most common variant to cause ESKD accounting for 25% of cases in this category in western communities. Chronic obstruction because of renal calculi is a relatively common cause of CKD in the tropics. Amongst elderly patients, CKD caused by renovascular disease is being diagnosed more frequently.

Pathologic conditions of diabetic nephropathy and CKD

The pathological features of CKD consist of a mixture of changes in the kidney, typical of the primary disease and those which are common to CKD of all types. As the disease progresses, the disease specific changes become less obvious, and the non-specific histopathological changes that come with advanced disease become more obvious.

For example, in diabetic nephropathy, early disease specific changes include glomerular basement membrane thickening and expansion of the mesangium and hyaline thickening of the afferent and efferent arterioles (Fig. 8.3). Usually, there is also superimposed hypertensive damage (thickening of small arteries and arterioles).

As diabetic nephropathy progresses, the non-specific changes of advanced CKD will start to dominate, which are characterised by progressive scarring of the glomeruli (glomerulosclerosis) and tubulointerstitium (tubular atrophy and interstitial inflammation and fibrosis) (Fig 8.4).

Consequences of CKD

The manifestations of CKD are protean and affect every organ system of the body (Fig. 8.5). They arise because the kidneys fail to perform their usual excretory, regulatory, metabolic, and biosynthetic functions. The current patient developed many of these problems. See Case 8.1: 2.

The uraemic syndrome refers to the composite clinical picture arising from the concurrent appearance of many of these manifestations, particularly those arising from the failure to excrete nitrogenous compounds (such as urea) and other 'uraemic toxins', many of which

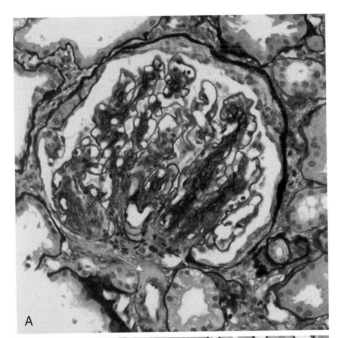

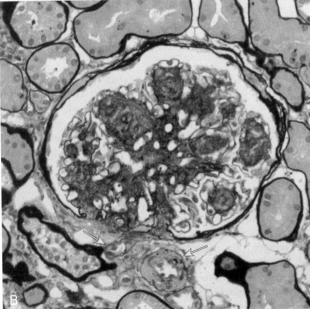

Fig. 8.3 Histologic changes. (A) Diabetic nephropathy with diffuse mesangial expansion and arteriolar hyalinosis (arrow). (B) Diabetic nephropathy with nodular mesangial expansion (Kimmelstiel–Wilson nodules) and concomitant hyalinosis of afferent and efferent arterioles (arrows). (from Najafian B, et al. 2015. AJKD Atlas of renal pathology: diabetic nephropathy. Am J Kidney Dis 66:e37.)

| Case 8.1 | Diabetic nephropathy and chronic kidney disease: 2 |

Diabetic kidney disease and disease progression

The diagnosis of diabetic nephropathy was discussed with Raylene, and her risk of progression was calculated. She was educated on the risk factors for acute kidney injury that she should avoid, and the benefits of interventions designed to slow the rate of progression of her chronic kidney disease. Her diabetes was better controlled with insulin titration and dietary advice. She was commenced on an ACE inhibitor which was uptitrated to bring her BP under control and was monitored for progression of kidney dysfunction, proteinuria, and the development of complications related to CKD.

Disease progression

Over the next few years, Raylene's kidney impairment continued to worsen slowly. She became progressively fatigued and developed anaemia. Her blood pressure became more difficult to control, as did her oedema. She developed mild pain in the long bones of her lower limbs and generalised pruritus. On one occasion, she presented with sudden shortness of breath, thought to be because of myocardial ischaemia. Her feet became numb, and a 2 cm ulcer developed on the plantar surface of her right hallux (big toe). The patient's symptoms were thought to be caused by complications of uraemia, affecting her bone marrow, bones, skin, central and peripheral blood vessels. Other symptoms related to progressive damage from diabetes with peripheral neuropathy and peripheral vascular disease.

The progressive decline of kidney function invites the following questions:

1. Why does this happen?
2. Can anything be done to prevent it?

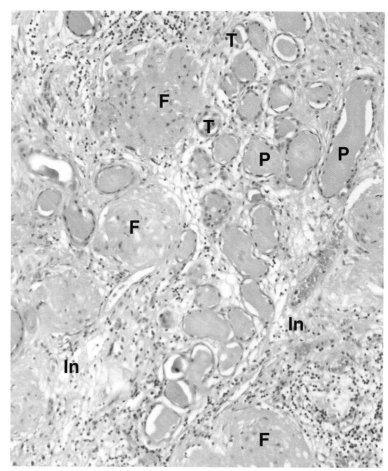

Fig. 8.4 Photomicrograph illustrating an end-stage kidney with glomerulosclerosis. In the cortex, the non-functioning or obsolescent glomeruli are replaced by avascular, acellular fibrous material (fibrosis) (F). The cortical tubules (T) also become shrunken and atrophic and the expanded interstitial spaces (In) undergo fibrosis; some atrophic tubules may become cystically dilated with casts of inspissated proteinaceous material (P) and resembles thyroid follicles, thus often called thyroidisation (from O'Dowd G., Bell S., Wright S. (2021). Wheater's Pathology: A Text, Atlas and Review of Histopathology, 6e. Oxford: Elsevier Ltd.).

remain poorly defined. In general, there is a poor correlation between the systemic concentration of most of these substances and uraemic symptomatology. In particular, fatigue, anorexia, nausea, vomiting, and pruritus (itch) are common uraemic symptoms, but drowsiness, neuropathy, and pericarditis can be seen when the condition is advanced.

It is sometimes difficult to differentiate symptoms of the primary disease (in this case, diabetes mellitus) from those of kidney failure, either because the symptoms are non-specific or because both diseases cause similar organ damage. For example, both diabetes and kidney failure can be complicated by myocardial and peripheral ischaemia, and by peripheral neuropathy. Shared symptoms may thus arise earlier in the course of diabetic CKD than would be the case with other primary diseases.

Fluid and electrolyte abnormalities

As CKD progresses, there is a failure to excrete salt and water adequately, leading to fluid retention and volume overload. Peripheral oedema commonly develops, and the patient may have all the clinical features of fluid over-

load; see Chapter 2. Whilst net retention of salt and water is usual, the capacity of the kidney to concentrate the urine and maximally reabsorb sodium is also impaired, so, paradoxically, the patient is at risk of volume depletion in the face of restricted intake of salt and water. Overall, the range of homeostatic responses to changes in salt and water intake is greatly narrowed in CKD.

Interesting facts

Nocturia is one of the earliest symptoms of CKD, first occurring when GFR is less than half normal. When this symptom has been present for some time prior to presentation, it is useful for differentiating chronic from acute kidney disease. It occurs because the loss of concentrating ability with reduced GFR means that obligate excretion of urinary solutes requires greater volumes of urine, particularly at night when urine concentration is normally maximal.

Hypertension occurs for several interlinked reasons: failure to excrete salt and water adequately, activation of the renin and angiotensin system because of reduced

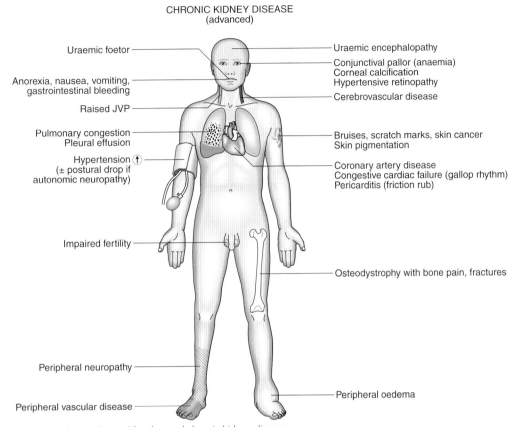

Fig. 8.5 Characteristic signs in a patient with advanced chronic kidney disease.

effective renal blood flow, resulting in systemic vaso-constriction and sodium retention, overactivity of the sympathetic nervous system, and endothelial dysfunction. Hypertension is involved in a vicious loop in the progression of kidney disease; hypertension is worsened by kidney impairment and is a major contributor to CKD progression.

Because of efficient renal adaptive mechanisms, hyperkalaemia (arising from a failure to excrete potassium) is usually a late manifestation of kidney failure. The renal adaptation consists of enhanced potassium secretion in the distal tubule. People with diabetes who are prone to develop hyporeninaemic hypoaldosteronism (see Chapter 4) are at particular risk of hyperkalaemia, and drugs used to block the RAAS system also increase potassium levels.

Acid base balance

CKD is associated with metabolic acidosis, which often occurs as the eGFR decreases below 30 mL/min. It is caused by a decrease in renal ammonium excretion and, initially, there tends to be a normal anion gap metabolic acidosis, but later in the disease process, an increase in anion gap occurs because of the lack of excretion of anions such as phosphate, sulphate, and urate. This gener-ally leads to mild metabolic acidosis, which contributes to renal bone disease, malnutrition, and possibly disease progression.

CKD-Mineral bone disease (CKD-MBD)

CKD-MBD refers to the systemic disorder of mineral and bone metabolism that almost universally occurs in moderate to advanced CKD. It arises because of a complex interplay between calcium, phosphate, parathyroid hormone, activated vitamin D, fibroblast growth factor 23, and klotho (Fig. 8.6).

There are two principal drivers of this disease process: impaired excretion of phosphate by the kidneys and a failure to transform vitamin D from inactive 25-OH vitamin D to its active form, 1,25-$(OH)^2$ vitamin D. As a result of these two defects in kidney function, an intricate network of events occur that result in CKD-MBD. In response to hyperphosphataemia, an osteocyte derived hormone called fibroblast growth factor 23 (FGF23) is produced, which acts to mitigate the high levels of phosphate by promoting increased phosphate excretion (through reduced proximal tubular phosphate reabsorption). However, at the same time, it also further inhibits the already compromised activation of vitamin D resulting in impaired intestinal absorption of calcium and

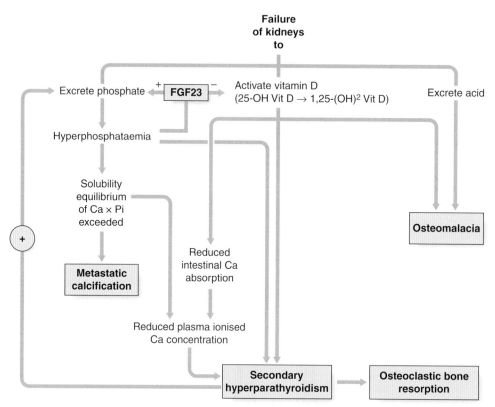

Fig. 8.6 Schema describing pathogenesis of CKD-MBD chronic kidney disease-mineral bone disease. FGF23, Fibroblast Growth Factor 23. See text for detailed description.

hypocalcaemia. Low calcium levels are also exacerbated by the formation of extracellular deposits of calcium and phosphate that occur because of high circulating phosphate levels.

Low calcium levels, high phosphate levels, and a lack of activated vitamin D all increase parathyroid hormone production, which acts to restore normal calcium levels in the blood at the expense of calcium from the bone. The dual outcomes of this complex interplay are osteoclastic bone resorption from secondary hyperparathyroidism, which in severe cases can cause pain and fracture, and calcium-phosphate deposition in vessels, which is likely to be one of the reasons for the increased risk of cardiovascular disease in patients with CKD.

CKD-MBD comprises a variable mix of hyperparathyroidism (causing osteoclastic bone resorption or osteitis fibrosa cystica), osteomalacia, adynamic bone disease, osteoporosis, and vascular disease. In rare circumstances, ischaemic injury because of small vessel occlusion in the skin can lead to ulcers (calcific uraemic arteriolopathy or 'calciphylaxis').

Anaemia

A common early symptom of CKD is fatigue. A significant contributor is normochromic normocytic anaemia resulting from the failure of erythropoietin production by the kidney. Erythropoietin is secreted predominantly as a glycoprotein of 165 amino acids by fibroblast-like interstitial cells in the kidney in response to anaemia and hypoxia. Its synthesis falls as renal scarring progresses, with a consequential fall in red cell mass as its stimulatory effect on the bone marrow is lost. The reduced capacity of the blood to carry oxygen because of deficiency of erythropoietin is a major cause of morbidity in patients with CKD, and management of this problem has been revolutionised by the availability of synthetic erythropoietin as replacement therapy. In contrast, white blood cells and platelets are normal in number, but their impaired function contributes to a predisposition to infection and a bleeding tendency, respectively.

Cardiovascular disease

Atheromatous vascular disease can impair circulation to all organs, in particular to the heart, brain, and lower limbs. Almost half of patients with ESKD die from cardiovascular events. In CKD, non-atheromatous vascular disease, including medial vascular calcification, reduced vascular elasticity, and consequent left ventricular hypertrophy and myocardial scarring, is much more common than in people without CKD. CKD-associated vascular disease arises owing to multiple factors in patients with kidney failure, including hypertension, dyslipidaemia, and metastatic calcification, sometimes aggravated by cigarette smoking.

Interesting facts

Over a 5-year period, 20%–25% of patients with stage 2 or 3 CKD die, usually from cardiovascular disease, whereas only 2% reach ESKD. The situation is similar for stage 4 CKD, where 45%–50% die in 5 years, yet only 20% progress to ESKD.

There are many other manifestations of CKD, some common and some rare. These are summarised in Tables 8.4 and 8.5 and illustrated in Fig. 8.5.

Case 8.1 Diabetic nephropathy and chronic kidney disease: 3

End-stage kidney disease

Raylene's renal failure continued to deteriorate, and she was started on several different drugs to control blood pressure, fluid retention, hyperphosphataemia, and acidosis. Her diet was adjusted to restrict salt, potassium, protein, and fluid intake.

Three years after her presentation with chronic kidney disease, she was started on haemodialysis and placed on the waiting list to receive a cadaveric kidney transplant.

Table 8.4 Main consequences of chronic kidney disease

Mechanism	Example	Consequence
Decreased excretion	Uraemic toxins, including nitrogenous wastes	Uraemic syndrome
	Salt and water	Volume overload, hypertension
	Phosphate	Hyperparathyroidism, metastatic calcification
	Acid	Metabolic acidosis
	Potassium	Hyperkalaemia
Decreased biosynthesis	Erythropoietin	Anaemia
	Activation of vitamin D	Osteomalacia, hyperparathyroidism
Altered metabolism	Dyslipidaemia	Atherogenesis
	Sex hormones	Abnormal reproductive function

Table 8.5 Organ system involvement in CKD

System	Main pathogenetic factors	Main consequences
Cardiovascular	Atheroma and medial vascular calcification	Occlusive vascular disease Increased systemic vascular resistance
	Salt and water retention	Hypertension, congestive cardiac failure
Bone	Secondary hyperparathyroidism	Pain, rarely fracture
	Osteomalacia	
	Osteoporosis	
Neuromuscular	Uraemic toxins	Sensorimotor peripheral neuropathy
		Autonomic neuropathy
		Encephalopathy
Blood	Erythropoietin deficiency	Anaemia
	Uraemic toxins	Impaired white cell and platelet function
Skin	Metastatic calcification	Pruritus, calcific uraemic arteriolopathy
	Sun exposure	Skin cancer
	Anaemia and 'uraemic toxins'	Sallow complexion
Reproductive	Abnormal regulation of sex hormones	Reduced libido, impaired fertility
Gastrointestinal	Uraemic toxins	Anorexia, nausea, vomiting, malnutrition
Serosal	Uraemic toxins	Pericarditis

DIABETIC NEPHROPATHY AND CHRONIC KIDNEY DISEASE

Principles of treatment

After establishing the cause and severity of CKD, management is directed towards detection and treatment of factors that may cause superimposed acute kidney injury, management of factors that contribute to the progression of CKD, and intervention when complications of CKD arise.

Management of progression of CKD

Once kidney impairment has become severe enough, the disease tends to progress through the various stages outlined in Table 8.2 to end-stage. This occurs even when the primary disease causing the kidney impairment has become inactive. However, if the primary disease becomes quiescent (either through natural or treatment-induced reparative processes) before kidney functional impairment and scarring have become critically severe, then CKD may not be progressive.

The factors causing CKD progression are not entirely clear, but several implicated factors are listed in Box 8.2. These factors are managed by disease specific treatments (e.g. insulin for the treatment of diabetic nephropathy; immunosuppressive medications for the treatment of glomerulonephritis) in addition to therapy aimed at the non-specific factors that promote progression of CKD regardless of the underlying cause.

Interesting fact

SGLT2 inhibitors are used to manage glucose levels in patients with type 2 diabetes but have also been found to have cardioprotective and renoprotective benefits, independent of their effects on blood glucose levels.

Managing BP is the cornerstone of therapy to slow the progression of CKD. Hypertension is both a cause and effect of CKD and affects most patients with CKD. Controlling hypertension manages to slow disease progression and reduce cardiovascular risk. Whilst non-pharmacological interventions are useful in reducing BP in CKD, they are rarely sufficient to control BP adequately. Patients with CKD and hypertension will often require a combination of antihypertensive medications to achieve BP reduction. When proteinuric, certain pharmacological therapies provide additional BP-independent renoprotective effect, and this must be considered when instituting therapy, but, on the whole, the benefit of blood pressure reduction appears to be independent of the agent used.

Proteinuria is not merely a manifestation of CKD but also an important factor leading to progressive kidney scarring. It is thought that reabsorbed protein causes tubular cell damage and leads to tubular cell production of cytokines that incite an inflammatory and fibrogenic response in the surrounding interstitium. The net effect of these and other factors is progressive scarring

Box 8.2 Factors causing the progression of CKD

Renal	Systemic
Continuing activity of the primary disease	Systemic hypertension
Intraglomerular hypertension	Smoking
Proteinuria	Obesity
Nephrocalcinosis (dystrophic and metastatic)	Dyslipidaemia

Box 8.3 Causes of acute deterioration of kidney function in patients with chronic kidney disease

Recurrence of the primary disease
Complications of the primary disease
Accelerated hypertension
Volume depletion
Cardiac failure
Sepsis
Nephrotoxins (radiocontrast, drugs*)
Renal artery occlusion
Urinary tract obstruction

*Including especially non-steroidal anti-inflammatory drugs and, in some situations, angiotensin-converting enzyme inhibitors and angiotensin receptor blockers (see Chapter 14).

of glomeruli and tubulointerstitial areas of the kidney. Antihypertensive agents that work to block the deleterious effect of the renin–angiotensin system (angiotensin-converting-enzyme (ACE) inhibitor; angiotensin receptor blockers) reduce proteinuria and slow progression of CKD whilst again having the added benefit of improving cardiovascular outcomes.

This non-specific progression of CKD needs to be distinguished from separate events that may lead to superimposed acute kidney injury: acute-on-chronic kidney disease (Box 8.3). For example, falls in extracellular fluid volume or blood pressure are commonly associated with an acute deterioration of GFR in a patient with otherwise stable CKD. When the abnormality can be corrected in a timely fashion, GFR should return to baseline. However, when the abnormality is sustained or cannot be corrected (e.g. with acute renal artery occlusion in a patient with renal artery stenosis), then GFR may not improve.

Management of consequences of CKD

The various fluid and electrolyte, and metabolic disturbances of CKD may respond well to dietary manipulation and drugs. For example, restricting excessive dietary protein, salt, potassium, phosphate, water, and saturated fats may be necessary at some stage. Hyperphosphataemia, metabolic acidosis, and sodium retention may be treated with phosphate binders,

Box 8.4 Principles of treatment of patients with CKD

Differentiate from acute kidney injury (see Table 8.1)
Establish cause (see Table 8.3)
Establish severity (see Table 8.2)
Seek and treat factors causing progression (see Box 8.2)
Seek and treat reversible factors (see Box 8.3)
Seek and treat complications (see Table 8.5)
Lifestyle changes (diet, exercise, cease smoking, avoid polypharmacy)
Planned transition to dialysis and transplantation (see Chapter 9)

sodium bicarbonate supplements, and loop diuretics, respectively. Erythropoietin (stimulating agents) and calcitriol may be given to replace deficiencies of those hormones. Smoking has been shown unequivocally to worsen atheromatous disease and promote the progression of kidney disease. Therefore, smoking should be stringently avoided, especially in patients with diabetes.

In most patients, CKD follows a predictable course. Thus, if appropriate, continuing surveillance for treatable complications and a planned transition to ESKD therapy (dialysis and transplantation) is possible. The principles of treatment of patients with CKD are summarised in Box 8.4.

Summary

1. Chronic kidney disease can be caused by several different medical problems. Diabetes is the most common cause of CKD, but hypertension and vascular disease are also common risk factors. Polycystic kidney disease and glomerulonephritis can also lead to CKD.
2. CKD tends to be asymptomatic until there has been considerable deterioration in kidney function, meaning that screening for kidney disease is important in high risk groups.
3. A staging system has been developed to allow uniform assessment of response to therapy and prognostication. The system combines the patient's level of eGFR and proteinuria to determine a CKD stage.
4. There are several potential consequences of CKD which relate to both the excretory and endocrine functions of the kidneys
5. The treatment of patients with CKD has various aspects. Specific treatment of underlying disease; non-specific treatment to slow the progression of disease; treatment of complications of CKD; management of cardiovascular risk factors.
6. Patients who develop CKD that progresses to ESKD will need to consider various management options: dialysis, kidney transplant, and supportive care. There are several variations of these treatment options, and each patient's needs are different.

Self-assessment case study

A 39-year-old woman with a 20-year history of type 1 diabetes mellitus was found to have an elevated serum creatinine. She described moderate nocturia for the past 4–5 years and swelling and numbness of her feet for 2 years. Fundoscopy revealed changes in the background and proliferative diabetic retinopathy. Her ankle jerks were absent, and she was moderately tender on digital compression of her tibiae. Her blood pressure was elevated.

Q1. Which of the following features suggests chronic rather than acute kidney disease (can answer more than one)?
  A. Nocturia for several months
  B. Anaemia
  C. Small echogenic kidneys
  D. Bone pain
  E. Intact ankle jerks

Q2. Which of the following clinical features occurs first as glomerular filtration rate falls in progressive chronic kidney disease?
  A. Oedema
  B. Anaemia
  C. Need for dialysis to sustain life
  D. Asymptomatic bone disease

Q3. Which of the following is the most common cause of chronic kidney disease in developed countries?
  A. Analgesic nephropathy
  B. Diabetes mellitus
  C. Polycystic kidney disease
  D. Glomerulonephritis
  E. Hypertension

Self-assessment case study answers

A1. A, B, C, D - These are all features of chronic kidney disease.
A2. D - An asymptomatic increase in PTH and PO4 are the earliest complications to occur related to CKD.
A3. B - Diabetes mellitus is the most common cause of ESKD in developed countries.

KIDNEY FAILURE AND REPLACEMENT OF RENAL FUNCTION

9

Chapter objectives

After studying this chapter, you should be able to understand:

1. What kidney functions can be replaced by dialysis and transplantation.

2. The principles and modes of dialysis.

3. How to prepare a patient for chronic dialysis.

4. The outcomes and complications of chronic dialysis.

5. The differences between dialysis for acute versus end-stage kidney disease (ESKD).

6. Modes of transplantation.

7. The principles of preparing a patient for transplantation.

8. Outcomes and complications of transplantation.

9. The principles of conservative management of ESKD.

Introduction

Renal replacement therapy refers to the treatment of a patient with advanced loss of renal function using dialysis and kidney transplantation. Dialysis may be required to replace kidney function temporarily in a patient with acute kidney injury (AKI) or long term in a patient with end-stage kidney disease (ESKD). Kidney transplantation may be used to replace kidney function in a patient with ESKD but is not used as a treatment of AKI. Patients with ESKD who have chosen to be cared for without dialysis or transplantation, should be managed via a renal supportive care pathway.

This chapter gives an overview of these forms of treatment based on consideration of two typical case histories.

Interesting facts
Currently, there are at least 2 million people with ESKD worldwide and more than 700 million people with early vascular disease and kidney dysfunction who are at risk of cardiovascular disease and ESKD.

Case 9.1	**Kidney failure and replacement of renal function: 1**

Roland Walkum is a 68-year-old man with chronic kidney disease (CKD) because of chronic glomerulonephritis. His renal function slowly deteriorated over 5 years until his glomerular filtration rate (GFR) fell to about 7 mL/min, and he developed symptoms of uraemia and fluid overload, including nausea and dyspnoea. He was otherwise a healthy man who did not wish to die from his kidney disease. When the options were explained to him, he opted to commence treatment with peritoneal dialysis (PD) as it best suited his lifestyle. A PD catheter was placed, and he was trained to perform continuous ambulatory PD at home. After dialysis was commenced, he was able to stop or reduce the dose of several medications that he had been taking to treat and prevent the complications of CKD. Apart from several episodes of peritonitis and exit site infection, he tolerated PD very well. After 4 years on PD, he slowly developed progressive oedema, which was unresponsive to changes in his dialysis regimen. An arteriovenous fistula was created in his left forearm, and he was switched to haemodialysis.

Several issues arise from this case history:

1. What are the different modes of dialysis delivery, and what factors govern the choice?
2. How should a patient be prepared for chronic dialysis?
3. What are the long term complications and outcomes of dialysis?

Replacement of kidney function

Once chronic kidney disease (CKD) has progressed to stage 5 (glomerular filtration rate (GFR) less than 15 mL/min/1.73 m^2), death from kidney failure will ensue in a relatively short timeframe unless some form of replacement of kidney function is provided.

Successful kidney transplantation can replace up to half of the total normal kidney function since a single kidney is transplanted. Potentially this is sufficient to adequately replace all functions of the normal kidney. In contrast, dialysis is able to replace only some of the functions performed by a normal kidney. It has the potential to replace most of the kidney's role in regulating fluid and electrolyte balance and to remove low molecular weight solutes but is only partially effective at regulating calcium and phosphate balance, controlling blood pressure, and removing larger solutes, and is unable to replace any of the hormonal and synthetic functions of the normal kidney (Box 9.1). As a consequence, supplementary dietary and drug treatment is required in nearly all patients on dialysis (Table 9.1).

Most of these supplementary therapies are required in progressively higher doses in patients with CKD as kidney function deteriorates. Once the patient commences dialysis, the need for supplemental therapy may disappear (e.g. sodium bicarbonate), diminish (e.g. some dietary restrictions, phosphate binders, and antihypertensives) or continue (e.g. erythropoietin, calcitriol). These changes depend on the extent to which dialysis can replace individual kidney functions (see Box 9.1).

Box 9.1 Replacement of kidney function by dialysis

Complete*	Partial**	Nil
Regulation of ECFV	Control of blood pressure	Metabolism of filtered proteins
Regulation of osmolality	Excretion of middle molecular range solutes	Synthesis of erythropoietin
Regulation of acid–base balance	Excretion of 'uraemic toxins'	Synthesis of renin-angiotensin
Regulation of potassium balance	Regulation of calcium and phosphate balance	Synthesis of their other local hormones
Excretion of low molecular weight solutes		Activation of 25 OH vitamin D

*Potentially these functions can be completely replaced by optimal dialysis but may require some supplementary therapy.
**Replacement of these functions usually requires additional drug therapy.
ECFV, Extracellular fluid volume.

Principles and modes of dialysis

Dialysis literally means the separation of a substance across a membrane. Clinically, it is used to refer to any process by which solutes (including drugs and toxins) are removed from the body fluids through an artificial intervention, using either an external circuit through which the blood is passed (haemodialysis (HD)) or the lining of the peritoneal cavity (peritoneal dialysis (PD)).

Haemodialysis

> **Interesting facts**
>
> HD was first used to save human life during World War II by a Dutch physician, Willem Kolff. From the 1960s, HD became more widely available because of the development of artificial shunts (by Belding Scribner) and arteriovenous fistulas (by Brescia and Cimino).

In HD, the patient's blood flows through an artificial kidney counter-current and is separated by a semipermeable membrane from dialysis fluid (Fig. 9.1). Solute removal from the body across the dialysis membrane occurs by diffusion down the solute's concentration gradient (best for low molecular weight solutes, less than 500 daltons) or convection in which solutes are dragged along with water (best for larger molecules, greater than 500 daltons). The amount of fluid and sol-

utes removed can be varied by regulating the flows of blood and dialysate and the pressures in the blood and dialysate compartments and using dialysis membranes with different permeabilities.

HD for patients with ESKD may be delivered in hospital, in a satellite unit specialising in dialysis or at home. In most patients, dialysis is delivered for 4 to 5 h, three times a week. This can replace approximately 10% of GFR. By increasing the hours of dialysis and, to a lesser extent, blood flow rates, dialysis delivery can be increased substantially. Some patients with very long dialysis hours (e.g. overnight dialysis, most nights per week) can achieve such good replacement of kidney function that the need for supplemental therapy (e.g. phosphate binders, anti-hypertensives, erythropoietin) can be obviated or greatly reduced.

Peritoneal dialysis

As an alternative to HD, PD can be used for patients with ESKD. In this situation, the peritoneal membrane, the endothelium of peritoneal blood vessels, and the supporting tissue between the two act jointly as the semipermeable membrane. Except in situations where HD is not available, PD is uncommonly used for the treatment of patients with AKI (Box 9.2). PD may be administered by machine, usually overnight (automated PD), or by manual exchanges during the day and night (continuous ambulatory PD, or CAPD).

Table 9.2 gives some data for the population of patients undergoing chronic dialysis in Australia in 2019.

Preparing a patient for dialysis

The best outcomes in dialysis can be achieved if the patient has a planned transition from the treatment of progressive CKD to dialysis, allowing for planned access creation and management of fluid and electrolyte issues leading up to dialysis initiation.

During stage 4 CKD (GFR 15–30 mL/min/1.73 m^2), patients should receive education about ESKD therapy so they can make an informed decision about the choice of modality, including information on the different dialysis modalities, home versus hospital options and consideration of transplant or supportive care as outlined later in this chapter. In the absence of medical and psychological contraindications, patient choice is the most important determinant of the initial mode of therapy. The patient's social and psychological wellbeing, suitability for home dialysis and suitability for PD versus HD needs to be assessed (Box 9.3). During this phase, it is necessary to correct reversible factors that preclude the dialysis modality chosen by the patient. The patient needs to be assessed for the presence of infectious diseases (hepatitis B & C, HIV, and multi-resistant organisms such as MRSA, VRE, ESBL) and, if they have no or insufficient

Table 9.1	Supplementary therapy
Function*	**Supplementary therapy**
Regulation of ECFV	Appropriate sodium and water intake; loop diuretic if passing urine
Regulation of osmolality	Appropriate water intake
Regulation of potassium balance	Dietary K restriction with HD, occasional use of K-binding resin (e.g. resonium); sometimes dietary K supplementation with PD
Regulation of calcium/ phosphate balance	Phosphate binders, calcitriol, calcimimetic drug
Regulation of magnesium	Avoid excessive magnesium intake
Synthesis of erythropoietin	Erythropoietin or its analogues
Synthesis of renin-angiotensin	Sometimes ACEi or ARB
Activation of 25-OH vitamin D	Calcitriol

*For other normal kidney functions (listed in Box 9.1), supplemental therapy is either unnecessary or not available.
ACEi, Angiotensin-converting enzyme inhibitor; *ARB,* angiotensin receptor blocker; *ECFV,* extracellular fluid volume.

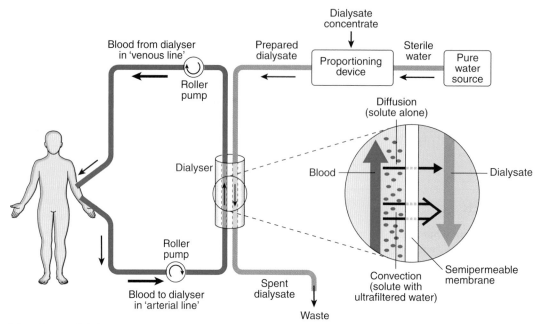

Fig. 9.1 Principles of haemodialysis.

Box 9.2 Modes of dialysis delivery

For AKI	For ESKD
Intermittent haemodialysis (HD)	HD – home, community house, satellite, or hospital
Continuous venovenous haemodialysis (CVVHD)	Automated peritoneal dialysis (APD)
Slow, low efficiency, daily dialysis (SLEDD)	Continuous ambulatory peritoneal dialysis (CAPD)
Acute peritoneal dialysis (uncommon)	

AKI, Acute kidney injury; *ESKD*, end-stage kidney disease.

Box 9.3 Relative medical contraindications to home

Peritoneal dialysis	Home haemodialysis
Previous abdominal surgery with adhesions	Vasculature unsuitable for arteriovenous fistula
Unrepaired abdominal hernia	Severe cardiovascular disease
Bowel diseases (e.g. diverticulitis)	Other severe medical conditions
Serious lung disease	
Abdominal obesity	

Table 9.2 Renal replacement therapy in Australia, 2019

Patients on dialysis		13,900
New patients (in 2019)		2100
PD	APD	10%
	CAPD	5%
HD	Facility (hospital, satellite, or community house)	75%
	Home	10%

APD, Automated peritoneal dialysis; *CAPD*, continuous ambulatory peritoneal dialysis; *HD*, haemodialysis; *PD*, peritoneal dialysis.

antibodies to hepatitis B, receive vaccination against hepatitis B. Their potential for receiving a kidney transplant also needs to be assessed.

In addition to patient preference, the modality of dialysis is determined by the presence or not of various medical, psychological, and social factors. For example, in patients with previous major abdominal surgery with peritoneal adhesions, unrepaired hernia, bowel conditions such as diverticulitis and severe respiratory insufficiency, PD may not be possible. In patients with blood vessels unsuitable for permanent vascular access and some medical comorbidities such as severe cardiovascular disease, HD may not be possible. In addition, PD is unable to deliver as much solute clearance as HD and may be less suitable for large patients with minimal or no remaining native kidney function.

Dialysis should be initiated before the patient has developed severe symptoms of kidney failure. Whereas dialysis is usually commenced when the patient's GFR has fallen to between 7 and 10 mL per min, other determinants of when to start dialysis than GFR *per se* are uraemic symptoms, worsening nutrition, poor blood pressure and fluid control and refractory metabolic complications of kidney failure (Box 9.4).

Box 9.4 When to initiate dialysis

GFR 5–10 mL/min, depending on symptoms
Uraemic symptoms
Malnutrition
Fluid overload and hypertension not responding to medical treatment
Refractory metabolic complications such as hyperkalaemia or metabolic acidaemia.

Interesting facts

Residual kidney function continues to deteriorate once a patient commences dialysis, more quickly with HD than PD because of the greater haemodynamic stressors associated with HD. Once residual kidney function is lost, some patients on PD need to transfer to HD.

Dialysis access

For PD, a catheter is placed in the peritoneal cavity (Fig. 9.2). The catheter usually exits the peritoneal cavity in the midline below the umbilicus, courses along a subcutaneous tunnel and exits the abdominal wall laterally. To reduce the risk of leakage of peritoneal fluid from the exit site, it is advisable for the catheter to be in place for 2 weeks prior to use. The catheter may be used earlier than this if urgent start dialysis is required, but PD catheters are subject to the risk of leakage of dialysate (and therefore the risk of infection), and initial dialysis needs to be small volume and delivered supine.

Permanent HD access is best achieved using an arteriovenous (AV) fistula in which an artery (frequently radial artery) is anastomosed end-to-side or side-to-side to a vein (cephalic vein in the case of radial artery) (Fig. 9.3). The vein becomes 'arterialised' because of the increased pressure and flow of blood through it and is suitable for recurrent cannulation after about 6 weeks. Alternatively, an AV graft may be constructed by the use of a synthetic conduit material or a harvested (e.g. saphenous) vein. In patients with poor peripheral blood vessels, especially when immediate access is required, it may be necessary to use a synthetic venous catheter, usually placed in the internal jugular vein and preferably with a subcutaneous tunnel to reduce the risk of catheter infection (Fig. 9.4).

Outcomes and complications of dialysis

Morbidity in dialysis patients arises from complications of the dialysis procedure itself, from inadequately controlled consequences of kidney failure, or from accompanying medical conditions. The most frequent complications of PD include infection (peritonitis, exit site infection, tunnel infection) or gradual failure of the peritoneal membrane to effectively transport solutes and water.

Complications of HD include infection, stenosis and thrombosis of the vascular access, problems during the HD procedure itself (e.g. hypotension) or problems occurring between treatments (usually because of excessive intake of water and solutes) (Box 9.5).

Intercurrent cardiovascular disease is common in patients with ESKD and a frequent cause of morbidity and mortality. The most common causes of death amongst dialysis patients are cardiac events (myocardial infarction and sudden death) and withdrawal from dialysis for various reasons (Table 9.3).

Dialysis for acute kidney injury

AKI (also known as acute renal failure) is common amongst hospitalised patients, particularly patients with multi-organ failure and patients with cardiac disease in intensive care and high dependency units. If AKI is severe enough, dialysis may be necessary until kidney function recovers. As these patients are frequently quite unwell, dialysis is often commenced at higher levels of GFR and with higher doses of dialysis than for patients with ESKD. Although complications of the dialysis procedure are relatively common (infection, cardiovascular instability), patient outcome is largely determined by the underlying disease. Dialysis partially replaces kidney function but, in general, does not affect the underlying disease or cause of kidney failure, nor does it hasten the recovery of kidney function. Patients with AKI may require dialysis for periods ranging from a few days to several weeks.

In a stable patient with AKI, HD may be delivered intermittently, as it is for patients with ESKD. However, many patients with AKI are quite unwell and are better dialysed with a slow continuous form of therapy which is characterised by greater cardiovascular stability. Most commonly, patients are dialysed continuously via catheters placed in large veins (continuous venovenous HD). As the blood is not arterial, an external pump is required to pump blood through the artificial kidney. Usually, dialysis is combined with filtration (convection) to allow optimal clearance of solutes, so-called haemodiafiltration. There is an increasing trend to use a dialysis treatment that combines the advantages of intermittent HD and continuous venovenous hemofiltration (CVVHD), so-called slow, low efficiency daily dialysis (SLEDD). Adequate removal of solutes and water can be achieved by dialysis for 8 to 12 h/day, allowing time for patients to attend investigations and receive other treatments whilst not on dialysis. PD is used infrequently for AKI, except in areas where the availability of HD is limited. This is related to the increased chance of infectious and mechanical complications with a newly inserted catheter and poor metabolic control because of initial small volume therapy.

Principles and modes of transplantation

Renal transplantation is a well-established form of treatment for ESKD, available in most parts of the developed world

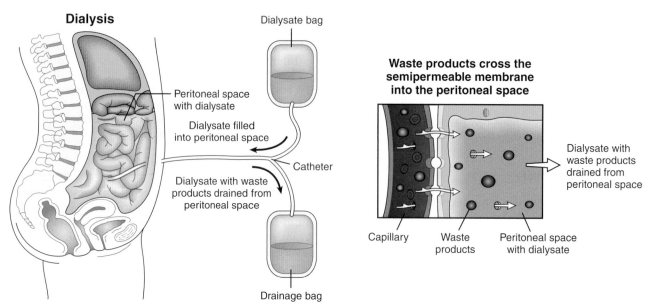

Fig. 9.2 Peritoneal dialysis catheter. The peritoneal membrane is a semi-permeable membrane allowing the transfer of both solute and water to the peritoneal cavity from the blood compartment (comprised of capillaries lining the peritoneal membrane). Solute comprises the 'waste products' accumulated in kidney diseases such as potassium, sodium, hydrogen ions, urea, and creatinine. On instillation of the dialysate bag fluid into the peritoneal cavity, solute transfers across the peritoneal membrane through diffusion, whilst water transfers across the peritoneal membrane because of osmosis (with the osmotic gradient conferred by the higher glucose concentration in dialysate fluid). Peritoneal dialysate fluid is instilled for several hours before being drained into a bag.

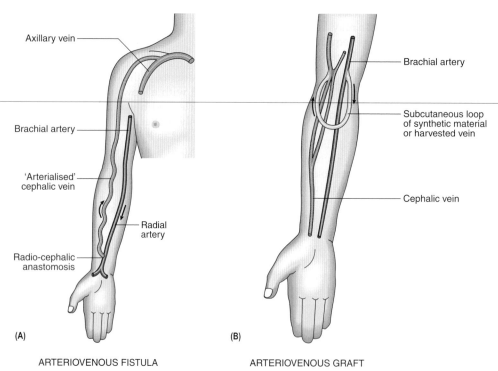

Fig. 9.3 (A) Arteriovenous fistula and (B) graft for haemodialysis.

and increasingly in some developing countries. Its successful delivery depends on access to high standards of care from a team involving transplant surgeons, nephrologists, immu-nologists, infectious diseases experts, and other personnel. The account given here introduces only some principles of the procedure and its consequences See Case 9.2: 1.

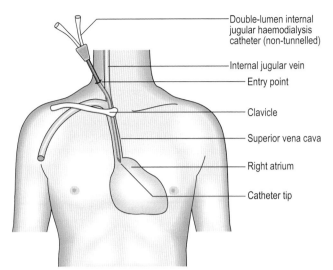

Fig. 9.4 Internal jugular catheter for haemodialysis.

Box 9.5 Common complications of chronic dialysis

Peritoneal dialysis (PD)

Infection – catheter exit site tunnel, peritonitis
Poor drainage of or leaking dialysate

Haemodialysis (HD)

Vascular access – infection, thrombosis, stenosis
Accidents during dialysis – blood loss, clotting of artificial kidney (dialyser)
Haemodynamic instability during dialysis

PD & HD

Insufficient dialysis
Inadequate nutrition
Fluid overload
Accelerated atherogenesis

Interesting facts

The first successful human kidney transplant was performed between identical twins in 1954. However, it was not until immunosuppressive therapy became available in the 1960s that transplantation became a routine clinical reality.

Modes of transplantation

Kidney transplants may be obtained from a living donor or a deceased donor. Living donors are either related by blood (e.g. parents, siblings) or are emotionally linked (e.g. spouse, close friend). Very occasionally 'altruistic' donation occurs from an unrelated living donor, but transplantation for profit (so called 'organ trafficking') is illegal. Living related donation has the potential advantage of greater histocompatibility and, therefore,

Table 9.3 Causes of death in ESKD patients

	Dialysis (%)	*Transplant (%)*
Cardiac	35	25
Withdrawal from treatment	35	5
Infection	10	15
Vascular	10	15
Malignancy	5	30
Miscellaneous	5	10

Case 9.2 — Kidney failure and replacement of renal function: 1

Cindy Lopez is a 50-year-old female with polycystic kidney disease. Her disease has been progressing slowly towards end-stage, and her latest glomerular filtration rate (GFR) was 20 mL/min/1.73 m². Apart from occasional macroscopic haematuria and kidney pain, she was asymptomatic. Her blood pressure, fluids and electrolytes were all well controlled by diet and medications. Cindy was not keen to have dialysis because her mother, who also had polycystic kidney disease, had died 15 years ago whilst on dialysis. Cindy has three brothers, two of whom are well with no kidney disease. Cindy is blood group A, as is one of her brothers; her other brother is blood group O. Cindy would like to receive a transplant from one of her brothers and not have dialysis.

This case raises the following questions:

1. Can she receive a kidney transplant without dialysis?
2. Would it be better for her to wait to receive a transplant from the deceased donor waiting list?
3. What are the likely outcomes of her transplantation?

potentially better outcomes, but the results of spousal donation are almost as good. Until recently, transplantation did not occur across ABO blood group incompatibilities. However, excellent long term results are now being achieved with ABO-incompatible transplantation, using plasma exchange and immunosuppression to remove the recipient's anti-donor blood group antibodies prior to transplantation. Kidney donation through an exchange programme, whereby a patient's living donor gives their kidney to a different patient in exchange for their donor giving theirs to the first patient, is a good option in situations where a better immunological match can be obtained. Living donation can occur either before dialysis or when a patient is already on dialysis. Transplantation prior to dialysis (so-called 'pre-emptive' transplantation) has the obvious advantage of avoidance of dialysis.

If there are no potential living donors, then the patient needs to commence dialysis and be placed on the waiting list to receive a transplant from a deceased donor. Deceased donor transplantation requires ABO blood group compatibility and histocompatibility. Preference is given to donor-recipient pairs that share major histocompatibility antigens and also to recipients who have been on the transplant waiting list for long periods. The number of patients awaiting transplantation is much greater than the number of available transplants, and so the number of patients on the transplant waiting list and the mean waiting time prior to transplantation are increasing steadily in most western countries.

Usually, one kidney is transplanted, extraperitoneally in the iliac fossa (Fig. 9.5). For a small number of patients with type 1 diabetes and kidney disease, the pancreas and kidney are transplanted at the same time.

Preparing a patient for transplantation

Factors that determine whether a patient is deemed fit enough to receive a kidney transplant include the operative risk, the risk of loss of the transplant because of technical and immunological reasons, and the risks associated with immunosuppression. The cardiovascular health of the patient is an important determinant of the safety of the anaesthetic and surgery and long term outcome. Age *per se* is not important, but in patients over 60 years old (or in people with long-standing diabetes), it is important to exclude significant cardiovascular disease. The risks of transplant loss relate to local factors (such as diseased iliac blood vessels, bladder abnormalities), recurrent disease in the transplant (such as can occur with focal segmental glomerulosclerosis and IgA glomerulonephritis) and heightened risk of rejection (as in a patient who is sensitised against donor antigens, has previously received a transplant, or is highly sensitised because of previous blood transfusions or pregnancy).

In patients with ongoing infection (including chronic hepatitis, HIV, latent tuberculosis) or heightened cancer risk, the need for immunosuppressive therapy to prevent transplant rejection may carry too great a risk of infection or malignancy.

If a patient is deemed fit for transplantation, then they submit a blood sample monthly to assess the development of immune responses, which would increase the risk of transplant rejection. As the waiting time for a kidney from a deceased donor is frequently quite prolonged, it is important that the patient's various risk factors are reassessed at regular intervals.

In patients who receive a living donor transplant, the processes of recipient assessment are similar. In addition, the likelihood of immunological response of the recipient to the donated kidney is more readily determined than with a deceased donor transplant.

In considering whether an individual is fit to donate a kidney, a prime consideration is whether the donation would increase the risk of deterioration in the remaining kidney. In a patient with a personal or family history of diabetes, hypertension or other diseases which may affect kidney function, the risk to the potential donor may not be acceptable. Potential donors need to have a total GFR of greater than 90 mL/min/1.73 m^2 (so that after donation, they are left with a GFR of at least half this amount) and no evidence of structural disease of the kidneys, urinary tract, and renal blood vessels; lesser GFR (80–89) may be acceptable if a full risk assessment determines that the potential donor has an acceptably low lifetime risk of kidney failure.

In the case of deceased donor transplantation, patients will receive only a few hours warning before the transplantation must proceed. In addition to the considerations above, they must have no acute health concerns, such as active infection. In the case of live donor transplantation prior to dialysis, the donation should occur prior to the development of significant symptoms of ESKD, usually when the GFR is about or greater than 7 to 10 mL/min/1.73 m^2.

Outcomes and complications of transplantation

With modern immunosuppression, transplant and recipient outcomes have improved markedly over the last couple of decades. The 1-year and 5-year survival for a deceased donor transplant in Australia is currently 95% and 80%, respectively, and patient survival is 95% and 90%. The outcomes after living donation are even better. The transplant may rarely be lost early because of surgical problems or acute rejection. Acute rejection now occurs in less than a quarter of patients during the first 12 months and accounts for less than 20% of grafts lost during that period. Patients at increased risk of acute rejection include those with a high percentage of antibodies against common histocompatibility antigens, donor-specific antibodies, and prior transplant loss from acute rejection. Transplants may be lost in the long term

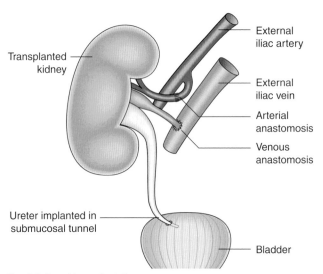

External iliac artery

Transplanted kidney

External iliac vein

Arterial anastomosis

Venous anastomosis

Ureter implanted in submucosal tunnel

Bladder

Fig. 9.5 Renal transplantation.

because of chronic rejection, nephrotoxicity of immuno-suppressive drugs (calcineurin inhibitors), recurrence of the disease which caused ESKD (such as glomerulone-phritis or diabetes) or patient death with a functioning transplant. Amongst the immunosuppressive agents, cal-cineurin inhibitors (such as cyclosporin and tacrolimus) can lead to progressive loss of graft function. So-called 'chronic allograft nephropathy' is multifactorial and is because of chronic immunological processes, calcineurin nephrotoxicity, and other factors.

Recipients of a kidney transplant remain on immu-nosuppressive medications for life since even late with-drawal will usually result in loss of the transplant by rejection. Commonly used immunosuppressive agents are listed in Table 9.4. The majority of patients receive three or four different agents initially, falling to two to three agents in lower doses after a year or so. Initial therapy frequently includes biological agents (anti-IL2 antibody or lympho-cyte depleting agents for those at high risk of transplant rejection). The reduction in immunosuppressive therapy over time is individualised, based on the patient's record of (or potential for) adverse events. Patient non-adherence to therapy is a major concern.

Interesting facts

Whilst the risk of many malignancies is increased in trans-plant recipients, no increased risk has been demonstrated with some cancers (including breast, prostate, and rectum).

Table 9.4 Immunosuppressive agents used to prevent kidney transplant rejection, and their common side effects

Drug class/example	Common side effects
Corticosteroids	
Prednisolone	Hypertension, osteopenia, dyslipidaemia, diabetes
Calcineurin inhibitors	
Cyclosporine	Nephrotoxicity, hypertension
Tacrolimus	Diabetes, hypertension, nephrotoxicity
mTOR inhibitors	
Sirolimus, everolimus	Poor wound healing, proteinuria, dyslipidaemia
Antiproliferative agents	
Azathioprine	Myelosuppression
Mycophenolate	Gastrointestinal disturbances, myelosuppression
T lymphocyte depleting agents	
Thymoglobulin	Myelosuppression
Agents that reduce T lymphocyte activation	
Basiliximab	Myelosuppression (mild)

mTOR, Mammalian target of rapamycin.

Immunosuppressive therapy increases the risk of infection and also malignancies. In 2019, malignancy accounted for almost 30% of transplant patient mortal-ity in Australia, whilst cardiac disease caused 25% and infection 15% of deaths (Table 9.3). During the first 3 to 6 months, patients receive agents to prevent the risk of bacterial infection (pneumocystis pneumonia and uri-nary tract infection), fungal infection (usually oral), and viral infection (such as CMV). BK virus infects both the transplanted graft and recipient's bladder, causes reduced graft function and even loss, and is managed with a reduction in immunosuppression and antiviral agents. Patients may have ongoing renal osteodystrophy and osteoporosis (from steroid therapy), which requires treatment with various agents such as bisphosphonates and vitamin D. Many patients also require chronic treat-ment for hypertension. Finally, as transplant function deteriorates, there may be a requirement for other treat-ments used for patients with CKD.

Interesting facts

Immunosuppressive therapy increases the risk of many infections. Post-transplant infections may also predis-pose to certain cancers (e.g. lymphomas associated with Epstein-Barr virus) and allograft dysfunction (e.g. BK virus).

Supportive therapy for advanced CKD

In patients approaching ESKD for whom dialysis is unlikely to prolong survival or improve quality of life, such as older patients with significant comorbid conditions, sup-portive treatment without dialysis should be considered. Supportive therapy is effective at prolonging quality of life and should also be directed at avoiding acute deterioration, delaying progression of CKD, reducing the complications of CKD, and treating comorbid conditions (Box 9.6).

To prolong and improve quality of life, therapy should include avoidance of nephrotoxins (e.g. drugs, intravenous radiocontrast), regular assessment of all medications to avoid unnecessary polypharmacy and nephrotoxicity, avoidance,

Box 9.6 Principles of supportive therapy for advanced CKD without dialysis

Avoid nephrotoxins, unnecessary polypharmacy and con-traindicated drugs
Optimise management of blood pressure and fluid status
Treat dangerous electrolyte abnormalities
Treat anaemia
Treat symptoms of uraemia
Consider continuation of therapy to slow CKD progression
Optimise social functioning using a multidisciplinary approach
Plan for a calm and dignified death with minimal suffering

or rapid reversal of AKI (e.g. from hypovolaemia or sepsis), treatment for specific symptoms of CKD, correction of dangerous electrolyte abnormalities, correction of anaemia, and specific measures to slow CKD progression.

Death from ESKD should be planned, peaceful, and dignified. As long as severe symptoms (in particular fluid overload) are avoided, then suffering should be minimal, and death occurs by progressive obtundation.

Summary

1. Kidney functions that can be replaced by dialysis include solute (electrolyte, acid-base, and uraemic toxin) and water clearance. Transplantation can, in addition, replace the endocrine functions of the kidney (erythropoietin production and vitamin D synthesis).
2. Dialysis relies on the principle of removal of solute and water through a semi-permeable membrane. Modalities include HD and PD. Preparation for dialysis should be commenced several months before it is needed.
3. Chronic dialysis is associated with morbidity arising from the dialysis procedure itself and associated comorbidities such as cardiovascular disease, anaemia, secondary hyperparathyroidism, and malnutrition.
4. Dialysis for AKI usually requires vascular access that is achievable in a short time (e.g. HD or acute PD via a catheter) versus ESKD (HD via a fistula or PD via a catheter).
5. Modes of transplantation includes kidney-only, kidney with pancreas/islet, or less commonly combined transplantation with liver and/or heart. Sources of transplant organs include live or deceased donors.
6. Transplantation is associated with much superior outcomes compared to dialysis. Complications include acute rejection, recurrent disease, chronic graft dysfunction associated with chronic antibody-mediated rejection/diabetes/hypertension/calcineurin toxicity. Causes of death include graft failure, cancer, and cardiovascular disease.
7. Conservative management of ESKD is appropriate in people who are unlikely to benefit from dialysis and focuses on symptom control.

Self-assessment case study answers

Answers to case study 9.2: Kidney failure and replacement of renal function: 1

Q1. Can she receive a kidney transplant prior to starting dialysis?

A1. Kidney transplant organs are sourced from either a live (related or unrelated) or deceased donor. In most countries, the allocation of a deceased donor kidney is only available to those already on dialysis or those with type 1 diabetes where a combined kidney-pancreas transplant is suitable. Therefore the most likely option is a kidney from a live donor.

Q2. Why are outcomes from a live donor transplant generally superior to those from a deceased donor?

A2. Transplantation from a live donor is almost always better than from a deceased donor. Waiting times on dialysis are usually a few years. Transplantation is associated with better survival than being on dialysis, so early transplantation is preferable. In addition, a live donation is a planned procedure, and so the donated graft kidney has a shorter time without blood supply (ischaemic time) than in deceased kidney donation.

Q3. What are the likely outcomes of kidney transplantation?

A3. Transplantation is associated with very good survival (>15 years on average, depending on the course of the disease). Rates of acute rejection causing graft failure are very low nowadays (<5%). Causes of graft failure include death because of other causes (cardiovascular disease and cancer being most common), chronic graft dysfunction (multifactorial, associated with chronic antibody-mediated rejection, calcineurin toxicity, vascular diseases such as hypertension or new-onset diabetes after transplantation). Patients with certain diseases such as glomerulonephritis and polycystic kidney disease also are at risk of recurrent disease.

Self-assessment questions and answers

After studying this chapter, you should be able to answer the following questions:

Q1. What are the different modes of dialysis delivery, and what factors govern the choice?

A1. The two modalities of dialysis are haemodialysis and peritoneal dialysis (PD). PD requires access to the peritoneal cavity using a specialised flexible catheter called a Tenckhoff catheter. PD is usually suitable as the first modality because of its ease of learning the technique for home use and association with better preservation of residual renal function. However, those with previous abdominal surgery or infection, hernias or severe obesity are less suitable for PD. In these cases, HD is better and is also generally superior to PD with solute clearance. HD can be trained in a home setting, but those not suitable (e.g. frailty or cognitive impairment) will need satellite or hospital HD. Those with peripheral vascular disease or cardiac disease may have more difficulties with HD.

Q2. How should a patient be prepared for chronic dialysis?

A2. If chronic dialysis is likely to be needed within the next few months, preparations should be commenced. This includes education regarding options for dialysis, transplantation and, if relevant, supportive care. Several weeks to months are usually required to create vascular access for HD, whilst access for PD requires a shorter time period.

Q3. What are the long term complications and outcomes of dialysis?

A3. Both PD and HD have a finite technique survival. PD may be complicated by infection (exit site or peritonitis) or technique failure because of sclerosis of the peritoneal membrane. HD may be complicated by problems with the AV fistula (thrombosis, infection, or excessive/deficient flow) or HD catheter (thrombosis, infection, or insufficient flow). Failure of one technique may require transition to the other technique. More often however, the patient is likely to succumb to associated disease, especially cardiovascular disease, but also sepsis or malignancy.

HYPERTENSION AND THE KIDNEY

Chapter objectives

After studying this chapter, you should be able to:

1. List some physiological determinants of arterial blood pressure and explain the role of the kidney in regulating these factors.

2. Discuss some mechanisms whereby abnormalities of the kidney may lead to hypertension (both essential and secondary forms).

3. Describe the pathologic conditions involved in end-organ damage because of hypertension.

4. Outline the principles of clinical and laboratory assessment of a patient presenting with hypertension.

5. Describe the mechanisms of action of the major classes of antihypertensive drugs.

6. Give the principles of management of a patient with renovascular hypertension.

Introduction

Arterial hypertension is the most prevalent chronic disorder of western populations and the most common preventable risk factor for cardiovascular disease. If untreated, it can result in a wide spectrum of morbidity and premature mortality, and, as such, its prevention and treatment are major goals for health care systems.

The kidney is involved both as a causative factor and as an organ of target damage in hypertension, and this chapter will outline some of its physiological and pathological features in relation to hypertension. The subject is a very large one, and the discussion here will necessarily be selective.

See Case 10.1: 1.

Determinants of normal blood pressure and role of the kidney

In its simplest form, the haemodynamic description of the systemic circulation can be reduced to the statement that the mean arterial blood pressure (BP) is the product of the cardiac output (CO) and the total peripheral resistance (TPR), that is,

$$BP = CO \times TPR$$

The CO itself is the product of the stroke volume times the heart rate, where the stroke volume is determined by the left ventricular filling volume and the force of contraction. Whilst a very wide range of physiological variables can influence BP through one or other of these parameters, and the relationship between them is, in fact, very complex, these formulas suggest several levels at which the function of the kidney may impact the final level of the BP. Some of these mechanisms are illustrated in Fig. 10.1.

The two main variables to be considered are the extracellular fluid (ECF) volume (which relates directly to the CO) and the degree of vasoconstriction of the arterial bed (which determines the TPR). Many aspects of renal function impinge on one or both of these variables. The following are some examples.

1. Anything causing a reduction of glomerular filtration rate (GFR) will lead to retention of salt and water, with consequent volume expansion.
2. Excessive salt reabsorption by the renal tubules will also lead to increased ECF volume.
3. Activation of the renin-angiotensin-aldosterone system has the capacity to influence both variables: angiotensin II is a potent vasoconstrictor and also enhances proximal sodium reabsorption, whilst aldosterone stimulates distal nephron sodium reabsorption.

Case 10.1 Hypertension and the kidney: 1

A case of deteriorating blood pressure control

Ross Schneider is a 72-year-old man who presents to his local doctor with 3 weeks of increasing headaches. He also mentions having generally been unwell for several months, with tiredness and increasing breathlessness on exertion. He is known to have had mild hypertension for over 25 years, but his blood pressure has been well controlled over this period of time, his current medication being the diuretic indapamide 2.5 mg daily. However, he has been living overseas with his son for the past 9 months and, during this period, has not had his blood pressure checked as regularly as usual. His past history also includes peripheral vascular disease, manifested 2 years previously by episodes of **claudication** in both calves on walking up hills. This symptom had eased after he stopped smoking, and no further investigation or treatment had been performed.

His family history includes hypertension in his father and one of his two sisters and ischaemic heart disease, which affected his father in his fifties. Mr. Schneider is a retired postal officer who smoked about 20 cigarettes per day from age 20 to 70 years. He drinks four or five beers (300 mL glasses) per day. He takes no medications other than his blood pressure tablets and says he complies strictly with these.

On examination, he looks rather tired and has a pulse rate of 90 beats/min. His blood pressure is 210/100, taken in the right arm in the seated position, and this is unchanged after 5 min of rest. The apex beat is found to be displaced 2 cm lateral to the mid-clavicular line and is thrusting (pressure-loaded) in character. Cardiac auscultation reveals a systolic ejection murmur and a loud aortic component of the second heart sound. A few soft **crepitations** are heard in the base of both lung fields. The abdomen is normal to palpation but, on auscultating over the right upper quadrant, a prolonged systolic **bruit** is heard. Peripheral pulses are difficult to feel below the popliteal in both legs. The optic fundi show thickening of arteriolar walls and **arteriovenous nipping**. Urinalysis shows protein + and no other abnormalities.

Two main issues arise for discussion from this presentation.

a. What was the basis of Mr. Schneider's original history of hypertension?

b. What has occurred to cause his blood pressure control to be dramatically impaired at this presentation?

---

4. The sympathetic nervous system likewise has dual actions: noradrenergic innervation of arteriolar vessels throughout the body leads to vasoconstriction and an increase in TPR, whilst noradrenergic nerve endings around the proximal tubule stimulate sodium and water reabsorption at that site.
5. The endothelium-derived peptide endothelin is a potent vasoconstrictor, and levels are elevated in renal failure.
6. The renal prostaglandins are one of several locally acting signalling mechanisms influencing

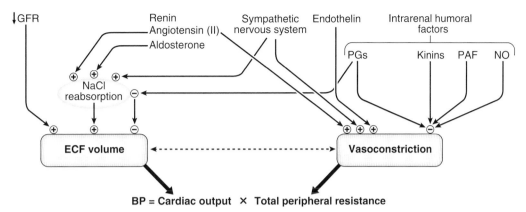

Fig. 10.1 Renal mechanisms involved in blood pressure control. Note that many interactions exist between the factors included in this schematic diagram. whilst extracellular fluid (ECF) volume and vasoconstriction are shown here as independent parameters, there is a direct interplay between these factors, as discussed in the text. 1 indicates a stimulating or enhancing influence, 2 indicates an inhibiting or suppressing effect; GFR, glomerular filtration rate; NO, nitric oxide; PAF, platelet-activating factor; PG, prostaglandins.

renal function in relation to hypertension. In this case, end products such as prostaglandin E_2 actually promote antihypertensive effects within the kidney, both by inhibiting salt and water reabsorption and hence promoting volume loss and also by causing vasodilatation within the kidney and elsewhere.

7. Several other vasodilator systems have been identified within the kidney: these include the renal kinin system resulting in the formation of the vasodilator bradykinin, and platelet-activating factor, nitric oxide, and other endothelial-based dilator systems.

It is important to emphasise that there is no simple relationship between disturbances in these factors and the generation of sustained arterial hypertension. Perturbations in any one system tend to be compensated by changes in other systems, and the critical role of central nervous system pathways modulating baroreceptor reflexes must be taken into account. Furthermore, a primary change in one major parameter, such as the ECF, can lead to secondary changes in the state of peripheral vasoconstriction so that the final pattern of haemodynamic disturbance is different from that which triggered the initial BP rise.

Pathogenesis of essential hypertension

These considerations may be relevant to the pathogenesis of so-called 'essential' hypertension, in which a specific underlying cause for increased BP cannot be defined in identifiable pathologic conditions in any organ system. This pattern, which would match the initial hypertensive history of our patient Mr. Schneider, may be associated with a genetic predisposition overlayed with environmental risk factors (Box 10.1) and the process of ageing. Whilst the precise pathogenesis of this condition has not been definitively established, a variety of physi-

Box 10.1 Risk factors for the development of high blood pressure (other than specific secondary forms of hypertension)

Non-modifiable

Family history
Inherited predisposition to essential hypertension
Specific inherited conditions (e.g. Liddle's syndrome, metabolic syndrome)

Potentially reversible

Lifestyle factors
Obesity (sleep apnoea)
Excessive salt intake
Excessive alcohol intake
Physical inactivity

Iatrogenic
Oral contraceptive pill use
Use of non-steroidal anti-inflammatory drugs
Steroid therapy
Excessive use of topical or systemic vasoconstrictor medications

ological disturbances are capable of leading to the endpoint of sustained hypertension, as shown in Fig. 10.2.

This model proposes three main pathways that may be disordered because of the impact of genetic and environmental influences. The development of sustained hypertension is likely to involve a complex interplay of these three pathways whereby the usual compensatory changes that would occur in response to abnormalities in one pathway are impaired or absent. For example, as we know, sodium regulation is crucial in maintaining blood volume. Increased sodium and water retention are usually associated with compensatory haemodynamic changes to maintain normal BP. The usual changes are a reduction in peripheral vascular resistance via the production of various vasodilators, in particular nitric oxide.

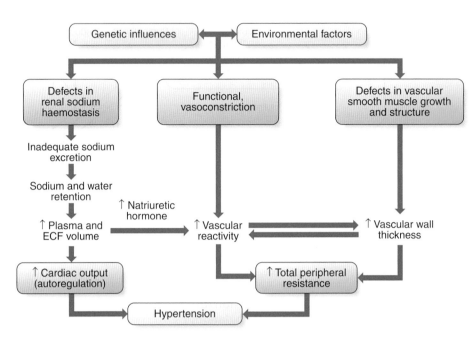

Fig. 10.2 This hypothetical model for the pathogenesis of essential hypertension implicates genetic and environmental factors in altering three major pathways of BP regulation in the development of sustained hypertension. (Modified from Kumar V Robbins and Cotran. Pathological basis of disease, seventh edition. Philadelphia: Saunders; 2004.)

If this response is absent or impaired, then hypertension will occur. Several other impaired responses may predispose to hypertension-endothelial dysfunction, activation of the renin-angiotensin-aldosterone system, natriuretic peptide deficiency, and activation of the sympathetic nervous system. These impaired responses may be related to genetic predisposition and modifiable environmental risk factors.

Of particular interest to the renal system are abnormalities of sodium regulation that are associated with hypertension. A genetic predisposition to increased sodium reabsorption is unlikely to be associated at this stage with a specific genetic defect, as essential hypertension is thought to be a polygenic disorder. However, several rare inherited syndromes have been defined, which are monogenic and tend to be associated with particular abnormalities of tubular sodium transport. Of recent interest is the definition of the cause of hypertension in Liddle's syndrome, in which BP elevation early in life is associated with evidence for volume expansion (suppressed renin and aldosterone levels). Here overexpression of the epithelial sodium channel in the apical membrane of the cortical collecting duct epithelium has been identified and linked to a specific gene defect. Similar but more subtle causes of increased tubular sodium avidity may underlie a wider spectrum of patients with familial hypertension. For example, in the 'metabolic syndrome,' in which hypertension is associated with obesity and insulin resistance, an increase in proximal tubular sodium-hydrogen exchange has been found.

Of the non-genetic factors, at least some of the reversible factors may operate through enhanced renal sodium retention. Certainly, the epidemiological and clinical evidence relating to a correlation between salt intake and hypertension is suggestive of a primary role for volume expansion (at least in genetically predisposed individuals).

The hypertension of common obesity may also be caused by volume expansion, possibly mediated by high insulin levels, which act to enhance proximal sodium reabsorption. Renal salt retention is also implicated in hypertension associated with a variety of medications, including oestrogens, non-steroidal anti-inflammatory drugs which interfere with prostaglandin synthesis, and corticosteroids.

ECF volume expansion also has an important role in the genesis of several forms of secondary hypertension; these are discussed later in this chapter.

Interesting facts

The epidemic of hypertension in modern human populations may relate to our evolutionary past as a species. Since our early terrestrial evolution occurred largely in salt-poor regions of the world such as Africa, physiological systems developed, which were salt-avid. Hence when dietary salt is plentiful in the modern world, particularly in the West, salt retention occurs, leading to volume expansion and hypertension.

The pathologic conditions of hypertension

Whatever the cause of a sustained increase in arterial BP, several forms of end-organ damage result from this haemodynamic change. As shown in Fig. 10.3, the kidneys are included among these target organs.

The fundamental pathologic conditions associated with hypertension is based on structural changes in the terminal radicals of the arterial tree, namely the small muscular arteries and arterioles. The repetitive mechanical stress associated with hypertension causes changes in all layers of the vessel wall, particularly in the media layer, where smooth muscle hypertrophy results in a thickening of

Hypertension target organs

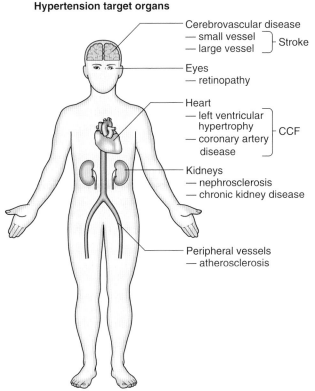

Fig. 10.3 End-organ damage in hypertension. CCF, congestive cardiac failure.

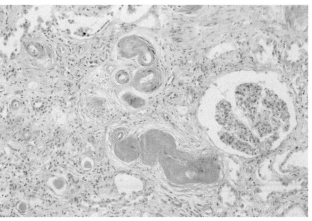

Fig. 10.4 Microscopic pathologic condition of the kidney in 'benign' essential hypertension. (From Klatt E.C. (2021). Robbins and Cotran Atlas of Pathology, 4e. Philadelphia: Elsevier Inc.).

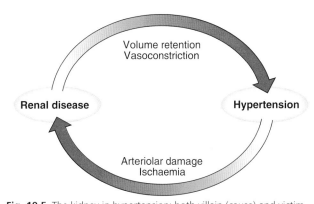

Fig. 10.5 The kidney in hypertension: both villain (cause) and victim (effect).

the arterial wall with concentric narrowing of the lumen. The internal elastic lamina becomes reduplicated and interrupted, and hyaline degeneration may occur in focal areas of the media where a glassy eosinophilic material accumulates. These changes, found in so-called 'benign' hypertension, are replaced in the more accelerated and severe variant known as 'malignant' hypertension by a more destructive severe form of vascular wall pathologic conditions, the characteristic lesion being that of fibrinoid necrosis. In all forms of sustained hypertension, the intima layer is also damaged and undergoes a proliferative response, which in larger vessels is associated with acceleration of the process of atherosclerosis.

These vascular lesions lead to various grades of ischaemia in the principal target organs, namely the brain, the heart, and the kidneys. Small vessel changes in the brain are reflected in the optic fundi, where progressive stages of vascular damage and retinal ischaemia can be observed directly (hypertensive retinopathy). In the heart, myocardial ischaemia develops and is aggravated by the development of left ventricular hypertrophy because of the chronic pressure load on that chamber. Within the kidney, ischaemia is manifested initially by wrinkling of the glomerular basement membrane. Hypertrophic and hyaline changes develop in the afferent arterioles, resulting in progressive atrophy and ultimately sclerosis of glomeruli (Fig. 10.4). In severe and neglected hypertension, this can lead to end-stage kidney disease

(see Chapter 8). Ischaemic changes also affect the tubules, which undergo atrophy, associated with interstitial inflammatory changes progressing ultimately to fibrosis. Eventually, the kidney as a whole undergoes contraction with a finely scarred surface ('nephrosclerosis').

It is clear that the kidney has an especially complex relationship to arterial hypertension. As mentioned previously (and to be developed further below), it is directly implicated in the cause and pathophysiology of some forms of hypertension, notably those in which definable renal disease provides the primary trigger for the development of high BP. Equally, however, it is an important end-organ of damage from hypertensive vascular disease, thereby setting up a vicious cycle of further aggravation of hypertension (Fig. 10.5). Intervention in this cycle by vigorous therapy to lower the BP and protect the kidney is thus a crucial task for clinicians caring for these patients.

See Case 10.1: 2.

Hypertension and the kidney: 2

Initial investigations

Mr. Schneider's physical examination revealed clear evidence for end-organ damage consistent with hypertensive effects. The displaced and prominent left ventricular impulse suggests the presence of left ventricular hypertrophy with some cardiac enlargement, and the pulmonary crepitations and recent history of breathlessness are consistent with early left ventricular failure. The history of claudication and finding of poor distal pulses in the legs suggest the development of peripheral vascular disease, whilst the finding of Grade II hypertensive retinopathy (thickened retinal arteriolar walls with arteriovenous nipping) implies hypertensive effects on small arterioles. The detection of + proteinuria on urinalysis is consistent with hypertensive damage to glomeruli and warrants further quantification.

The initial investigations performed on Mr. Schneider reveal the following results.

Plasma biochemistry:

Sodium 135 mmol/L

Potassium 4.1 mmol/L

Chloride 99 mmol/L

Bicarbonate 29 mmol/L

*Urea 9.2 mmol/L

*Creatinine 180 µmol/L.

These levels had been normal when last checked 3 years previously.

Random blood glucose is 6.8 mmol/L, and the lipid profile is normal. A chest X-ray shows a moderately enlarged heart (principally the left ventricle) and bilateral pulmonary congestion. Electrocardiography shows evidence of left ventricular hypertrophy with non-specific ST segment changes.

These data were interpreted as evidence for renal and cardiac damage resulting from his hypertension.

Whilst waiting for these initial investigation results, Mr. Schneider's doctor initiated some changes in his therapy, having made the assessment that he had experienced a marked deterioration in his level of blood pressure control. He urged the patient to discontinue all alcohol intake, reduce his salt intake, continue with his diuretic medication, and begin taking amlodipine 2.5 mg daily. He asked to review him in 3 days time. He explained that he suspected that some new problem had arisen, causing his hypertension to become exacerbated and that he thought some further investigations would be required.

Issues for further consideration at this point include:

1. What clues are there as to the cause of Mr. Schneider's deterioration in blood pressure control?

2. What are the appropriate next steps in his management?

*Values outside the normal range; see Appendix.

Principles in the management of hypertension

In a patient presenting for the first time with hypertension, management consists of three general steps:

1. Ensure accurate reproducible BP measurements with multiple observations, including the use of ambulatory BP monitoring and home BP monitoring where appropriate. See Clinical skills for how to measure BP.
2. Baseline investigations to assess end-organ damage (particularly in the heart and kidney), to quantitate other vascular risk factors (particularly plasma lipid profile), and to screen for major causes of secondary hypertension as clinically appropriate (see below).
3. Initiation of lifestyle modification (Box 10.1) ± pharmacological treatment.

This staged approach can be accelerated in situations in which the BP is severely elevated at presentation (>160/100) or where there is clinical evidence of organ-threatening complications such as heart failure, renal impairment or neurological symptoms or signs. In practice, in the absence of specific clinical clues, the 'screening' investigations in the second step can be limited to urinalysis to detect renal parenchymal disease and plasma biochemistry to detect renal failure or electrolyte changes suggestive of endocrine hypertension. Further investigations are initiated when abnormalities are detected on these preliminary tests, taken in conjunction with clinical information.

The selection of an appropriate antihypertensive medication depends on the properties of the available agents (including cost), patient characteristics and comorbidities, guided by information from relevant published clinical trials. A summary of some key features of the available drugs is given in Table 10.1. The most commonly used agents are currently from three classes, drugs interfering with the renin-angiotensin system, including angiotensin-converting enzyme (ACE) inhibitors and A-II receptor blockers, thiazide diuretics and calcium channel blockers.). Frequently, drugs are given in combination to reduce side effects and oppose secondary compensations, which can reduce the effectiveness of a single agent. One of the most effective such combinations is a low dose diuretic together with an ACE inhibitor or A-II receptor blocker.

Interesting facts

Before the middle of the 20th century, hypertension was commonly ascribed to an over-excited emotional state, and treatments usually included central nervous system sedatives such as barbiturates.

Deterioration in BP control

When a patient who has been stabilised on an antihypertensive treatment regimen experiences a deterioration in BP control, as did Mr. Schneider, several possibilities

Table 10.1 Overview of main classes of antihypertensive drugs

Class	Example drug(s)	Advantages	Disadvantages
Thiazide Diuretics	Chlorothiazide	Useful in coexistent CCF, adjunctive action with other agents	Electrolyte/metabolic side effects, allergies
Beta-blockers	Metoprolol (beta-1 selective)	Beneficial in IHD	Fatigue, insomnia; may worsen asthma, heart block, PVD, lipids
Alpha-blockers	Prazosin	Metabolically neutral	Postural hypotension
Calcium channel blockers* a. Non-dihydropyridine b. Dihydropyridine	(a) Verapamil (b) Nifedipine	Can be easily combined with other first-line agents (although avoid beta-blockers and non-dihydropyridines because of risk of heart block)	(a) May cause constipation, worsen heart block/CCF; (b) Cause flushing, oedema
ACE inhibitors	Captopril	Beneficial in CCF, reduce proteinuria, conserve kidney function	Cough, angio-oedema, reduce GFR in renal artery stenosis, hyperkalaemia
A-II receptor blockers	Losartan	Beneficial in CCF, reduce proteinuria, conserve kidney function	As for ACE inhibitors, but less cough
Nitrates	Isosorbide mononitrate	Systolic BP control	Headache
Aldosterone antagonist	Aldactone	Resistant hypertension or primary hyperaldosteronism	Androgen effects Hyperkalaemia
Centrally acting drugs	Methyldopa, clonidine		Drowsiness, depression
Direct-acting vasodilators	Hydralazine, moxonidine		Reflex tachycardia, oedema

*Representative drugs are shown for the two main classes of calcium channel blockers: (a) the non-dihydropyridines; and (b) the dihydropyridines. ACE, angiotensin-converting enzyme; A-II, angiotensin II; CCF, congestive cardiac failure; GFR, glomerular filtration rate; IHD, ischaemic heart disease; PVD, peripheral vascular disease.

Box 10.2 Causes of deterioration in blood pressure control

- Poor treatment adherence (compliance)
- Commencement of interacting medications (e.g. NSAIDs)
- Lifestyle changes (weight gain, excessive salt, or alcohol intake)
- Superadded secondary hypertension (especially renovascular or renal parenchymal disease)

NSAIDs, non-steroidal anti-inflammatory drugs.

must be considered (Box 10.2). The patient's adherence to the recommended treatment regimen must always be checked since poor compliance is a relatively frequent phenomenon, especially when the medications used are associated with unwelcome side effects. Occasionally, the inadvertent co-prescription of an interacting medication may be the cause; the best example here is the commencement of a non-steroidal anti-inflammatory drug that promotes salt and water retention and will elevate the BP in predisposed individuals. Occasionally, there has been a progressive slide into poor lifestyle habits which raise the BP, such as weight gain beyond ideal body weight or excess intake of salt or alcohol.

An important consideration, however, is the possibility that a form of secondary hypertension has become superimposed on what was originally essential hypertension.

Secondary hypertension

The principal causes of secondary hypertension are illustrated in Fig. 10.6. One of these causes may be defined soon after presentation in a patient with newly diagnosed hypertension and should be considered in scenarios outlined in Box 10.3 or following a period of resistance to therapy or deterioration in BP control in a patient with established hypertension. It should be emphasised that around 10% of all hypertensive patients have hypertension secondary to a defined pathologic condition in a specific organ system. Whilst causes other than those shown in Fig. 10.6 need to be considered in special patient groups (e.g. coarctation of the aorta in hypertensive children, pre-eclampsia in pregnant women, thyroid disease, obstructive sleep apnoea and selected medications), the most commonly encountered causes of secondary hypertension arise from conditions in the adrenal gland or the kidney.

Adrenal causes

Adrenal lesions causing hypertension may arise either in the adrenal cortex or medulla.

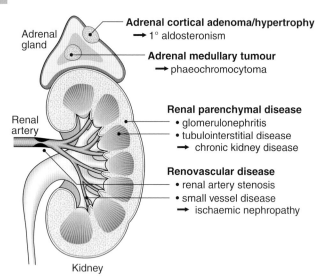

Fig. 10.6 Principal causes of secondary hypertension.

Box 10.3 Patients at high risk for secondary causes of hypertension

- Acute rise in BP in a patient with previously stable readings.
- Age <30, particularly in the absence of family history.
- Evidence of end organ damage on diagnosis of hypertension
- Severe hypertension (BP > 180/120 mmHg).
- Resistant hypertension (hypertension that is not controlled despite 3 antihypertensive agents, including one diuretic).

The adrenal cortex can be the site of an aldosterone-secreting adenoma, resulting in primary aldosteronism or Conn's syndrome. In this condition, autonomous production of aldosterone by the tumour leads to sustained salt and water retention by the kidney, with volume expansion and secondary vasoconstriction, which sustains the hypertensive state, as previously discussed. This condition may be accompanied by hypokalaemia, reflecting the action of aldosterone in enhancing renal potassium excretion. Whilst low serum potassium, usually accompanied by an elevated bicarbonate concentration, may act as a useful clue to the presence of an aldosterone excess state, these electrolyte abnormalities are not universally found in cases of primary aldosterone overproduction, and screening should occur for this condition in all patients whose hypertension is consistent with Box 10.3. One screening approach depends on the measurement of plasma aldosterone and renin concentrations, using a high aldosterone: renin ratio as a signal for further adrenal investigation, but can be challenging because of the effects of various medications on renin levels. Primary aldosteronism can also arise from hyperplasia of both adrenal cortices, sometimes because of an inherited defect in adrenal corticosteroid biosynthesis.

When the adrenal adenoma or cortical hypertrophy is associated with autonomous secretion of the glucocorticoid hormone cortisol, Cushing's syndrome results, hypertension being one of the principal clinical manifestations. Other clues here are bodily habitus changes associated with glucocorticoid excess, accompanied by hyperglycaemia and hypokalaemia and alkalosis (see also *Systems of the Body: The Endocrine System*).

The adrenal medulla may also give rise to tumours causing hypertension, in this case, phaeochromocytoma, secreting the catecholamines adrenaline (epinephrine), noradrenaline (norepinephrine) and related metabolites. These tumours can also arise in neural crest-derived tissue outside the adrenal gland. Characteristically they are associated with labile hypertension, with spasms of vasoconstriction and organ ischaemia related to bursts of catecholamine release. However, a significant proportion of these tumours are accompanied by sustained hypertension without such dramatic episodic changes in the peripheral circulation. The investigation is based on an index of suspicion, leading to 24 hour urine collections for measurement of catecholamines and their metabolites, followed by computed tomography (CT) imaging of the adrenal gland. Radioisotope scans with specialised tracers (e.g. 68Ga-DOTATATE) can be useful in localising extra-adrenal phaeochromocytomas. The pathophysiology of hypertension in this condition relates to intense catecholamine-induced vasoconstriction rather than primary volume expansion. The cornerstone of treatment before operative removal of the tumour is effective alpha-blockade using agents such as phenoxybenzamine.

Renal causes

The kidney can be the cause of secondary hypertension by one of two fundamental mechanisms: via activation of the renin-angiotensin system in renal ischaemia because of renovascular disease or through non-renin-dependent mechanisms in renal parenchymal disease, both in its early stages and in end-stage renal failure.

The mechanisms involved in the various forms of renal hypertension are best illuminated through some classic experiments first performed by Goldblatt in the 1930s (Fig. 10.7).

When the renal artery supplying one kidney of an animal is clipped so that the lumen is reduced by more than 70%, the animal develops hypertension. The mechanism of the initial phase of BP rise is dependent on the activation of secretion of renin from the clipped kidney, largely because of the fall in perfusion pressure in the afferent arterioles beyond the obstructed artery (see Chapter 2). Within the first few weeks after production of this lesion, the BP can be normalised by agents interfering with the action of angiotensin II, verifying that vasoconstriction produced by this peptide is the main mechanism for hypertension. The ECF volume does not undergo significant change in this phase, partly because

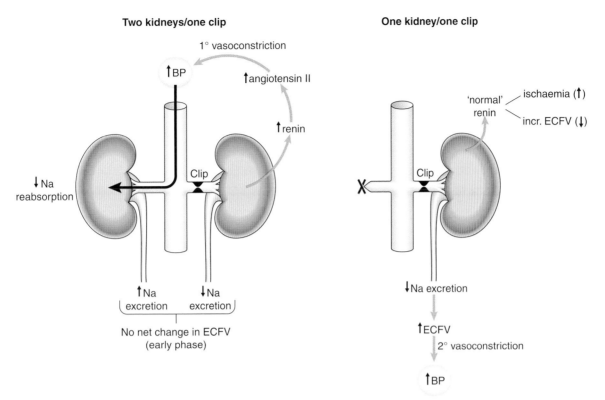

Fig. 10.7 Pathophysiology of renovascular hypertension (Goldblatt models). The two experimental models shown here represent extreme illustrations of the role of vasoconstriction (early phase of two kidney/one clip model) and volume expansion (one kidney/one clip) in the generation of hypertension during renal ischaemia (see text for details). BP, blood pressure; ECFV, extracellular fluid volume.

the reduction in sodium excretion from the clipped kidney is compensated by an increase in sodium excretion from the unclipped kidney. This is because of the effect of the increased BP in the unclipped kidney to inhibit salt and water reabsorption in proximal tubules on that side (so-called 'pressure natriuresis'). After some months, however, the increased BP becomes resistant to the action of angiotensin inhibition but does respond to a reduction of ECF volume. This is because of the long term effects of sustained hypertension on the blood vessels of the unclipped kidney, where obliterative changes lead to glomerular damage and reduced excretion of salt and water from that side. That is, the initial vasoconstriction-mediated hypertension has been replaced by a volume-dependent pattern.

When a similar experiment is performed in an animal in which one of the kidneys has been removed, clipping the renal artery of the remaining kidney also leads to the development of hypertension, but in this case, both the early phase and the long term phase of hypertension are dependent on an expanded ECF volume. This is because the overall reduction in total GFR promotes volume retention to occur early in the model, counteracting the ischaemia induced stimulus for renin release and triggering hypertension through secondary vasoconstriction via mechanisms described earlier in this chapter. This model provides a basis for understanding the hypertension of advanced kidney disease in which volume expansion is nearly always present.

Renal artery stenosis

Renal artery stenosis occurs in one of two main pathological forms.

Fibromuscular dysplasia (FMD) is a congenital condition in which the development of the media or adventitia layer of the renal artery (and sometimes other arteries) is abnormal, leading to an irregular narrowing of the lumen, often in a 'beaded' pattern. Typically affecting young women in the second or third decade of life, this is one of the classic causes of secondary hypertension in a young patient and, when unilateral, is usually detected in the phase of high renin release from the affected kidney. Intervention to correct the stenosis frequently results in restoration of normal BP and protection of renal function.

The more common cause of renal artery stenosis is that because of **atherosclerosis,** affecting patients in older age groups. In this condition, the atherosclerotic pathologic condition, which may also affect other vascular beds, involves one or both renal arteries, frequently producing a relatively focal stenosis (Fig. 10.8). Whilst there is often no special clue to the presence of this underlying lesion, the clinician's index

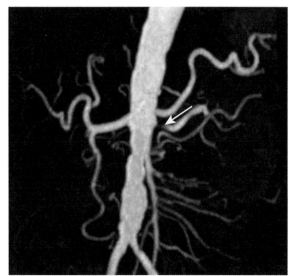

Fig. 10.8 Intra-arterial digital subtraction arteriogram showing left-sided atheromatous renal artery stenosis (From Ralston S.H. et al (2018). Davidson's Principles and Practice of Medicine, 23rd ed. Oxford: Elsevier Ltd.).

Table 10.2 Methods of renal artery imaging

Technique	Comments
Digital subtraction angiography	The intra-arterial method is the gold standard; the intravenous approach lacks adequate resolution
	Requires use of contrast agent (may reduce GFR)
Spiral CT angiography	Good 3D images; uses intravenous contrast (often high volumes required)
Magnetic resonance angiography	Avoids contrast agent; accurate only for main (proximal) vessels, expensive, limited availability
Renal artery Doppler–ultrasound scan	Operator-dependent; variable sensitivity/specificity
Radionuclide renography with captopril	Poor anatomical resolution but sensitive detection of functional stenosis via GFR effects
GFR, glomerular filtration rate.	

of suspicion that stenosis is present is raised by the following:

1. The relatively sudden appearance of hypertension in an older person.
2. The development of resistance to usual antihypertensive medications or an abrupt deterioration in BP control in a patient with previously stable hypertension (as in our current case).
3. Severe hypertension in an older patient is associated with progressive deterioration of renal function.

Careful clinical, biochemical, and radiological analysis is necessary to define the presence of renal artery stenosis in selected patients, and the pathophysiological assessment and appropriate management of such patients is frequently a complex matter. Three basic components are involved in the overall assessment:

1. What is the morphology of the lesions in the renal artery (or arteries)?
2. What is the role of the renal artery stenosis in the pathogenesis of the patient's hypertension at this time?
3. What is the influence of renal arterial disease on overall renal function?

Several imaging modalities, summarised in Table 10.2, may be used to define the anatomy of the renal arteries. Whilst intra-arterial digital subtraction arteriography (Fig. 10.8) is the gold standard for the definition of renal artery lesions, recent technical advances have made alternative less invasive procedures such as CT angiography attractive alternatives.

Whilst intervention is effective in controlling BP in patients with FMD, the evidence behind intervention for those with atherosclerotic RAS is less convincing.

Case 10.1   **Hypertension and the kidney: 3**

Further investigations and management

Three factors in Mr. Schneider's case led his doctor to initiate a further investigation for renal artery stenosis. First, a bruit over the upper abdomen had been heard on clinical examination, suggestive (but not diagnostic) of critical narrowing in a renal artery or another branch of the abdominal aorta. Second, he had recently developed clinical evidence for significant peripheral vascular disease, suggestive of a widespread process of advanced atherosclerosis. Third, his serum creatinine had risen over recent years, suggesting some cause of impaired glomerular perfusion.

After referral to a consultant nephrologist, further studies were performed that confirmed this suspicion. A renal ultrasound demonstrated that both kidneys were slightly reduced in size at 8 cm in length. A CT renal angiogram demonstrated 90% stenosis in the proximal segment of the right renal artery, with only minor luminal irregularities in the left renal artery but significant atheromatous disease in the abdominal aorta. A discussion was had about the risk/benefit ratio of performing a procedure to revascularise the artery, and it was decided to continue with aggressive cardiovascular risk reduction and blood pressure control.

These patients should be treated with aggressive cardiovascular risk reduction and BP control and intervention reserved for individualised cases with severe disease at risk of progressive chronic kidney disease (see Case 10.1: 3).

Renal parenchymal disease

Hypertension in renal parenchymal disease has multiple possible origins. In the phase before the advanced loss of kidney function has occurred, one important factor may be the loss of vasodilator substances generated normally by healthy renal tissue. This may lead to unopposed systemic vasoconstriction. However, as renal functional impairment progresses, the dominant mechanism is undoubtedly retention of salt and water because of the inadequate GFR, leading to expansion of the ECF volume and hypertension through secondary vasoconstrictive mechanisms. Thus, the great majority of patients approaching end-stage kidney disease or on dialysis have volume-dependent hypertension, which can be difficult to control until salt and water are removed from the ECF by diuretics or a form of dialysis.

In a minority of patients with advanced renal disease (<10%), the pathological processes within the kidney cause it to act as an ongoing source of renin release, producing hypertension via angiotensin-induced vasoconstriction. In individual patients, activation of the sympathetic nervous system appears to play a role in the pathogenesis of hypertension in renal failure, and in these cases, high circulating levels of catecholamines are found. See Case 10.1: 3.

Summary

1. Hypertension is a very common condition that results in significant morbidity and mortality
2. The majority of people who suffer from hypertension have 'essential hypertension'.
3. Around 10% of patients will have an underlying cause of their hypertension – 'secondary hypertension'.
4. Hypertension is a common risk factor for cardiovascular disease, and other cardiovascular risk factors should be assessed and managed in conjunction with controlling blood pressure.
5. There are several investigations for secondary causes of hypertension, and it is important to understand their limitations.
6. Management of hypertension should include lifestyle modification and non-pharmacological therapy prior to initiating BP-lowering drugs unless the hypertension or cardiovascular risk is severe and warrants pharmacological treatment from the outset.
7. There are several major classes of antihypertensive drugs, each offering different effects, appropriate in different conditions and associated with different side effects.

Clinical skills 10.1

As we have discovered, hypertension is very common, but the development of hypertension is almost always asymptomatic. It is therefore important that all adults should have their BP measured at each clinic visit, and if found to be high, further BP measurements should be taken to confirm the diagnosis.

So, having the skills to accurately measure BP is very important:

- The patient should be sitting quietly for 5 min before taking the BP.
- Ensure the BP cuff when wrapped around a patient's upper arm is at heart level and should be the correct size for the patient.
- BP should be measured on both arms on the initial visit, to rule out vascular abnormalities, and both sitting and standing, to exclude orthostatic hypotension.

- BP is recorded as two numbers: the systolic pressure, which is the pressure on the arteries as the left ventricle contracts and the diastolic pressure, which is the pressure on the arteries when the heart is at rest.
- When the cuff is inflated to the point that the brachial artery is occluded, no noise is heard through the stethoscope placed over the brachial artery, just below the cuff. As the cuff is gradually deflated, blood flow is re-established, and tapping sounds can be heard that signify systolic pressure. As the pressure falls further, the tapping ceases signifying diastolic pressure.
- As outlined in the text, BP readings should be repeated on two to three separate occasions to provide an accurate estimation of BP, but the readings should also be performed two to three times at each sitting, particularly if an automated BP cuff is used.

Self-assessment case study

A 52-year-old woman is referred for assessment of resistant hypertension. She has had raised blood pressure for only 5 years, during which time a variety of medications have been tried to control the blood pressure, with limited success. Treatment with a thiazide diuretic was partly effective but produced severe hypokalaemia (plasma potassium *2.4 mmol/L) and had to be discontinued. Even in the absence of diuretic treatment, the plasma potassium is generally in the range 2.9–3.6 mmol/L. Currently, imperfect blood pressure control has been achieved using the beta-blocker atenolol,

the ACE inhibitor enalapril, the alpha-blocker prazosin and the calcium channel blocker amlodipine.

After studying this chapter, you should be able to answer the following questions:

Q1. What is the most likely cause of secondary hypertension in this patient?

A. Atherosclerotic renal artery stenosis

B. Cushing's syndrome

C. Primary aldosteronism

D. Fibromuscular dysplasia

Self-assessment case study – con'd

Q2. When investigating for this condition, which of the antihypertensives that have been prescribed is most likely to result in a falsely elevated plasma aldosterone to renin ratio?
A. Atenolol

B. Enalapril
C. Prazosin
D. Verapamil

Self-assessment case study answers

A1. A patient who presents with hypokalaemia in association with hypertension is most likely to have primary aldosteronism. Hypokalaemia can occur because of severe renal artery stenosis or fibromuscular dysplasia because of secondary hyperaldosteronism, but this is more unusual. Cushing syndrome is an uncommon cause of hypertension.

A2. Atenolol causes a reduction in renin excretion, thereby often resulting in a false-positive plasma aldosterone to renin ratio. Enalapril causes an increase in renin, thereby resulting in frequent false-negative results. Prazosin and verapamil are not thought to impact on renin or aldosterone readings and are therefore commonly used medications when investigating for primary aldosteronism.

PREGNANCY AND THE KIDNEY

11

Chapter objectives

After studying this chapter, you should be able to:

1. Describe the anatomical changes that occur in the renal tract in normal pregnancy.

2. Understand the importance of diagnosis and treatment of urinary infection in pregnancy.

3. Demonstrate an understanding of the physiological alterations in pregnancy in fluid volume, renal plasma flow, glomerular filtration rate, and blood pressure, and the mechanisms by which they occur.

4. Describe the 'normal' changes in plasma biochemistry seen during pregnancy and the mechanisms that underpin these changes.

5. Define the various categories of hypertensive disorders encountered in pregnant women.

6. Describe the systemic abnormalities that occur in pre-eclampsia.

7. Demonstrate an understanding of the approach to the management of hypertension in pregnancy.

Introduction

The renal system undergoes several important structural and functional changes during normal pregnancy. These have implications for understanding several common complications of pregnancy and interpreting the results of laboratory and imaging investigations during pregnancy.

This chapter will survey these changes and introduce some important complications of pregnancy relating to the urinary tract, including the hypertensive disorders of pregnancy.

Structural changes in the urinary tract during pregnancy

Pregnancy induces changes in almost every organ system of the body, generally as an adaptive process to provide the best outcome for both mother and foetus. A key factor in supporting placental blood flow is the expansion of maternal blood volume, which leads to increased cardiac output. Because of the increased intra- and extravascular volume, the kidneys enlarge by up to 70%. However, the most striking anatomical change in the urinary tract during pregnancy is dilatation of the pelvicalyceal system and the ureters (Fig. 11.1). Generally, the right side is affected more than the left. These changes develop in the first trimester and progress such that by the third trimester, more than 90% of women will have dilated ureters and pelvicalyceal systems. The changes persist for up to 3 months post-partum. Hence images of the kidneys in the first 3 months post-partum should be interpreted with caution.

In general, these anatomical changes are completely asymptomatic. However, a small number of women will develop transient loin pain, which may sometimes be severe. However, the urine is sterile and few or no red blood cells are observed. Treatment should be expectant as symptoms will generally resolve post-partum.

The cause of the dilated urinary tract is debated. Some obstruction of the urinary drainage system occurs at the pelvic brim, where the enlarged uterus may cause partial ureteric compression. Engorged vessels, for example, a dilated ovarian venous plexus, uterine veins, or iliac vessels, may also contribute to ureteric obstruction. Hormonal changes, including increases in oestrogen, progesterone, prostaglandins, and relaxin, may also decrease smooth muscle contractility in the urinary tract and promote dilatation. The dilatation of the urinary tract in pregnancy contributes to the increased incidence of asymptomatic bacteriuria and pyelonephritis in pregnant women because of impaired urine drainage and the resultant urinary stasis.

Case 11.1 — **Urinary tract infection in pregnancy: 1**

Anne Farrell is a 26-year-old woman who presents in her first pregnancy at 8 weeks gestation for her first antenatal review. She has previously been well, apart from a history of recurrent urinary infection in her late teenage years. These had occurred at the time she began to be sexually active. They were generally treated with short courses of antibiotics. She had no episodes of upper urinary tract infection. No radiological investigations of her urinary tract had been performed. However, her renal function was determined to be normal. Her only recent symptom has been some urinary frequency which she ascribed to early pregnancy, but she has not experienced dysuria. On examination in the clinic, her blood pressure is 95/60 mmHg, pulse rate 96/min, and urinalysis demonstrates blood, nitrites, and leucocytes. The examination is otherwise normal. A midstream urine (MSU) examination is reported to show 10–100 × 10^6/L erythrocytes and 100 × 10^6/L leucocytes, with a bacterial count of 10^8/L and a pure growth of *Escherichia coli* sensitive to both ampicillin and cephalosporins. Having found an asymptomatic urinary infection in this pregnant patient, we should consider the normal anatomical changes that occur in the renal system during pregnancy that may predispose to complications such as urinary tract infection.

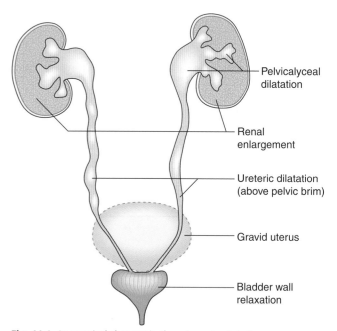

Fig. 11.1 Anatomical changes in the urinary tract during pregnancy.

Pelvicalyceal dilatation

Renal enlargement

Ureteric dilatation (above pelvic brim)

Gravid uterus

Bladder wall relaxation

Case 11.1 — Urinary tract infection in pregnancy: 2

Initial treatment

Anne is treated for 1 week with cephalexin 500 mg QID. One week later, her MSU revealed a further *E. coli* infection, still sensitive to cephalosporins. She remains asymptomatic and is concerned about the possible effects of both infection and antibiotics on the pregnancy and her unborn child.

This raises the questions:

1. What are the risks of untreated asymptomatic bacteriuria in pregnancy?
2. How should recurrent infection in pregnancy be treated?
3. What are the preferred antibiotics to use in pregnancy?

Urinary tract infection in pregnancy

Pregnant women are at greater risk of urinary tract infection than usual because of physiological changes that occur during this state. As the uterus enlarges, pressure on the bladder can cause urinary retention and hormonal changes relax the ureters and cause accumulation of urine in the bladder. Urinary infection has been associated with several maternal and foetal complications, including pre-term delivery, increased caesarean section rates, pre-eclampsia, and intrauterine growth retardation. Pregnant women with asymptomatic bacteriuria or cystitis are also more likely to progress onto the more dangerous urinary complication of pyelonephritis. Hence, detection and treatment of urinary infection in pregnancy is mandatory and this is one of the few situations where asymptomatic bacteriuria should be treated.

The collection of a clean sample of midstream urine (MSU) can be problematic in pregnancy. Furthermore, increased excretion of leucocytes can occur in pregnancy because of contamination of the urine by physiological vaginal discharge. Hence pyuria may be present without necessarily signifying infection.

Between 2% and 10% of women have asymptomatic bacteriuria, the incidence being similar in the pregnant and non-pregnant population. During pregnancy, 40% of untreated patients with asymptomatic bacteriuria will develop an acute symptomatic infection. Hence treatment is recommended. The choice of drug is determined by the sensitivity of the organism. Cephalosporins or ampicillin/amoxicillin are generally used as first-line agents. A single course of antibiotics is recommended with a follow-up urine culture 1 week later and then at 4 weekly intervals throughout the pregnancy. Up to 25% of patients will relapse during the pregnancy, and of these, less than 5% will have their infection cleared by a further course of therapy. If not cleared by a second course of antibiotics, in general, patients should be treated with a prophylactic nightly dose of antibiotic, either amoxycillin or a cephalosporin, for the duration of the pregnancy.

Acute cystitis occurs in approximately 2% of pregnancies. Symptoms are similar to those occurring in non-pregnant women, but as pregnancy itself can also be associated with frequency, the symptoms can be misinterpreted. Treatment and follow-up are the same as for asymptomatic bacteriuria.

Acute pyelonephritis is more likely to follow from lower urinary tract infection in pregnant than non-pregnant women because of the anatomical changes observed in the urinary tract in pregnancy. Symptoms are identical to those observed in non-pregnant patients. Treatment is dictated by the severity of the illness and may include rehydration and parenteral antibiotics – guided by sensitivities and antibiotics suitable for pregnancy. Renal imaging is often difficult to interpret because of the normal anatomical changes in pregnancy and thus should generally be deferred until at least 3 months post-partum in patients with recurrent infection or pyelonephritis.

In choosing an antibiotic for use during pregnancy, sulphonamides should be avoided, particularly in the last four weeks of pregnancy, because of the increased risk of newborn hyperbilirubinemia and kernicterus. Nitrofurantoin should also be avoided in the latter stages of pregnancy as it may be associated with neonatal haemolysis and birth defects. Trimethoprim–sulphonamide combinations and tetracyclines should not be used throughout the pregnancy because of possible teratogenicity and the effects on teeth and bones, respectively. There have been few studies using quinolones in pregnancy, but as these drugs have been documented to cause arthropathy in immature animals of various species, they should be avoided in pregnancy.

Case 11.1 — Urinary tract infection in pregnancy: 3

Further treatment and outcome

Anne was treated for 10 days on this occasion with ampicillin 500 mg QID. However, 1 week later her MSU again demonstrated a pure growth of *E. coli*. Hence, following a further 10 days course of treatment, this time with cephalexin 500 mg QID, she was asked to take 500 mg cephalexin nocte as a prophylactic measure for the remainder of her pregnancy. Monthly MSUs did not show any recurrence, and she delivered at term without complication. At review 3 months post-partum, she had no evidence of urinary tract infection, and a renal ultrasound was normal.

Renal physiology changes in pregnancy

Changes in fluid volume during pregnancy

Approximately 10 to 14 kg of weight gain occurs in normal pregnancy, which is primarily because of an increase of 7 to 9 L of water, of which 6 to 7 L is estimated to be extravascular and 2 L intravascular. Plasma volume expansion starts

Box 11.1 Factors influencing Na excretion during pregnancy

Decreased Na excretion	Increased Na excretion
Increased tubular Na reabsorption (via glomerulotubular balance)	Increase in GFR
	Hormones promoting Na loss:
Increased Na-retaining hormones:	Progesterone
Aldosterone	Vasopressin
Deoxycorticosteroid	Oxytocin
Oestrogens	Prostaglandins
Prolactin	Natriuretic hormone
Renin/angiotensin	Melanocyte stimulating hormone
Human placental lactogen	
Physical factors:	Physical factors:
Increase in ureteric pressure	Decreased serum albumin
Ureteroplacental shunt	Decrease in renal vascular resistance
Exaggerated influence of posture	

The net effect of these changes is considerable net retention of Na.

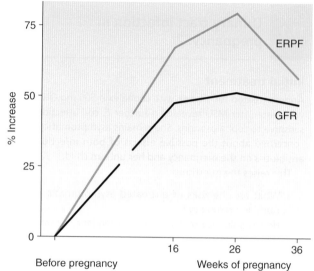

Fig. 11.2 Changes in effective renal plasma flow and glomerular filtration rate (GFR) during pregnancy.

in the first trimester, peaks at 32 weeks and continues till term. Hence hypervolaemia is present and results in an enhanced cardiac output of about 30% to 40% above pre-pregnant levels, which supports placental perfusion. The interstitial fluid volume also increases because of decreased oncotic pressure, consequent on a low serum albumin concentration secondary to dilution. Approximately 950 mmoL of Na are retained in normal pregnancy because of the net effect of the many haemodynamic, hormonal, and physical changes that occur. These are summarised in Box 11.1.

Changes in renal plasma flow and glomerular filtration rate

In the normal pregnant woman, the effective renal plasma flow increases by up to 80% from conception to mid-pregnancy and then falls in the third trimester to 50% to 60% above baseline (Fig. 11.2). The glomerular filtration rate is increased by about 50% at the end of the first trimester and can be maintained at that level until one month post-partum. Therefore, the increased glomerular filtration rate (GFR), plasma urea and creatinine fall. Thus, a plasma creatinine regarded as 'normal' in a non-pregnant individual may signify kidney impairment in a pregnant person. The calculation of GFR by the MDRD or CKD-EPI formulae (see Chapter 5) has been reported to significantly underestimate GFR in pregnancy and should not be used to monitor kidney function.

Osmoregulation in pregnancy

Very early in pregnancy, plasma osmolality decreases to about 10 mosm/kg below the non-pregnant norm, an

occurrence thought to be related to vasodilation, arterial underfilling, and subsequent antidiuretic hormone (ADH; vasopressin) release. In fact, there is a resetting of the osmostat in pregnancy, with the osmotic thresholds for ADH release and thirst decreasing during the initial weeks of pregnancy. However, plasma ADH concentrations are usually kept normal in pregnancy because of increased metabolism. The placenta produces vasopressinase, which is capable of inactivating circulating ADH and can directly metabolise ADH *in situ*. Hence the placenta is thought to be responsible for at least one-third of ADH metabolism in pregnancy. The result of these changes is that mild hyponatraemia in pregnancy is common and occasionally made more severe by other non-osmotic ADH stimuli such as nausea and pain.

Renal tubular function in pregnancy

Some changes in plasma and urine biochemistry during pregnancy are summarised in Table 11.1.

Plasma uric acid concentrations decrease by 25% to 35% during early pregnancy because of an increase in GFR and a decrease in proximal tubular reabsorption. As pregnancy progresses, excretion progressively falls, and hence plasma uric acid levels gradually increase towards normal non-pregnant levels. In pregnancies complicated by pre-eclampsia (see below), plasma uric acid concentration may be elevated because of enhanced renal reabsorption of uric acid, although this is not used as a diagnostic marker. Its presence is, however, considered to be a risk factor for adverse maternal and foetal outcomes.

Glucose excretion is commonly increased in normal pregnancy, with excretory rates normalising to zero within a week of delivery. Hence the glycosuria observed in a proportion of pregnant women does not in itself suggest a diagnosis of diabetes mellitus. Aminoaciduria similarly may be observed in pregnancy. Up to 2 g of amino

Table 11.1 Changes in blood and urine biochemistry during normal pregnancy

Blood	Effect of pregnancy
Plasma uric acid	↓
Plasma sodium	↓
Plasma potassium	N to ↓
Plasma bicarbonate	↓
Serum creatinine	↓
Arterial pCO_2	↓
Arterial pH	↑
Urine	
Glucose excretion	↑
Amino acid excretion	↑
Potassium excretion	↓
Calcium excretion	↑
Magnesium excretion	↑
Citrate excretion	↑

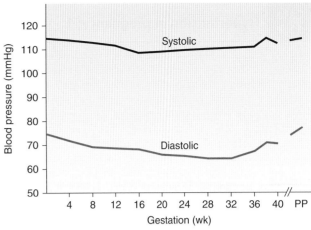

Fig. 11.3 Changes in blood pressure during normal pregnancy. PP, post-partum.

acid may be excreted daily, which generally has few clinical consequences. It is considered that the increased GFR increases the filtered load of glucose and amino acids, and the proximal tubules do not have the capacity to increase their reabsorptive rates to match.

Acid-base regulation is altered in pregnancy. The blood concentration of hydrogen ions decreases by 2 to 4 mmol/L in early pregnancy and this change is sustained until delivery. Blood concentrations of bicarbonate similarly fall by about 4 mmol/L such that a normal plasma bicarbonate level in pregnancy is between 18 and 22 mmol/L. Thus the average arterial pH in pregnancy is 7.44 compared to 7.40 in the non-pregnant individual. The mild alkalosis is primarily respiratory in origin as progesterone induces an increase in respiratory rate, which reduces the arterial pCO_2 from an average value of 40 mmHg to approximately 32 mmHg during pregnancy.

The regulation of potassium excretion by the kidney is significantly altered in pregnancy. It would be expected that the high levels of aldosterone and other mineralocorticoids during pregnancy, and lower blood concentrations of hydrogen, would lead to increased renal excretion of potassium. However, this is not observed, and indeed there is net retention of potassium in pregnancy, although plasma potassium concentration generally remains normal or slightly decreased. The conservation of potassium has been ascribed to progesterone.

A net increase in urinary calcium excretion occurs in pregnancy, again attributed to the increase in filtered load of calcium which is not matched by a parallel increase in tubular calcium reabsorption. However, no increase in renal stone formation is seen in pregnancy because of parallel increases in urine flow rate and urinary excretion of citrate and magnesium (known

inhibitors of stone formation) and acidic glycoproteins, including Tamm-Horsfall protein, which inhibit calcium oxalate deposition.

There is an increase in the amount of protein in the urine, mostly consisting of Tamm-Horsfall proteins, with a small amount of albumin and other circulating proteins. This relates to the rise in GFR, although other glomerular changes may also occur. Abnormal proteinuria in pregnant women is defined as protein levels of greater than 300 mg/24 h (equivalent to a urinary protein to creatinine ratio of 30 mg/mmol), which is twice the normal limit in non-pregnant women

Blood pressure and pregnancy

Blood pressure decreases early in normal pregnancy, with diastolic values typically 5 to 10 mmHg below pre-pregnancy values by the second trimester (Fig. 11.3). In the third trimester, blood pressure generally returns towards normal, signifying a return of normal vasomotor tone. Since cardiac output increases, the drop in blood pressure reflects a marked decrease in peripheral vascular resistance, due in part to vasodilation in the uteroplacental bed. However, vasodilation also occurs in other organ systems such as the kidney and skin. Vasodilation occurs despite increases in systemic levels of renin and angiotensin II, signifying a loss of responsiveness to the pressor effects of angiotensin II. Conversely, there is a normal pressor response to catecholamines in pregnancy. Increased production of prostaglandins (particularly by the pregnant uterus) and nitric oxide are considered to mediate the decrease in maternal vascular resistance observed in pregnancy (see Case 11.2: 1).

Hypertension in pregnancy

Hypertension in pregnancy is diagnosed when the systolic blood pressure (SBP) is >140 mmHg and/or diastolic

Case 11.2 Hypertension in pregnancy: 1

Denise Gill, a 36-year-old primigravid schoolteacher, presented for her first antenatal visit at 9 weeks gestation. An ultrasound done by her GP the previous week demonstrated a dizygotic twin pregnancy. She had been well in the past but, when questioned, admitted that on being checked for prior prescriptions for the oral contraceptive pill, her blood pressure was generally 'on the high side'. However, no treatment had been suggested. Her younger sister had recently developed pre-eclampsia in her first pregnancy, necessitating delivery at 36 weeks. Her mother had no history of pregnancy-related illness, but her grandmother had 'toxaemia' requiring bed rest for 6 weeks prior to the birth of her mother. She was a non-smoker, drank little alcohol, had recently commenced 'pregnancy' vitamins, but otherwise took no regular medications.

On examination, her body mass index was 30 kg/m^2. Her blood pressure was 140/90 mmHg on repeated measurements, using a large cuff in both right and left arms. Examination of the optic fundi revealed minor arteriovenous nipping but no other abnormalities. Urinalysis was negative.

Denise was provided with a sphygmomanometer and instructed how to measure her blood pressure at home and return in one month with records of twice-daily BP measurements. Baseline 'pregnancy' blood tests (full blood count, blood group, rubella, hepatitis, syphilis, and HIV serology) and an MSU had already been taken by her GP and were all normal. Additional blood tests were requested to assess her renal function, liver function and uric acid.

Denise was concerned about the implications of having 'borderline' hypertension in pregnancy, the potential risks to her and her unborn baby, and whether lifestyle modifications would help control her hypertension.

Box 11.2 Classification of hypertension in pregnancy (International Society for the Study of Hypertension in Pregnancy).

- De-novo hypertension
  - Gestational hypertension
  - Pre-eclampsia
- Chronic hypertension
  - Essential hypertension
  - Secondary hypertension
- Pre-eclampsia superimposed on chronic hypertension
- White coat hypertension
- Masked hypertension

Pre-eclampsia

Pre-eclampsia is generally detected initially because of hypertension and proteinuria. However, it is a multisystem disorder in the mother with features shown in Fig. 11.4. Pre-eclampsia additionally has significant foetal manifestations and consequences, manifesting as intra-uterine growth retardation and rarely foetal death. A serious deterioration in the mother's condition is marked by the occurrence of a seizure, often accompanied by a decrease in the level of consciousness. This turn of events is termed eclampsia.

Interesting facts

Eclampsia comes from the Greek word eklampsis, meaning a sudden flashing. It was introduced when it was believed that seizures in pregnancy occurred without any pre-existing disorder and hence came 'like a flash of lightning'. It is now known that eclampsia generally follows some degree of preceding pre-eclampsia, although the duration may be brief. Both pre-eclampsia and eclampsia used to be considered forms of 'toxaemia' of pregnancy.

The criteria for the diagnosis of pre-eclampsia are shown in Box 11.3. Note that oedema is not one of the diagnostic criteria of pre-eclampsia as it is often seen in otherwise normal pregnancy. Similarly, an elevation in plasma uric acid is not included in the criteria but remains a useful marker.

Pre-eclampsia may rarely occur prior to 20 weeks gestation in patients with hydatidiform mole, multiple pregnancy, foetal triploidy, prothrombotic disorders, or renal disease. Other disorders may present with some of the features observed in pre-eclampsia: these include acute fatty liver of pregnancy, HELLP syndrome (haemolysis, elevated liver enzymes, low platelet count), anti-phospholipid antibody syndrome, thrombotic thrombocytopaenia purpura, and haemolytic uraemic syndrome. The differential diagnosis is

BP is >90 mmHg. The consistency of the readings should be documented with several measurements over several hours. Blood pressure is measured in the seated position with the feet supported, using an appropriately sized cuff. Approximately 10% of primigravidae will develop gestational hypertension (see below), and 7% will develop pre-eclampsia. A small proportion of women will manifest signs and symptoms of hypertension or pre-eclampsia predominantly in the immediate post-partum period.

The various forms of hypertension in pregnancy are shown in Box 11.2.

Gestational hypertension

Gestational hypertension is hypertension arising in pregnancy after 20 weeks gestation without any other features of pre-eclampsia, that resolves post partum.

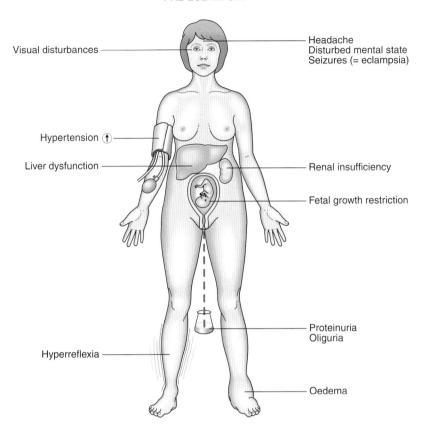

PRE-ECLAMPSIA

Visual disturbances

Headache
Disturbed mental state
Seizures (= eclampsia)

Hypertension ⊕

Liver dysfunction

Renal insufficiency

Fetal growth restriction

Proteinuria
Oliguria

Hyperreflexia

Oedema

Fig. 11.4 Clinical features of pre-eclampsia.

Box 11.3 Definition of pre-eclampsia

Hypertension arising after 20 weeks gestation plus the new onset of at least one of the following:

- Proteinuria (spot urine protein to creatinine ratio of >30 mg/mmol)
- Renal insufficiency (plasma creatinine greater than 90 μmol/L or oliguria)
- Liver disease (defined as raised transaminases)
- Neurological signs (hyperreflexia with clonus; headaches with hyperreflexia and/or visual disturbances; altered mental state)[1]
- Haematological disturbances (low platelet count, disseminated intravascular coagulation, haemolysis)
- Uteroplacental dysfunction (such as foetal growth restriction, abnormal umbilical artery doppler analysis, or stillbirth)

[1]The occurrence of seizures defines the onset of eclampsia.

Box 11.4 Risk factors for the development of pre-eclampsia

- Primigravida
- Multigravida pregnant by a different partner
- Maternal age greater than 40 years
- Prior pre-eclampsia in a pregnancy by the same partner
- Family history of pre-eclampsia
- Multiple pregnancy
- Obesity
- Renal disease
- Essential hypertension
- Diabetes
- Autoimmune disease, particularly systemic lupus erythematosus, and the anti-phospholipid syndrome
- Thrombophilia
- Severe alloimmunisation

made based on the constellation of clinical and laboratory findings.

Factors marking pregnant women at increased risk of pre-eclampsia are listed in Box 11.4. However, it should be noted that severe pre-eclampsia can occur, particularly in the primigravid individual, with no other risk factors. Current views on the cause and pathogenesis of pre-eclampsia consider that the condition arises because

of a combination of genetic and environmental factors resulting in abnormal placentation. Although there is a clear familial element in the development of the disease, the mode of inheritance remains elusive. The incidence of pre-eclampsia is increased in women who live at high altitudes and in areas of low socioeconomic status, suggesting that as yet undefined environmental factors may also influence pre-eclampsia development.

Pathologically, the maternal spiral arteries supplying blood to the fetoplacental unit fail to develop into sac-like flaccid vessels, retaining a muscular arteriole phenotype leading to decreased placental perfusion and placental ischaemia.

It is now clear that ischaemic placentas produce antiangiogenic factors, such as a soluble receptor for vascular endothelial growth factor and a placental growth factor called sFlt-1, which may be the link between disordered implantation and maternal symptoms of pre-eclampsia. Most of the maternal features of the condition (see Fig. 11.4) are associated with vascular endothelial dysfunction and/or vasoconstriction in the various organ systems affected by the disease process, although much remains to be discovered of the precise mechanisms involved.

The HELLP syndrome (haemolysis, elevated liver enzymes, low platelets) is a severe manifestation of pre-eclampsia.

Chronic hypertension

Essential hypertension is defined as high blood pressure in those women already on antihypertensive drugs, or when systolic BP >140 mmHg and/or diastolic BP >90 mmHg pre-conception or in the first half of pregnancy with no underlying cause. Secondary hypertension is defined as in the non-pregnant population, that is hypertension associated with an underlying condition, particularly renal parenchymal, renovascular, or endocrine disorders.

White coat hypertension, that is hypertension in the presence of a clinician but not observed in ambulatory or home BP assessments, is associated with an increased risk of pre-eclampsia.

Masked hypertension, that is hypertension present on home BP assessment but normal in the clinic, is a form of chronic hypertension usually only found when a patient has unexplained abnormalities consistent with target organ damage from hypertension but no apparent hypertension. Its prevalence and significance in pregnancy are unclear, and routine assessment for this condition is not recommended unless other target organ manifestations such as chronic kidney disease (CKD) are present.

Pre-eclampsia superimposed on chronic hypertension

The presence of chronic hypertension is a risk factor for the development of pre-eclampsia. In patients with chronic hypertension, the development of proteinuria, increasing blood pressure, right upper quadrant pain signifying liver involvement, neurological symptoms, or intrauterine growth restriction (IUGR) should be considered highly suggestive of superimposed pre-eclampsia.

Case 11.2 — Hypertension in pregnancy: 2

Initial treatment

Denise returned at 12 weeks gestation and remained feeling well. Her blood pressure readings had consistently been between 120/70 mmHg and 140/90 mmHg. Her plasma creatinine was 60 µmol/L, liver function tests normal, and her plasma uric acid was 0.20 mmol/L. Her risk factors for developing pre-eclampsia complicating chronic hypertension were explained, i.e. twin pregnancy, obesity, pre-existing hypertension, and her positive family history. She was advised to return to the clinic every 4 weeks but to continue monitoring her blood pressure at home and advise if it was increasing to over 140/90 mmHg.

At 28 weeks gestation, she presented with worsening hypertension up to 150/100 mmHg but no proteinuria. She was monitored in a day stay obstetric unit. Foetal movements and heart sounds were present, and foetal growth was assessed as normal. Repeat blood tests were taken, including an oral glucose tolerance test, and were found to be normal. Her plasma uric acid was 0.36 mmol/L, but other blood test results were normal. She was commenced on treatment with labetalol 100 mg bd and asked to return for review in 1 week.

Denise is now concerned that she has developed pre-eclampsia and asks about the effect of medication on the foetus, the likelihood of premature delivery and whether she should stop work as it has been particularly stressful of late.

Management of hypertension in pregnancy

The management of hypertension in pregnancy needs to take into account both maternal and foetal factors. It should be noted that controlling the blood pressure does not in itself cure pre-eclampsia, but it is indicated to avoid maternal cerebrovascular and cardiovascular complications.

Patients with gestational or chronic hypertension can usually be managed in the outpatient setting.

Antihypertensive therapy is generally instituted to reduce the risk of maternal pulmonary oedema, stroke, and placental abruption. For those reasons, severe hypertension (SBP >160 mmHg and/or DBP >110) should always be treated and rapid-acting antihypertensive medication is required. Agents commonly used are oral nifedipine, IV hydralazine, or IV labetalol. In general, SBP should be gradually lowered to ensure maternal safety and protect foetal circulation. Continuous cardiotocography (CTG) monitoring of the foetal circulation should be undertaken when parenteral agents are used to lower critically elevated blood pressure in this setting.

Managing mild to moderate hypertension should follow similar principles. There is some controversy about BP readings at which to commence therapy and BP targets, but decisions should be made that prevent the morbidity of hypertension whilst ensuring adequate foetal circulation. Obstetric units have individualised protocols for the use of oral antihypertensive agents during pregnancy, and in general, shorter-acting, 'older' antihypertensive agents are used. These include the beta-blocker labetalol, centrally-acting agents like alpha-methyldopa, and others such as hydralazine, nifedipine, verapamil, and prazosin. Longer-acting beta-blockers, such as atenolol, are not recommended as they have been shown to be associated with impaired foetal growth, hypoglycaemia, and bradycardia. Angiotensin-converting enzyme inhibitors and angiotensin receptor blockers should not be prescribed during pregnancy since their use, particularly during the third trimester, has been linked with the development of foetal growth retardation, oligohydramnios, neonatal renal failure, and death. Antihypertensives utilised in pregnancy are also considered safe when breastfeeding. Hypertension in pregnancy does not generally preclude the opportunity to breastfeed.

Once a diagnosis of pre-eclampsia is made, the stage of gestation, the degree of maternal organ dysfunction, and foetal well-being all need to be considered in determining subsequent management. If eclampsia has developed, the seizure should be terminated with the use of IV magnesium which also provides prophylaxis against further convulsions, the blood pressure controlled, and immediate delivery arranged. In impending eclampsia, when premonitory neurological signs are present, the use of IV magnesium sulphate can be considered.

In general, if either the mother or foetus is at risk of significant complications as a consequence of hypertensive disease in pregnancy, delivery should be considered, particularly when the foetus is mature. General indications for delivery in this context are given in Box 11.5 (Also see Case 11.2: 3).

Follow-up of patients with hypertension in pregnancy

In patients with severe pre-eclampsia, maternal complications may develop for up to 5 days post-partum. Hence vigilance in monitoring is required. As blood pressure settles, antihypertensives may be withdrawn. Immediately after delivery, there may be a reduction in blood pressure because of blood loss and the use of epidural anaesthesia, but hypertension may later reappear. Review is undertaken 3 months post-partum to ensure that blood pressure has settled and urinalysis is normal, and if laboratory tests have not normalised post-delivery, these should be reassessed. Investigations for an underlying thrombophilia state, renal disease or autoimmune disease are not routinely undertaken but should be per-

Box 11.5 General indications for delivery in hypertensive disorders of pregnancy

- Pre-eclampsia occurring at term
- Accelerated hypertension uncontrollable on treatment
- Deteriorating renal or liver function
- Progressive thrombocytopenia
- Neurological complications suggesting imminent eclampsia
- Placental abruption
- Foetal compromise

Case 11.2 Hypertension in pregnancy: 3

Further treatment and outcome

Denise was followed up regularly, her labetalol was increased to maximal doses, and hydralazine was added to her treatment over the next 8 weeks. At 36 weeks gestation, she presented complaining of headache and swollen ankles. The examination showed her BP to be 170/110 mmHg. She had moderate oedema, proteinuria and two beats of ankle clonus. A CTG of both foetuses showed a normal pattern.

She was given 5 mg hydralazine intravenously, which brought her blood pressure down to 160/100 mmHg, but over the next 90 min, it again increased to 175/105 mmHg. Her blood tests showed a platelet count of 162×10^9/L (previously 250×10^9/L), uric acid 0.46 mmol/L, AST 70 IU/L, with other blood tests normal. Her urine protein to creatinine ratio was 424 mg/mmol. Caesarean section was arranged as planned, as one twin had consistently been in a breech position. Epidural anaesthesia resulted in a fall in blood pressure to 130/80 mmHg, and an uneventful caesarean delivery occurred. Following delivery, her blood pressure remained well controlled on oral medication, and her drug treatment was progressively weaned. She was advised to follow-up her blood pressure with her general practitioner and return for a review in 3 months.

She was concerned about her ability to breastfeed and, although not an immediate priority, about her risks in a future pregnancy.

formed in women with recurrent or early and severe pre-eclampsia. Women with pre-eclampsia are at high risk of future cardiovascular disease, and efforts should be made in the follow-up of these women to identify and address cardiovascular risk factors through lifestyle and pharmacological therapy.

Recurrence in subsequent pregnancies occurs in up to a quarter of patients with pre-eclampsia, particularly if it develops early in the pregnancy. Low dose aspirin has been demonstrated to reduce the incidence of pre-eclampsia and is indicated in those women with a high baseline risk, such as those with chronic hypertension, CKD, or previous pre-eclampsia. In addition, if a thrombophilia trait is identified, anticoagulation with heparin or low molecular weight heparin throughout the pregnancy may be recommended.

Recurrent gestational hypertension generally indicates the future development of chronic hypertension. Recent studies have suggested that patients with a history of pre-eclampsia are more likely to develop insulin resistance, impaired vascular compliance, and renal disease. However, whether these comorbidities are independent of the factors that predispose to pre-eclampsia is yet to be determined (see Case 11.2: 4).

Pregnancy in patients with pre-existing kidney disease

Fertility progressively declines in patients with CKD. If conception occurs, maternal and foetal outcomes can be compromised, particularly in the presence of co-existent hypertension, greater than 1 g proteinuria/day or if the pre-conceptual plasma creatinine is greater than normal (90 µmol/L). In these circumstances, there is an increased risk of severe pre-eclampsia, foetal growth restriction, premature delivery, and perinatal mortality.

CKD in the population of childbearing age is likely to be because of reflux nephropathy, polycystic kidney disease, diabetic nephropathy, lupus nephritis or IgA nephropathy. In those with reflux nephropathy, assessment for asymptomatic bacteriuria should occur at least on a monthly basis; those with diabetes need strict glycaemic control, and in those with a history of lupus nephritis, the disease should preferably be quiescent for 6 months prior to conception.

Most women with CKD who become pregnant have mild disease, and pregnancy usually does not affect the renal prognosis. In patients with more significant kidney impairment (i.e. CKD stages 3–5), pregnancy may lead to an accelerated decline in kidney function, which will persist in about half of patients post-pregnancy. The risk of reduced renal function is lessened with strict blood pressure control.

Conception in patients on dialysis is rare but possible. Around 80% of dialysis associated pregnancies are pre-term, and pre-eclampsia can be difficult to diagnose. Successful pregnancies are more likely with frequent dialysis and more intensive anaemia management than in non-pregnant patients.

Pregnancy following transplantation occurs relatively frequently. The optimal timing for pregnancy

Case 11.2	Hypertension in pregnancy: 4 follow-up

Denise returned 14 weeks post-partum, breastfeeding, feeling well, and enjoying her twins. Her blood pressure was 140/90 mmHg. Her blood tests had returned to normal, and she had no proteinuria. Given the early gestation of her presentation, the likelihood that she had chronic hypertension was explained; she was advised to lose weight, increase her exercise pattern and have regular checks of her blood pressure. Simple investigations were performed to exclude a secondary cause of hypertension.

following transplantation is 18 to 24 months post-transplant when the immunosuppressive regimen is stable, assuming good kidney function. Pregnancy outcomes are generally good for patients with good graft function and no hypertension or proteinuria. Preferred immunosuppressive regimens in pregnant patients include steroids, azathioprine, cyclosporine, and tacrolimus. Mycophenolate mofetil is not advised in pregnancy.

Summary

1. Several important anatomical and physiological changes occur in the kidneys during pregnancy.
2. Asymptomatic bacteriuria is associated with several adverse foetal and maternal outcomes during pregnancy and should be treated.
3. Cystitis and pyelonephritis are more common in pregnant women and need to be treated with antibiotics appropriate for pregnancy.
4. There are several chronic and de-novo disorders of hypertension that can occur in pregnancy.
5. Pre-eclampsia is a common and serious condition that can affect both foetal and maternal outcomes.
6. Women who have had a hypertensive disorder of pregnancy should be followed up post-partum to ensure that abnormal parameters have resolved and to discuss future pregnancy and cardiovascular risk.
7. Women with CKD should be counselled on their risks of pregnancy prior to conception.
8. The risk of CKD in pregnancy depends on the degree of renal dysfunction, degree of proteinuria, presence of hypertension and cause of CKD.

Self-assessment case study

Betty is a 22-year-old woman who has a history of pre-eclampsia that occurred at 34 weeks in her first pregnancy. She presented with proteinuria, hypertension that required management with two agents and an ultrasound suggesting IUGR. She had a caesarean section at 35 + 2 weeks when a CTG trace suggested foetal distress and delivered a 1.8 kg baby girl.

She has returned to see you 2 years later – her blood and urine tests have returned to normal, and thrombophilia tests are normal. She asks you about the risks of having another pregnancy and what can be done to reduce the chance of developing pre-eclampsia again.

Q1. You can advise her that:

A. She will not develop pre-eclampsia again as this only occurs in first pregnancies

B. She will definitely develop pre-eclampsia again as she had it in her first pregnancy

C. If she falls pregnant with a different partner, her risk of pre-eclampsia is the same compared to the same partner.

D. She has an increased risk, compared to the general pregnant population, of developing pre-eclampsia again

Q2. To reduce her risk of recurrent pre-eclampsia, you advise her that there is evidence to support:

A. Low dose aspirin at night from early pregnancy

B. Therapeutic anticoagulation from early pregnancy

C. High dose fish oil from early pregnancy

D. Vitamin E prior to conception

Self-assessment case study answers

A1. Pre-eclampsia is more common in initial pregnancies but can also occur in subsequent pregnancies, although this is not universal for women who have had pre-eclampsia in their first pregnancy. A change of partner can alter the risk of developing pre-eclampsia in subsequent pregnancies but does not eradicate the risk. Women who have had pre-eclampsia in one pregnancy have a small chance of developing pre-eclampsia in subsequent pregnancies.

A2. Low dose aspirin at night has been demonstrated in multiple trials and meta-analyses to reduce the incidence of pre-eclampsia; anticoagulation is beneficial for women with anti-phospholipid disease; fish oil and vitamin E have been shown not to be of benefit in these circumstances.

URINARY TRACT OBSTRUCTION AND STONES

12

Chapter objectives

After studying this chapter, you should be able to:

1. Recognise the principal causes of loin pain.

2. Recognise the principal causes of haematuria.

3. Understand the pathophysiology of urinary tract obstruction.

4. Discuss the complications of urinary tract obstruction.

5. Discuss the investigation and principles of treatment of urinary tract obstruction.

6. Describe some common types of urinary tract stones and outline their forms of presentation and management.

Introduction

Loin (also termed flank) pain may arise because of a pathologic condition in the nerves radiating from the spinal cord, vertebral column, paraspinal and lumbar muscles, and retroperitoneal organs such as kidneys, abdominal aorta, and pancreas. The simultaneous presence of haematuria strongly suggests that the loin pain is caused by a pathologic condition in the kidneys or ureters. If loin pain and/or haematuria are present, then it is necessary to consider whether urinary tract obstruction is also present. The following case history describes a patient with a renal calculus (stone) causing loin pain, haematuria, and urinary obstruction. See Case 12.1: 1.

Differential diagnosis of loin pain and haematuria

Any back or retroperitoneal structure may give rise to back pain (Box 12.1). Pain arising from the spasm of a tubular or hollow organ, such as the ureter, is referred to as colic. The severity and radiation of this patient's pain were typical of renal colic, although pain of a similar distribution could occur because of compression or involvement of a nerve root. The extension of the pain into his right groin and inner right thigh is explained by the movement of the pathologic condition down the ureter (Fig. 12.1). Kidney pain arises because of rapid stretching or inflammation of the kidney capsule, whereas pain arising from the renal pelvis or ureter is caused by distension and excessive peristaltic contractions.

Macroscopic (or frank) haematuria may arise from lesions anywhere within the urinary system, including the kidney itself, the renal pelvis, ureter, bladder, and urethra (see Chapter 13). As few as 5×10^6 red cells per millilitre (1 μL of blood per millilitre of urine) can be detected visually as red-coloured urine.

Macroscopic haematuria needs to be distinguished from the following:

1. Red discolouration of urine caused by certain dyes, occasional drugs (e.g. rifampicin) and foods (e.g. beetroot).
2. The presence of haem pigment in the case of intravascular haemolysis (haemoglobin from red blood cell lysis) or rhabdomyolysis (myoglobin from muscle breakdown).
3. Bleeding outside the urinary tract (e.g. perineum or vagina).

The relationship of the blood to urine helps to distinguish bleeding involving the bladder or above (uniform discolouration of urine) from that arising from the urethra (blood separate or mixed with urine).

Box 12.1 Principal sites of the pathologic conditions that lead to loin pain

- Spinal nerve roots
- Vertebral column
- Paraspinal and lumbar muscles
- Kidneys
- Renal pelvis/ureters
- Abdominal aorta
- Pancreas

Case 12.1 Urinary tract obstruction and stones: 1

Loin pain and haematuria

Kevin Whiteside is a 63-year-old man who presented to the Casualty department of his local hospital with a 6-h history of right-sided pain and smoky (reddish-grey) urine. The loin pain was situated at the level of the first three lumbar vertebrae and radiated around the right side of his abdomen. After several hours it radiated further into his right testis and the upper medial aspect of his right thigh. The pain was constant and very severe. His right kidney was ballotable and very tender. See Clinical Skills in Chapter 13 for how to ballot kidneys. He was afebrile, sweating, and pale. His blood pressure and the remainder of his physical examination were normal. Urinalysis was strongly positive for blood.

The main features in this patient's history were the presence of severe loin pain and macroscopic haematuria. The haematuria suggested strongly that the pain originated in the urinary tract rather than other potential sites.

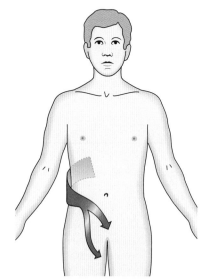

Fig. 12.1 Site of renal colic. Renal colic typically radiates from the loin around to the lower quadrant of the abdomen and the upper medial thigh on the same side.

Table 12.1 Differential diagnosis of red urine

	With loin pain	Uniform discolouration of urine	Haem pigment on dipstick	Red blood cells in urine	Casts and protein in urine	Predominantly dysmorphic red blood cells
Foods and dyes (e.g. beetroot)	–	+	–	–	–	–
Drugs (e.g. rifampicin)	–	+	–	–	–	–
Pigmenturia (haemolysis or rhabdomyolysis)	–	+	+	–	–	–
Non-urological bleeding	–	–	+	+	–	–
Urethral bleeding	–	–	+	+	–	–
Renal, ureteric, or bladder tumours	–*	+	+	+	–	–
Calculi or infection	+	+	+	+	–	–
Renal parenchymal lesion (glomerulonephritis or interstitial nephritis)	±	+	+	+	+	+

*Ureteric and bladder tumours may cause pain because of obstruction.

Haematuria arising from the kidney parenchyma (glomeruli or interstitium) tends to be accompanied by proteinuria and casts, whereas bleeding arising from renal tumours or lesions in the renal pelvis or below may be isolated or (particularly with infection) associated with pyuria (white blood cells in the urine). Moreover, most red blood cells arising from kidney parenchymal lesions have an abnormal morphology (best appreciated by phase contrast microscopy), whereas those from renal tumours or more distal lesions have a normal biconcave appearance (Table 12.1). Red cells may also be damaged by urine of high osmolality (which causes cell shrinkage) or low osmolality (causes cell swelling and haemolysis). With brisk bleeding, there may be frank blood with little urine.

Macroscopic haematuria arising from tumours tends to be painless, whereas that arising from calculi or infection is usually associated with pain. Occasionally, crystals (microcalculi) can cause pain and macroscopic haematuria. Renal calculi are discussed in more detail later in this chapter and urological tumours in Chapter 13.

See Case 12.1: 2.

Imaging of the urinary tract

As outlined in Chapter 1 (in the context of urinary tract infection), there are multiple investigations from which to choose to image the urinary tract. These are summarised in Table 12.2. Each has particular attributes, so the choice depends on the suspected diagnosis and the question to be answered.

In the investigation of loin pain and macroscopic haematuria, adequate information can usually be obtained from simple investigations. As 90% of renal calculi

are radio-opaque, the abdominal X-ray (KUB, kidney–ureter–bladder series) is a useful first test (Fig. 12.2). Ultrasonography is cheap, non-invasive and requires no radiation and provides useful information about renal size, renal mass lesions (in particular cysts), and renal pelvic and ureteric dilatation (Fig. 12.3). Increasingly, an abdominal computed tomography (CT) scan is performed relatively early in the investigation of possible abnormalities of the urinary tract to define the site and cause of urinary tract obstruction (Fig. 12.4). A CT-KUB (usually 'low-dose' to minimise radiation dose) is the investigation of choice to evaluate suspected urinary calculi. MRI scan of the kidneys is occasionally required in instances where iodinated contrast is not able to be used to evaluate a renal mass by CT scanning – such instances include where there is a high risk of contrast allergy or contrast-induced acute kidney injury.

Interesting facts

Ultrasonography is useful for demonstrating hydronephrosis and hydroureter. The kidney, pelvis, and ureter may appear dilated when the bladder is full of urine, so it is standard practice to repeat the examination after the bladder has been emptied.

Pathophysiology of urinary tract obstruction

The presence of renal pelvic dilatation (hydronephrosis) on the current patient's ultrasound scan indicates a partial or complete obstruction to urinary flow; there was no hydroureter, consistent with the obstruction being caused by the calculus at the level of the pelvic-ureteric junction (PUJ). Stones of 5 mm or greater in diameter are unlikely to pass

Urinary tract obstruction and stones: 2

Obstruction

As the pain was typical of renal colic, Kevin was suspected of having a renal calculus. A plain abdominal X-ray was arranged; this demonstrated a large radio-opaque lesion lying to the right of the L2/L3 vertebrae (Fig. 12.2). An abdominal ultrasound demonstrated dilatation of the right renal pelvis (hydronephrosis) above a hyperechogenic, shadowing lesion (renal calculus) with normal thickness and echogenicity of the right kidney (Fig. 12.3).

The imaging of the patient's renal tract demonstrated a renal calculus causing blockage of urinary flow. These findings give rise to the following questions:

(a) What are the different modalities for imaging the urinary tract? Which are the best for a patient with a suspected renal calculus?

(b) Why do renal calculi occur?

(c) What are the consequences of urinary tract obstruction caused by a renal calculus?

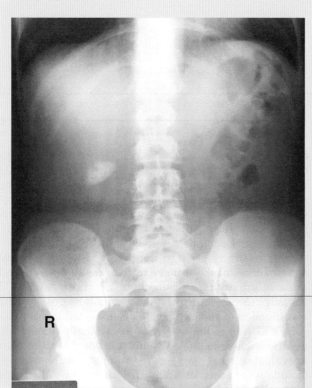

Fig. 12.2 Plain abdominal X-ray of the current patient showing a radio-opaque calculus near the second and third lumbar vertebrae on the right.

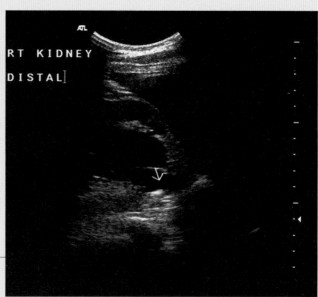

Fig. 12.3 Ultrasound scan of the right kidney of the current patient showing dilatation of the renal pelvis and an echogenic lesion (arrowed) at the pelvic-ureteric junction, associated with an acoustic shadow beneath it. The denser an object is in relation to water, the brighter it appears on ultrasound (echogenic). Note how the contents of the renal pelvis (urine) appear black, that is, non-echogenic.

beyond this level spontaneously. As with any hollow organ, the obstruction could be because of an extrinsic, intramural, or luminal lesion. In this case, the obstruction is because of a calculus obstructing at the PUJ. Common causes of urinary tract obstruction are shown in Fig. 12.5.

The patient's age and gender, and clinical setting often allow accurate prediction of the cause of obstruction. For example, in an elderly male, obstruction is commonly because of prostatic enlargement, whereas in an elderly female, it might be because of a gynaecological tumour. Obstruction may be bilateral, in particular with lesions of the bladder or urethra, when it poses a particular risk of causing renal failure.

As a result of urinary flow obstruction, resting intraluminal pressure rises (from 1 up to 80 mmHg) and

leads to proximal functional and structural changes. Ureteral peristalsis increases in frequency and amplitude initially. The ureter and renal pelvis dilate (Fig. 12.6), and, with persistent obstruction, peristalsis diminishes and becomes disorganised, and intraluminal pressure falls. It is notable that ureteral and renal pelvic dilatation does not always mean the patient has renal tract obstruction, for example women may have urinary tract dilatation from poor bladder emptying for functional reasons such as an underactive bladder (poor detrusor contraction). Conversely, urinary tract dilatation may not occur with obstruction because of the inability of the renal pelvis to expand, e.g. patients with retroperitoneal fibrosis.

Table 12.2 Imaging of the urinary tract

Test	Particularly useful for:	Cost
Plain abdominal X-ray	Radio-opaque calculi	+
Plain renal tomogram	Renal size and outline	+
Intravenous pyelogram*	Renal size, outline, and function (nephrogram) Renal pelvis, ureter, and bladder (excretory phase)	++
Retrograde pyelogram*	Bladder visualisation by cystoscopy**, ureter, and renal pelvis	++++
Antegrade pyelogram*	Obstructed renal pelvis and ureter	+++
Ultrasonography	Renal cysts, size, and pelvis	++
Dynamic isotope scan†	Renal blood flow, differential function, and outflow	++
Static isotope scan†	Renal size and scars	++
CT scan (± contrast)	Renal mass lesions, non-radio-opaque calculi	++
Spiral CT	Renal artery anatomy	++
Magnetic resonance imaging	Renal mass lesions	++++
Magnetic resonance angiography	Renal arterial flow	++++
Positron emission tomography	Renal mass lesions	++++

*A pyelogram is an X-ray image of the renal pelvis.
**Cystoscopy is an endoscopic examination of the bladder performed prior to contrast injection up the ureters.
†'Dynamic' isotopes (e.g. diethylenetriamine pentaacetate) are filtered and excreted by the kidney, whereas 'static' isotopes (e.g. dimercaptosuccinic acid) are taken up by renal cells.

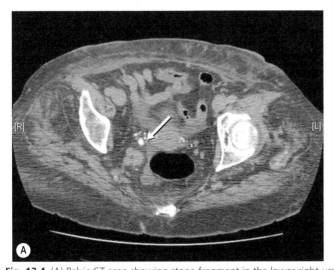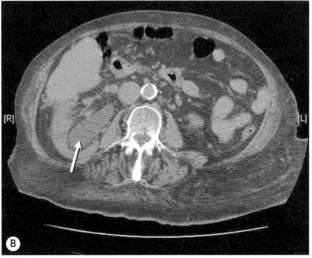

Fig. 12.4 (A) Pelvic CT scan showing stone fragment in the lower right ureter (arrow). (B) Abdominal CT scan showing dilated right renal pelvis (arrow) above an obstructing calculus.

The pressure effects are transmitted to the kidney and lead to a range of structural and functional changes (Box 12.2). As might be predicted, the distal tubular function becomes compromised with impairment of the following:
1. water and sodium reabsorption
2. urinary concentration
3. acid and potassium secretion.

After an initial phase of compensatory vasodilatation, glomerular filtration rate (GFR) and renal blood flow fall because of a combination of the back-pressure effects and release of locally active vasoconstrictor hormones (in particular thromboxane A_2 and angiotensin II), which alter intrarenal haemodynamics (Fig. 12.7).

These functional changes may be reversible with relief of acute obstruction, or partially reversible or irreversible with prolonged obstruction, leading to renal scarring. Characteristically, with the relief of obstruction and, therefore, the passage of urine, the distal functional defects may manifest clinically. This is called postobstructive diuresis, caused by an osmotic and physiological diuresis because of the excretion of retained water,

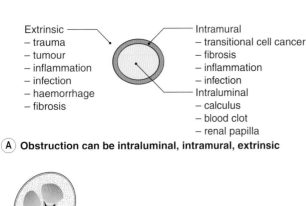

Extrinsic
– trauma
– tumour
– inflammation
– infection
– haemorrhage
– fibrosis

Intramural
– transitional cell cancer
– fibrosis
– inflammation
– infection
Intraluminal
– calculus
– blood clot
– renal papilla

(A) **Obstruction can be intraluminal, intramural, extrinsic**

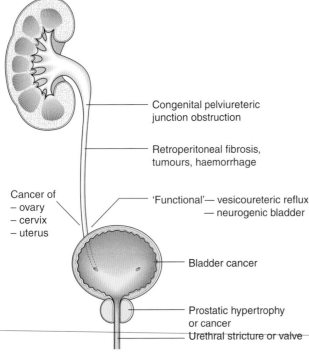

Congenital pelviureteric
junction obstruction

Retroperitoneal fibrosis,
tumours, haemorrhage

Cancer of
– ovary
– cervix
– uterus

'Functional'— vesicoureteric reflux
— neurogenic bladder

Bladder cancer

Prostatic hypertrophy
or cancer

Urethral stricture or valve

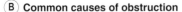

(B) **Common causes of obstruction**

Fig. 12.5 Sites and causes of urinary obstruction.

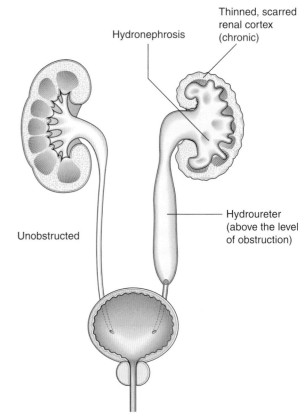

Hydronephrosis

Thinned, scarred
renal cortex
(chronic)

Unobstructed

Hydroureter
(above the level
of obstruction)

Fig. 12.6 Structural consequences of urinary tract obstruction.

Box 12.2 Functional consequences of urinary tract obstruction

- Reduced glomerular filtration rate
- Reduced renal blood flow (after an initial rise)
- Impaired renal concentrating ability
- Impaired distal tubular function
- Nephrogenic diabetes insipidus
- Renal salt wasting
- Renal tubular acidosis
- Impaired potassium secretion
- Post-obstructive diuresis

sodium, and urea. A persistent defect in collecting duct function involving impaired aquaporin 2-mediated water reabsorption (a form of nephrogenic diabetes insipidus; see Chapter 3) contributes to postobstructive diuresis. Renal scarring occurs over a period of weeks because of the effects of pressure and the release of chemoattractant and fibrogenic cytokines, such as osteopontin and monocyte chemoattractant protein 1, and transforming growth factor β, respectively.

With unilateral, slowly progressive and/or partial obstruction, the symptoms and clinical and laboratory signs of obstruction may not be obvious.

Renal calculi

Renal calculi (stones) are a common cause of loin pain, haematuria, and urinary tract obstruction. Some 90% of calculi are radio-opaque and so may be detected by plain radiography, as with the current patient.

Common types of renal calculi are listed in Table 12.3. An illustration of the physical characteristics of specific types of stone is given in Fig. 12.8. Urinary stasis, caused by poor urine output or obstruction, is an important pathogenic factor in the formation of most stones. Other factors relevant in particular cases include altered urinary pH, low concentration of naturally occurring stone inhibitors (e.g. citrate), infection (especially with microorganisms that split urea to form ammonia), and excess urinary excretion of the substances which form stones owing to excess dietary intake, systemic overproduction, or release, and/or reduced renal reabsorption. Calculi usually form in the calyces of the kidneys but can also form in the bladder.

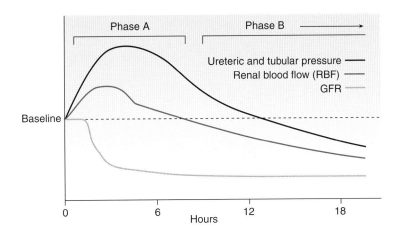

Pathophysiology of changes

	Intraluminal pressure	RBF	GFR
Phase A	↑ ...due to : Obstruction ↑ Peristalsis	↑ ...due to : Vasodilatation — prostacyclin — prostaglandin E$_2$	↓ ...due to : ↑ Intratubular pressure
Phase B	↓ ...due to : Disorganized peristalsis Dilation of tubules and ureter	↓ ...due to : Vasoconstriction — angiotensin II — thromboxane A$_2$	↓ ...due to : — continuing obstruction — vasoconstriction

Fig. 12.7 Functional consequences of acute urinary tract obstruction. GFR, glomerular filtration rate.

Table 12.3 Renal calculi

Composition	Percentage	Radio-opaque	Appearance	Crystal shape	Pathogenesis
Calcium oxalate	60	+++	Small, smooth, or spiky	'Back of envelope' or dumb-bell	Hyperparathyroidism, hypercalciuria, hypocitraturia, hyperoxaluria, hyperuricosuria
Calcium phosphate	20	+++	Slightly larger, more friable	Elongated	High urine pH because of distal renal tubular acidosis
Uric acid	<10	–	May be large	Rhomboidal	Low urine pH, hyperuricosuria
Struvite (MgNH$_4$PO$_4$)	<10	++	Staghorn	'Coffin lid'	Infection with urease-producing microorganisms, causing high urine pH
Cystine	<5	+	Pale yellow, may be large	Hexagonal	Cystinuria

The current patient's calculus was causing obstruction of urinary flow and was too large to pass to the bladder spontaneously. This raises the question of what would happen if the obstruction were not relieved and how should the stone be treated. These issues will be addressed in the last section of this chapter.

See Case 12.1: 3.

Interesting facts

Some kidney stones, particularly those that fill the renal pelvis (staghorn calculus), can be quite large; these include stones that are composed mainly of uric acid, struvite, or cystine. The largest kidney stone is reported to have weighed 1.36 kg!

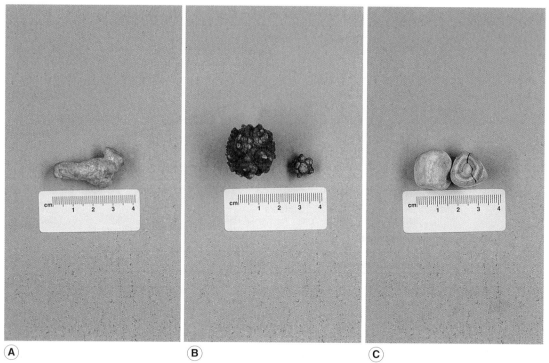

Fig. 12.8 Macroscopic appearance of renal calculi. (A) Staghorn calculus (forming a cast of the calyces and renal pelvis); (B) spiculated (spiked) stones of calcium oxalate ('mulberry' stones or 'jackstones'); (C) lamellated (layered) bladder stones, mainly of uric acid. (Courtesy the Department of Urology, Concord Hospital.)

| Case 12.1 | Urinary tract obstruction and stones: 3 |

Infection and treatment

Over the next 24 h, the patient became febrile (39 °C), with rigours and increased left loin pain. The peripheral white cell count rose to *15.0 × 10^9/L with predominant neutrophilia. It was felt that infection had developed proximal to the obstructing stone.

The patient was started on intravenous antibiotics and, on the same day, was taken to the operating theatre. Here the stone was manipulated by ureteric instrumentation back into the renal pelvis, and a ureteric stent was placed to relieve the obstruction. (A stent is a narrow tube that is placed within the ureter to maintain its patency.) Between 50 and 100 mL of purulent fluid passed through the ureter when the stent was placed. The patient improved over the next few days.

Four weeks later, he underwent extracorporeal lithotripsy (shattering of calculus using external shock waves) and subsequently passed several of stone fragments (Fig. 12.9). These were analysed and shown to consist predominantly of calcium and oxalate.

With stasis of urinary flow, microorganisms are not flushed out and can multiply. The addition of infection to the patient's clinical picture turned this into a condition that required emergency treatment.

*Values outside the normal range; see Appendix.

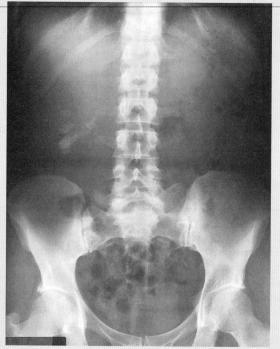

Fig. 12.9 Plain abdominal X-ray showing stone fragments after extracorporeal lithotripsy of the stone shown in Fig. 12.2.

Interesting facts

Bladder stones are much less common than kidney stones but are usually painful and can cause urinary tract obstruction. Factors that lead to bladder stones include foreign bodies, infection (such as schistosomiasis) and alterations in diet. One famous case of bladder stones was that of East Anglia (now the Eastern part of modern England) man Samuel Pepys (1633–1703), who underwent open lithotomy (without anaesthetic) and survived!

Principles of treatment

With urinary tract obstruction, the main principle of treatment is to relieve the obstruction to prevent functional and structural damage to the kidney (Table 12.4). If left untreated for a period of weeks, this damage becomes irreversible. However, with superadded urinary infection, the patient may become septicaemic and develop pyonephrosis (an infected obstructed kidney) with rapid renal destruction: these conditions require emergency treatment. Stones less than 5 mm in diameter usually pass spontaneously, whereas larger stones may require surgical intervention. Depending on their size, position, and composition, they may be treated with a combination of lithotripsy (to fracture the stone into fragments), endoluminal extraction (from within the urinary tract lumen), or open surgical removal.

Where possible, the pathogenesis of stone formation in a particular patient should be determined to guide appropriate treatment measures to prevent further stone formation. The pathogenesis can usually be inferred from a dietary history, history of fluid intake, information about familial occurrence, urinary culture, and a 'metabolic screen' of plasma and urine. The main components of the metabolic screen are determined by the usual or expected composition of the stone (see Table 12.3) and known promoters and inhibitors of stone formation. They include plasma calcium and uric acid, urinary pH, calcium, uric acid, oxalate, citrate, sodium, magnesium and, in some cases, cystine. General advice for stone formers should include increased fluid and reduced salt intake.

Interesting facts

It used to be thought that reducing dietary calcium intake might reduce the incidence of kidney stones. However, a large epidemiological study showed that dietary calcium restriction was actually associated with increased stone formation! This probably occurred because there would be less intestinal calcium to bind

Table 12.4 Principles of treatment of renal calculi

Emergency	Narcotic analgesics for pain relief Long-acting alpha-adrenergic receptor blocking and calcium-channel blocking drugs to relieve ureteric spasms and promote stone passage Correction of fluid and electrolyte disturbances Intravenous antibiotics for systemic or intrarenal infection Relief of obstruction to treat infection and preserve renal function
Remove calculus	Endoluminal procedure, lithotripsy, or open operation
Determine pathogenesis	Stone analysis Fluid intake and dietary history Family history for genetic factors Serum and urinary 'metabolic screen'
Prevent further calculi	Increased fluid intake (e.g. 2.5–3 L/day) Modification of diet (lower dietary sodium and freely absorbed phosphorous intake for all) Specific treatment of metabolic abnormality

oxalate, leading to greater absorption of oxalate across the bowel and therefore increased urinary excretion of oxalate. Other changes in diet may have unrecognised effects on stone risk. For example, increased dietary fructose increases the risk of stone formation.

Summary

1. Loin pain is commonly because of disease affecting the kidneys and ureters, and spinal nerve roots, vertebral column, paraspinal and lumbar muscles, and rarely abdominal aorta and pancreas.
2. Haematuria is because of glomerular or non-glomerular causes (the latter including conditions such as cancer, stones).
3. Urinary tract obstruction leads to pain, proximal structural and functional changes, and scarring if prolonged. Common causes include stone disease, cancer, and extrinsic obstruction (e.g. pelvic tumour).
4. Urinary tract stones are commonly made of calcium salts, but other types (e.g. struvite, cystine) should also be considered. Management includes acute treatment of the stone (relief of obstruction, surgical reduction of size often by laser lithotripsy) and managing the underlying cause of stone formation.
5. Management of stones includes acute treatment of the stone (relief of obstruction, surgical reduction of size often by laser lithotripsy) and managing the underlying cause of stone formation.

Self-assessment case study

A 75-year-old man presented with an inability to pass urine for 12 h. He had a 3-year history of increasing problems in passing urine (micturition). He noted difficulty in initiating micturition, a weak urinary stream and post-micturition dribbling. In the past, he had had an episode of macroscopic haematuria associated with dysuria and fever. On examination of his abdomen, there was fullness and tenderness in the suprapubic area. His serum creatinine was twice the upper limit of normal.

After studying this chapter, you should be able to answer the following questions:

Q1. What is the most likely explanation for his acute history of difficulty in passing urine?

Q2. What is the likely explanation for the previous episode of dysuria, macroscopic haematuria, and fever?

Q3. Explain why his serum creatinine was elevated.

Q4. What is the best test to confirm the diagnosis?

Q5. What are the main principles of treatment in this situation, and why?

Self-assessment case study answers

A1. The failure to pass urine for 12 h is probably caused by complete obstruction of urinary flow. The suprapubic signs suggest bladder enlargement and therefore indicate that the obstruction to urinary flow is likely to be at the level of the bladder neck or urethra. The longer history of difficulty in passing urine is typical of chronic obstruction because of prostatic enlargement.

A2. Urinary tract infection, either in his prostate (prostatitis) or above because of bacterial overgrowth occurring with urinary stasis.

A3. The chronic and then acute obstruction of urinary flow leads to high intraluminal pressures and disordered peristalsis above the level of obstruction. GFR falls as a combined result of this back-pressure, superimposed intrarenal haemo-

dynamic changes (mediated by vasoactive hormones) and the subsequent development of renal scarring.

A4. Renal tract ultrasonography, which in this case should show an enlarged prostate, a full bladder and distension of the ureters and renal pelvis. In addition, there may be renal scarring if the obstruction has been longstanding.

A5. Relief of urinary tract obstruction using a bladder catheter and (subsequently) prostatectomy to prevent renal scarring and superimposed infection. In addition, there are likely to be fluid and electrolyte disturbances that may require immediate correction. In milder cases, patients with large prostates may benefit for a 5-alpha-reductase inhibitor, sometimes in combination with an alpha blocker.

Self-assessment questions and answers

Q1. Abnormalities of what structures can give rise to loin pain?

A1. Spinal nerve roots, vertebral column, paraspinal and lumbar muscles, kidney capsule, renal pelvis, ureters, abdominal aorta, pancreas.

Q2. How can the red urine occurring with haemolysis be distinguished from that occurring with haematuria?

A2. Haem pigment is detected on urinalysis with both, but red blood cells are present on urine microscopy only with haematuria.

Q3. Describe the pathophysiology behind changes in renal blood flow and GFR during the first 24 h after acute obstruction.

A3. Initial vasodilatation is caused by the release of vasodilatory prostaglandins. Subsequent vasoconstriction is principally caused by the release of angiotensin II and thromboxane A2. A fall in GFR is initially because of a rise in intraluminal pressure and is subsequently caused by vasoconstriction.

Q4. List the chemical composition of five types of renal calculi.

A4. Calcium oxalate, calcium phosphate, uric acid, struvite, cystine.

RENAL MASSES, CYSTS, AND URINARY TRACT TUMOURS

13

Chapter objectives

After studying this chapter, you should be able to:

1. Give the differential diagnosis of a renal mass.
2. List some risk factors for the development of renal cell carcinoma.
3. Describe the common presenting features of renal cell carcinoma.
4. Outline the principles of management of renal cell carcinoma.
5. Understand the presentation and natural history of polycystic kidney disease.
5. List some risk factors for the development of bladder cancer.
6. Describe the common presenting features of bladder cancer.
7. Outline the principles of management of bladder cancer.

Introduction

Many of the disorders described in earlier chapters of this book are based on pharmacological, inflammatory, haemodynamic, or toxic disturbances to normal renal function. However, the kidneys themselves and the lower urinary tract may also be the site of malignant tumours; hence the differential diagnosis of presentations such as haematuria and loin pain must always consider and actively exclude this possibility. This important fact will be highlighted by the two clinical cases discussed in this chapter (see Case 13.1: 1).

Differential diagnosis of a renal mass

Whilst a renal cell carcinoma (RCC, traditionally known as a Grawitz tumour) is the most common cause of a renal mass detected on computed tomography (CT) scan, a variety of other possibilities has to be considered since not all such masses require surgical treatment. The differential diagnosis is given in Box 13.1.

Occasionally the history and the presence of other clinical findings may give a clue as to one of the alternative diagnoses, but the most useful information to diagnose kidney cancer is obtained from the features of the mass on the CT scan image itself. RCC usually shows considerable heterogeneity within the lesion, with marked enhancement on contrast injection, reflecting the high vascularity of the tumour. Other features, especially in tumours larger than 3 cm, may include calcification and internal septa.

In most cases, as in Mr. Parkinson, diagnosis of RCC is based on the CT image alone, with pathological confirmation being obtained following operative resection of the kidney. It may occasionally be helpful to perform a percutaneous biopsy or fine-needle aspiration of the lesion, especially where the diagnosis is in doubt or where the patient is elderly or at high risk for operation.

Cysts are benign when simple (filled only with clear fluid and having a well-defined spherical border), but if imaging detects features suggesting that a cyst is complex, patients may be managed with active surveillance or resection. Polycystic kidney disease is generally easy to diagnose, given the multiplicity of cysts in both kidneys (and sometimes the liver), as well as the associated hypertension and progressive chronic kidney disease (CKD), and in many cases, the pattern of dominant inheritance in the family history. Genetic testing is also available in many centres.

Of other conditions listed in Box 13.1, lymphoma and secondary malignancies can usually be diagnosed in association with systemic features, whilst nephroblastoma affects children. Urothelial cell carcinoma of the renal pelvicalyceal system and ureter may shed dysplastic or malignant cells into the urine where they can be detected by cytology.

Renal mass: 1

Robert Parkinson is a 64-year-old man who was referred to a urologist because of an abnormal abdominal CT scan. This had been ordered by his local doctor, whom he had visited 3 weeks earlier because of obvious blood-staining in his urine. This had occurred about one week after being started on treatment with warfarin for atrial fibrillation. He had no significant recent or past problems in the urinary tract, although, on questioning, he did comment on a vague ache in the right loin, which he had noted particularly since he started on warfarin. He had been treated for hypertension with a calcium channel blocker for 12 months but was otherwise quite well. He has a 40 pack-year smoking history but ceased 4 years ago because of pressure from his wife.

On examination, he was overweight at 88 kg and was in atrial fibrillation with a ventricular rate of 86/min. The blood pressure was 158/88, and there were no signs of heart failure. There was central abdominal obesity, but no organ enlargement could be detected, and the kidneys were not bimanually palpable or ballotable. Genital and rectal examinations were normal. Urinalysis showed blood +++, protein trace.

The CT scan ordered by his local doctor showed a 10-cm mass in the lower zone of the right kidney, highly suggestive of renal cell carcinoma (Fig. 13.1).

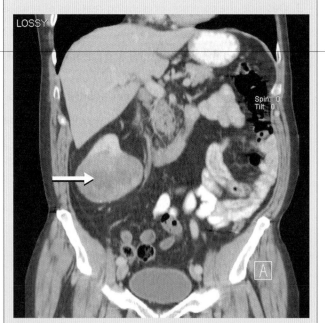

Fig. 13.1 CT scan after contrast infusion showing large mass replacing lower pole of the right kidney (arrow), suggestive of renal cell carcinoma. Note that the left kidney is not seen in this section plane.

Box 13.1 Differential diagnosis of a solitary renal mass

Malignancy
- Renal cell carcinoma
- Nephroblastoma (Wilms' tumour)
- Urothelial cell carcinoma of renal pelvis
- Lymphoma
- Secondary neoplasm

Benign tumour
- Adenoma
- Oncocytoma
- Angiomyolipoma

Cyst
- Isolated cyst
- Polycystic kidney disease

Infection
- Complicated pyelonephritis
- Abscess (bacterial, tuberculous, fungal)

Of the benign tumours, angiomyolipoma is a common tumour that is sometimes associated with the congenital condition tuberous sclerosis and shows fat within the lesion on a CT scan. Incompletely resolved pyelonephritis, especially when associated with partial obstruction by a stone, can lead to the formation of a yellowish mass (xanthogranulomatous pyelonephritis).

Simple cysts

Simple cysts are the most common type of cysts found in the kidneys. They are fluid-filled sacs that originate from the surface of the kidney and are acquired rather than inherited. The presence of renal cysts increases after the age of 40, with around 50% of people over the age of 50 having one or more cysts. They are almost always identified incidentally. Simple cysts rarely require treatment, although occasionally they may become infected requiring antibiotic therapy or can cause a mass effect requiring aspiration.

Case 13.1 Renal mass: 2

Further investigations and treatment

The urologist arranged for a full evaluation of Mr. Parkinson for presumed renal cell carcinoma prior to contemplating surgery to remove his right kidney. Full blood count was normal, and plasma biochemistry showed normal electrolytes with a creatinine of 105 μmol/L, indicating an eGFR of 72 mL/min/1.73m^2 (stage 2 CKD). Liver function tests and calcium/phosphate levels were normal. Urine culture yielded no growth of microorganisms, and urine cytology was negative for atypical or malignant cells. Chest X-ray showed changes suggestive of chronic airways disease, and a chest CT did not detect metastatic disease. The original abdominal CT was closely reviewed with a radiologist who found no evidence of extrarenal metastases or inferior vena cava invasion.

Following anaesthetic and cardiology review, Mr. Parkinson was prepared for surgery by temporary replacement of warfarin with heparin, which itself was discontinued in the perioperative period. He underwent a laparoscopic right nephrectomy without complications. The kidney and its contained tumour mass were submitted to anatomical pathology for further examination, which confirmed the diagnosis of renal cell carcinoma, clear cell type (Fig. 13.2).

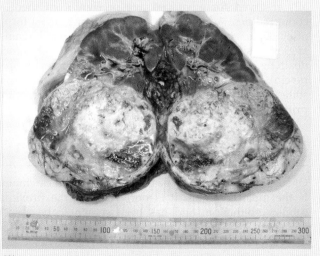

(A)

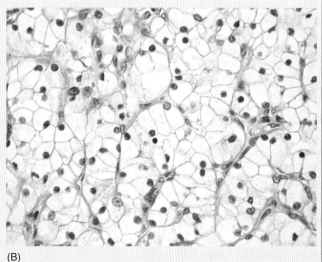

(B)

Fig. 13.2 (A) Macroscopic cross-section of the kidney containing renal cell carcinoma. (B) Histopathology of clear cell renal carcinoma. The tumour is highly vascular, and the malignant cells are characterised by prominent, clear cytoplasm (haematoxylin and eosin stain, original magnification 600x).

It is important when a cyst is found that it is adequately accessed radiologically to confirm its benign nature, meaning that it will not require further imaging or intervention. However, if there are any features of the cyst that suggest that it is complex, then further imaging, active surveillance or occasionally aspiration may be required to assess the risk of malignancy, most commonly RCC (see Case 13.1: 2).

Renal cell carcinoma

Epidemiology and risk factors

RCC is more common in men than women, typically presenting between 40 and 70 years of age, and is statistically associated with smoking and obesity. Certain occupational exposures, notably metals and solvents, have also been implicated. The risk is also increased in CKD, especially with cyst formation. Inherited conditions such as von Hippel–Lindau disease and tuberous sclerosis have a high rate of RCC formation, up to 35% in the former condition.

Interesting facts

RCC is sometimes called a Grawitz tumour after Paul Grawitz, a German professor of pathology of the late 19th–early 20th century who described the condition in detail. He mistakenly thought that these tumours arose from displaced adrenal tissue, and the term 'hypernephroma' was coined to describe them.

Presenting features

RCC is commonly asymptomatic and detected incidentally following the performance of an abdominal ultrasound or CT scan for another condition. Other presentations include macroscopic haematuria (provoked by anticoagulation therapy in the present case), loin pain, and detection of an abdominal mass. With larger tumours, systemic features may develop, such as fever, weight loss, and anaemia. A variety of specific paraneoplastic syndromes may occasionally be associated with RCC because of the secretion of humoral substances. These manifestations include hypercalcaemia (because of parathyroid-related peptide), hypertension (because of renin), hepatic dysfunction, myopathy, and polycythaemia (because of erythropoietin), though this is less common than anaemia. Up to 10% of patients with RCC will develop venous thromboembolism, and up to 20% will present with tumour extension into the renal vein, inferior vena cava, or atrium.

Interesting facts

The incidence of RCC has more than doubled in the developed world over the last 30 years, and this may be due in part to ascertainment bias. In an era when abdominal ultrasound and CT scanning are readily ordered to assess a range of abdominal complaints, renal cancer is commonly detected incidentally at a relatively early stage before any symptoms related to it have arisen.

Staging and treatment

Staging involves establishing the anatomical extent of disease, which is an important determinant of treatment approach and prognosis. Relevant factors include the size of the primary tumour, the presence of invasion of adjacent tissues, particularly the renal vein or vena cava, involvement of regional lymph nodes, and the presence of distant metastases. Tumours measuring less than 4 cm are labelled small renal masses consistent with stage 1a RCC, these tumours usually have a slow growth rate (1–3 mm/year) and 25% of these lesions are benign, needing a carefully balanced management approach.

Surgical resection is the recommended treatment for all tumours measuring greater than 4 cm (stage 1B and above), but in the most advanced cases, and even with metastatic disease, surgery may assist in the control of local symptoms. A radical nephrectomy (with the adjacent adrenal gland and regional lymph nodes) performed minimally invasively by robotic or laparoscopic means, or open surgery is recommended when removing a kidney for malignant reasons. Nephron-sparing approaches such as partial nephrectomy may be used when the primary tumour is small, when there are multiple primary tumours, or when there is pre-existing renal impairment or a solitary kidney. Radiofrequency ablation is an alternative nephron-sparing technique usually reserved for advanced age or significant medical comorbidities. Advanced RCC is resistant to most forms of cytotoxic chemotherapy, but therapy targeted against angiogenesis, checkpoint pathways (e.g. programmed death ligand-1) and cell cycle (mammalian target of rapamycin) are now considered standard of care for metastatic disease, sometimes accompanied by excision of the primary tumour.

Pathology

Of several histological types of RCC, clear cell carcinoma is the most common. It is derived from the proximal tubular epithelium and has been shown to be associated with a mutation in the *von Hippel–Lindau* gene in most sporadic cases as well as the eponymous hereditary form. Tumours are usually highly vascular because of the local induction of angiogenic factors. Less common types are papillary, chromophobe and collecting duct RCCs and oncocytomas.

Prognosis

Most patients present with disease localised to the kidney or with regionally invasive disease, and the 5-year survival in these groups is relatively good, around 90% and 75%, respectively. The presence of distant metastases reduces the 5-year survival to 10% to 30%. Prognosis is worse at any tumour stage for a higher grade on histopathology.

> ### Interesting facts
>
> Despite their high vascularity, the kidneys are rarely the site of metastasis from other malignancies. However, carcinomas of the lung or breast and melanomas can occasionally be associated with secondary renal tumours.

Polycystic kidney disease

Polycystic kidney diseases are the most common cause of hereditary end-stage kidney disease (ESKD) and are either autosomal dominant or recessive. Autosomal dominant polycystic kidney disease (ADPKD) and autosomal recessive polycystic kidney disease (ARPKD) are monogenic diseases that are caused by cilia abnormalities. ADPKD is a relatively common disease that mostly presents in adults, whereas ARPKD is rarer and often presents perinatally or in early childhood, with a more severe form of polycystic kidney disease, progressing to early end-stage kidney disease.

Autosomal dominant polycystic kidney disease

ADPKD is estimated to affect 1:500 to 1:1000 people and to be the fourth most common cause of end-stage kidney disease. Patients tend to require renal replacement therapy towards the end of their fifth decade, and kidney failure is caused by the replacement of normal tissues with cystic tissue. Remaining glomeruli hypertrophy and hyperfiltrate to compensate for a reduction in filtration, but eventually, too many nephrons have been replaced by cystic tissue, and ESKD ensues.

The *PKD1* gene is located on chromosome 16p13.3, whilst the *PKD2* gene is located on chromosome 4q22. Mutations of *PKD1* are more common (85% of ADPKD) with more severe disease and earlier progression to end-stage kidney disease when compared to patients with mutations of *PKD2*. Mutations of both genes, however, are responsible for very similar phenotypes of disease by causing abnormalities in cilia related proteins, polycystin 1 and 2, respectively.

In addition to the usual issues related to progressive CKD, clinical manifestations of ADPKD relate either to the presence of cysts in the kidney or extrarenal problems. Ballotable kidneys generally suggest the presence of polycystic disease (see Clinical skills - how to ballot kidneys). The presence of cysts can cause significant pain and an ultrasound to investigate renal angle pain is a common way that ADPKD is diagnosed. Cyst infection and haemorrhage into a cyst can also present with fever or haematuria, respectively, and pain. Renal stone formation is more common in patients with ADPKD, so it should also be considered in this population when pain is present. Extrarenal manifestations of ADPKD include liver and pancreatic cysts, which tend to be asymptomatic unless hepatic enlargement causes early satiety and malnutrition; cerebral aneurysms, which may rupture; cardiac valve disease, classically mitral valve prolapse, and diverticular disease.

Diagnosis tends to be made by imaging. Genetic testing is not required for diagnosis and, in fact, is not commonly used because of the difficulties in examining the large *PKD1* gene. It is used occasionally in genetic counselling prior to pregnancy or for family members who are potential living kidney donors with equivocal scans.

Treatment at present involves standard management of renal risk factors and, in particular, the use of RAAS blockade for hypertensive therapy. The vasopressin 2 receptor antagonist tolvaptan has been found to slow the development of cysts and to slow the rate of kidney function decline, although hepatotoxicity and polyuria can limit its tolerability. Renal transplantation may require the removal of one or both kidneys to make space for a transplanted kidney.

Differential diagnosis of microscopic haematuria

Microscopic haematuria may arise from renal parenchymal disease or pathologic disease affecting the structures of the urinary collecting system (renal pelvis, ureters, bladder, urethra), most commonly infections, stones, or tumours. As discussed in the previous chapter, clues to a source in the collecting system structures include the absence of significant proteinuria or urinary casts, normal morphology of the excreted red cells, and no associated renal function impairment or hypertension. A non-renal source is also suggested where there are associated features of bladder inflammation (dysuria and frequency) or other lower urinary tract symptoms (incontinence, hesitancy, urgency of micturition).

However, it is important to recognise that no indirect clues can reliably exclude urinary tract malignancy, and full evaluation with imaging and appropriate follow-up investigations including cystoscopy or monitoring should be performed where doubt as to the cause of haematuria persists (see Case 13.2:1).

Case 13.2 **Bladder cancer: 1**

Philip Carpenter is a 59-year-old man who consulted his local doctor for a pre-retirement medical examination. He had been working in a rubber factory for most of his working life and had been well except for two episodes of pneumonia in the past 5 years, probably related to his long-standing history of cigarette smoking.

Physical examination was unremarkable except for the presence of some nicotine staining of the fingers and scattered inspiratory crepitations heard in both lung fields. Urinalysis revealed blood 1+, but no protein or other abnormalities.

The doctor arranged for a urinary tract ultrasound to be performed, as well as urine microscopy and full blood count and biochemistry. The ultrasound revealed two normal sized kidneys and no abnormalities in the renal outlines or the bladder. The prostate was not enlarged, and the bladder emptied normally. Urine microscopy revealed 80 red blood cells per microlitre, and these were of normal morphology. There were no urinary casts and no increase in white cell excretion; urine culture was negative. Full blood count and biochemistry profile were normal, with a plasma creatinine of 90 μmol/L.

Mr. Carpenter was referred to a urologist for further evaluation.

Urothelial cell carcinoma of the bladder

Epidemiology and risk factors

Malignancy affecting the urothelial (previously known as the transitional cell) lining of the bladder frequently arises because of environmental exposure to carcinogens or chronic irritants excreted in the urine. Tobacco smoking is by far the most commonly implicated risk factor. Some occupations at increased risk include workers in paint, dye, rubber, or other chemical industries. The incidence is also increased in patients with analgesic nephropathy and those previously treated with cyclophosphamide or pelvic irradiation. The age and gender predominance are similar to those for RCC.

> **Interesting facts**
>
> Particular industrial chemicals have been firmly linked with bladder cancer. Aromatic amines, such as benzidine and beta-naphthylamine, which are used in the dye industry, can cause bladder cancer. Other industries that carry high risks include those that produce rubber, leather, textiles, and paint products. This known association of various industrial chemicals with bladder cancer has led to strict measures to limit occupational exposure, as well as close monitoring of factory workers in these industries for early disease. This involves the regular sampling of urine to detect blood, abnormal epithelial cells, and other markers of early transitional cell carcinoma.

Presenting features

Most patients present with haematuria, either asymptomatic and microscopic as with Mr. Carpenter, or with macroscopic haematuria sometimes associated with clot colic or other features of ureteric obstruction. In general, macroscopic bleeding is associated with more locally advanced disease, whilst voiding symptoms (frequency, dysuria, urgency) can be a feature of carcinoma in situ affecting the normal function of the bladder detrusor muscle or sphincter.

Staging and pathology

CT imaging with contrast known as a CT intravenous pyelogram (CT IVP) and cystoscopic examination form the basis of the staging of bladder cancer or urothelial lesions of the renal pelvis and ureter, although a renal tract ultrasound may reveal a bladder mass or polyp. CT scanning may provide information as to extravesical extension or lymph node involvement, as well as evidence of metastatic disease further afield. It is important to recognise the limitations of CT to identify lesions within a hollow organ such as the bladder and cannot define the depth of invasion into the bladder wall, for which cystoscopic examination ± excision biopsy is required. Cystoscopy also provides an opportunity for ureteric catheterisation and retrograde pyelography ± ureteric sampling for cytology where upper tract lesions are suspected. Ureteroscopy and biopsy are required for histological diagnosis.

Histopathology shows malignant proliferation of the urothelial cell epithelium and determines pathological staging by revealing the depth of invasion of the bladder wall: lesions may either be exophytic (papillary) and non-invasive or may invade into the submucosa, the lamina propria or into the underlying smooth muscle layer. This latter finding is of greatest significance in determining therapy, as it indicates a need for cystectomy, as well as prognosis. Prognosis is also influenced by histological grading into low-grade and high-grade tumours, based on nuclear atypia and degree of pleomorphism (see Case 13.2: 2).

Treatment and prognosis

Bladder cancer is especially prone to recurrence, which affects more than 50% of patients who have superficial (non-invasive) disease at first presentation. Patients, therefore, need to undergo surveillance cystoscopies to detect recurrence. Once detected, or if the patient is at high risk of recurrence, adjuvant intravesical chemotherapy or immunotherapy is used with caution to monitor local and systemic reactions.

Bladder cancer: 2

Investigations

The urologist noted the occupational history and suspected bladder cancer. He referred Mr. Carpenter for a urinary tract CT scan with contrast and also ordered urine cytology on three early morning specimens. The CT scan showed no abnormalities, but the urine cytology was positive in all samples for atypical urothelial cells (Fig. 13.3).

The following week, cystoscopy using a flexible fibreoptic cystoscope was performed under local anaesthetic. The appearances were of a pedunculated tumour with frond-like surface structures (papillae), suggestive of bladder urothelial cancer (Fig. 13.4). This was resected under general anaesthetic using a rigid cystoscope. The histopathology confirmed low-grade papillary transitional cell carcinoma, with no invasion of the lamina propria or muscularis propria (bladder muscle layer) (Fig. 13.5).

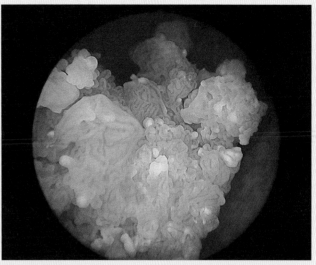

Fig. 13.4 Cystoscopic appearance of low-grade papillary bladder cancer.

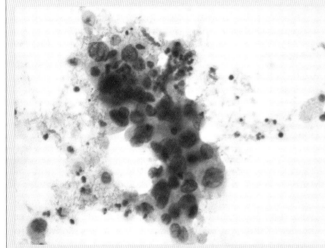

Fig. 13.3 Urine cytology showing atypical urothelial cells. The atypical cells have enlarged hyperchromatic nuclei, with irregular nuclear borders and an increased nuclear/cytoplasmic ratio (Pap stain, original magnification 600x).

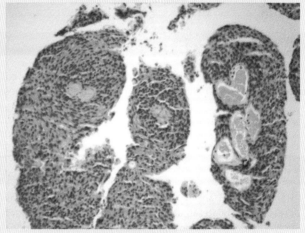

Fig. 13.5 Resected low-grade papillary transitional cell carcinoma of the bladder. The carcinoma has a papillary architecture being composed of central fibrovascular cores surrounded by atypical cells (haematoxylin and eosin stain, original magnification 200x).

Interesting facts

Bacillus Calmette-Guérin (BCG) is a vaccine that was originally used to prevent tuberculosis. It is made from a weakened strain of *Mycobacterium bovis* and has been used for many years to treat superficial bladder cancer. It is applied intravesically and controls local disease by a combination of direct cytotoxicity and by stimulating the immune system to attack the cancer cells.

Despite appropriate initial treatment of superficial disease, in some 15%–20% of patients, the disease will progress to invasion into the bladder muscle layer or beyond. When this occurs, radical cystectomy is recommended if the patient's age and general condition make this an appropriate decision. This major procedure involves fashioning a urinary diversion system, using either an isolated segment of the bowel, usually an ileal conduit (non-continent diversion, requiring a collection bag) or by forming a pouch or 'neobladder' allowing for intermittent voiding (continent diversion). Both systems are prone to a variety of mechanical and metabolic complications, and close follow-up care is required. An alternative to surgery for elderly patients with significant comorbidities is a course of treatment with radiotherapy and chemotherapy.

Survival in bladder cancer depends on the initial stage and histological grade of the tumour and the effectiveness of surveillance and adjuvant intravesical therapy in preventing recurrence of superficial disease. A 5-year survival of over 90% can be expected with non-recurrent superficial disease or 70%–80% if transurethral resection of a primary tumour is followed by intravesical BCG for recurrent superficial disease. Invasive disease requiring cystectomy or radiotherapy has a 5-year survival in the range of 10%–60%.

Case 13.2 Bladder cancer: 3

Follow-up and treatment

Following his initial operation, Mr. Carpenter underwent 3-monthly check cystoscopies. At the third of these, a recurrent mucosal tumour was detected, which was resected per urethram. Following a 2-week healing period, he was started on a 6-week course of adjuvant therapy with weekly intravesical BCG installations. He was made aware of the ongoing risk of developing invasive bladder cancer and agreed to continue with close surveillance of his bladder and upper urinary tract.

Other urinary tract tumours

A range of other benign and malignant tumours can arise in the structures of the urinary tract, and these are of special significance for the function of the renal system if they lead to urinary tract obstruction. Most important in this regard are the conditions affecting the prostate gland, which surrounds the origin of the urethra at the base of the bladder in males. Reference has already been made in the previous chapter to benign prostatic hypertrophy and prostate cancer as causes of urinary tract obstruction, and indeed of renal failure when the condition is not recognised or undertreated. Further discussion of these conditions is beyond the scope of this book.

Summary

1. Several different conditions can present with a renal mass
2. Environmental exposure are important considerations when taking a history from a patient with a renal mass
3. Microscopic haematuria is a common presentation of a renal or bladder mass, but glomerular causes of haematuria also need to be considered
4. RCC may be found incidentally, via the local effect of the tumour or because of several specific paraneoplastic phenomena
5. ADPKD is a cause of end-stage kidney disease in about 5% to 10% of cases
6. Patients with ADPKD may have extrarenal manifestations

Clinical skills - how to ballot kidneys

Normal kidneys are not able to be felt or balloted, and the presence of bilateral ballotable kidneys generally suggests polycystic kidney disease or unusually amyloidosis. A unilateral kidney tumour may also be balloted.

Balloting kidneys is part of the abdominal examination. Place your right hand on the lower border of the upper left quadrant perpendicular to the orientation of the body. Press the hand in firmly and hold it steady with some pressure. Put your left hand underneath the patient directly underneath your right hand. Keeping your right hand still, push your left hand up into the patient's back quickly as though you are throwing a ball to your other hand. If there is a ballotable kidney, you should be able to feel it gently float up and hit your right hand. You may need to repeat this action a couple of times to convince yourself that you have felt the kidney.

Move to the other side of the abdomen and again place your right hand on the top of the abdomen, on the lower border of the right upper quadrant. This side is slightly more awkward because you need to twist your hand around so that it is facing you. Again, push your right hand in firmly and use your left hand underneath to 'throw' the kidney up to your right hand.

This can be a tricky skill to learn, and it is really useful to see a patient with large polycystic kidneys to learn the process. The mistakes that medical students most commonly make when balloting are not pressing down firmly enough with the right hand and moving both hands at once rather than keeping the right hand still and moving only the left hand. It takes some practice!

Self-assessment case study

A 45-year-old woman presents to her general practitioner for a routine review. She is found to be hypertensive and, on further review, has signs suggestive of mitral valve prolapse and bilateral ballotable kidneys. She is referred for a renal ultrasound and is found to have multiple bilateral renal cysts.

After studying this chapter, you should be able to answer the following questions:

Q1. What is the most appropriate first-line agent to manage her blood pressure?

A. Beta-blocker

B. Angiotensin-converting-enzyme (ACE) inhibitor

C. Alpha-blocker

D. Calcium channel blocker

Q2. The woman recalls that her father, who also had polycystic kidney disease, collapsed and died at the age of 56. You should advise that she undergo:

A. Carotid artery Dopplers

B. Renal artery Dopplers

C. Cerebral artery imaging

D. Retinal artery imaging

Self-assessment case study answers

A1. (B) Angiotensin-converting-enzyme (ACE) inhibitor. The patient appears to have ADPKD with hypertension. RAAS blockade with an ACE inhibitor has been found to slow the rate of deterioration of renal function in addition to controlling blood pressure, whilst the other antihypertensives will not have this additional benefit.

A2. (C) Cerebral artery imaging. Berry aneurysm with subarachnoid haemorrhage (SAH) can be an extrarenal manifestation of polycystic kidney disease. ADPKD patients with a personal or family history of SAH or a family history of sudden death should be investigated for the presence of an aneurysm.

DRUGS AND THE KIDNEY

Chapter objectives

After studying this chapter, you should be able to:

1. Describe the mechanisms of renal excretion of drugs in patients with normal and impaired kidney function.

2. Recognise characteristics of a drug that will increase its action and/or toxicity in patients with impaired kidney function.

3. Identify patients in whom drug dosage should be modified in light of kidney disease, changes in total body water or protein binding, which will affect the distribution or toxicity of the drug.

4. Describe the common mechanisms that underlie nephrotoxic insults to the kidneys.

5. Understand the natural history of the common forms of drug-induced nephrotoxicity.

6. Describe some preventative therapies and monitoring procedures that should be put in place before prescribing potentially nephrotoxic drugs.

Introduction

Many drugs are excreted by the kidney through glomerular filtration, tubular secretion, or a combination of these processes. Conjugated metabolites produced by the liver are also excreted by the kidney. Reduced renal clearances in patients with kidney disease may result in the accumulation of drugs and their metabolites, with an increased risk of toxicity. Renal dysfunction may also affect the distribution of the drug in the body by altering total body water or the metabolism or protein binding of the drug, which in turn may modify its therapeutic and adverse effects.

In addition to the effect of pre-existing kidney dysfunction on drug excretion and metabolism, many drugs may themselves directly influence kidney function through:

1. Effects on volume status or renal haemodynamics that may alter the glomerular filtration rate (GFR).

2. Accumulation of the drug or its metabolites causing direct toxicity to the kidney.

Mechanisms to 'protect' the kidney from nephrotoxic insults and maintain cellular integrity exist, but these are likely to be impaired in the presence of chronic kidney disease, which further predisposes to drug nephrotoxicity. The list of potential agents contributing to acute kidney injury is extensive and includes the use of traditional medicines in some geographical areas. Hence a careful history should be undertaken with respect to both pre-scribed and complementary medicines in the investigation of an abrupt decrease in kidney function.

This chapter will discuss the factors and mechanisms influencing drug excretion by the kidneys in patients with both normal and abnormal kidney function in Part A. In Part B, the physiological and cellular basis for drug-induced nephropathies will be considered.

See Case 14.1: 1.

Part A

Effect of kidney impairment on drug excretion

Principles of drug dosing

The dosage of a drug and the frequency with which it is given requires an understanding of both its pharmacodynamics and pharmacokinetics. Pharmacodynamics refers to the relationship between drug dose, plasma concentration and the effect of the drug. Pharmacokinetics describes the parameters of absorption, distribution, and excretion of the drug: these factors determine the dose that should be administered and the dosage interval required to maximise the effectiveness of the drug and minimise side effects. Many patient-related factors will influence the pharmacodynamics and pharmacokinetics, which should be reflected in both the dosage and timing of drug administration.

Case 14.1 Drugs and the kidney: 1

Too much digoxin?

Mrs. Beverley Johnson is a 71-year-old woman who has been under treatment from her general practitioner for heart failure for several years. She has underlying ischaemic heart disease and suffered an acute myocardial infarction affecting the anterior wall of the left ventricle at the age of 68. Since that time, she has been treated with an angiotensin-converting enzyme (ACE) inhibitor (lisinopril 5 mg daily) and a diuretic (furosemide (frusemide) 40 mg twice daily), in addition to aspirin, a statin and a beta-blocker.

Recently Mrs. Johnson's condition deteriorated, with increased shortness of breath and fatigue. After admission to the local hospital's emergency department, she was found to have developed atrial fibrillation and was started on digoxin 0.25 mg daily. Ten days after returning home from this admission, she called her general practitioner to visit her because she had been experiencing increasing nausea with three episodes of vomiting since her discharge.

On examination, Mrs. Johnson looks pale and uncomfortable but is haemodynamically stable (blood pressure 130/80, pulse 86 beats/min, still in atrial fibrillation). She appears a little dry and weighs 56 kg (usual weight 57–58 kg). The doctor checks the records, which reveal that Mrs. Johnson's biochemistry (at the time of her recent admission) showed normal electrolytes, but slightly increased plasma concentrations of urea (*9.5 mmol/L) and creatinine (*140 μmol/L), reflecting some kidney impairment presumed to be caused by vascular disease and poor cardiac output.

The doctor now suspects that digoxin toxicity has developed and takes blood for a serum digoxin level as well as electrolytes and renal function. She is advised to stop taking the digoxin until he gets the results.

This case raises the following questions:

1. How is the kidney involved in the metabolism and excretion of drugs?
2. What characteristics of a drug are likely to predict whether the kidney has a primary role in determining its plasma concentration?
3. What patient characteristics influence the metabolism and excretion of a drug under normal circumstances?
4. How and when should drug dosing be modified in the presence of kidney impairment?

Before we consider the specifics of Mrs. Johnson's clinical problem, it is useful to consider the general principles involved in the normal metabolism and excretion of a drug that will influence its prescription.

---

*Values outside the normal range; see Appendix.

An important pharmacodynamic concept is that the response to a drug is related to its concentration, either in plasma or tissue. The classic relationship between dose and effect is demonstrated in Fig. 14.1A. It is clear from this relationship that a minimal concentration of a drug is necessary to achieve the desired effect and that once a certain level of drug is reached, no further therapeutic effect is gained. However, if higher concentrations of the drug are obtained, then toxicity may ensue. The overlap between toxic and beneficial effects is referred to as the therapeutic index. For some drugs, there is a large difference between the drug levels at which maximum efficacy is achieved, and toxicity develops (Fig. 14.1B). In these circumstances, dosage modification is not generally needed with kidney impairment, even if the drug accumulates to high levels (e.g. penicillin). However, other drugs have a narrow therapeutic index, which means that toxicity occurs at a level close to the maximal efficacy (Fig. 14.1C). It is in these circumstances that blood levels of the drug, generally taken just before the next planned dose, are most useful to ensure that efficacy is maintained and the risk of toxicity minimised. This is the case, for example, with digoxin.

Altered pharmacokinetics in renal disease

As described above, pharmacokinetic factors determine the plasma concentration achieved after a drug is administered. These factors include the absorption of the drug, its distribution in body fluids and tissue, and its excretion. All of these steps may be altered during kidney disease, although the greatest effect is on excretion.

Gastrointestinal absorption

The amount of drug absorbed from the gastrointestinal tract largely depends on the characteristics of the drug rather than patient-related factors. However, in patients with kidney impairment, the absorption of drugs from the gastrointestinal tract may be reduced because of gastric stasis, reduced gastric acidity, and concurrent treatment with phosphate-binding drugs, which will also bind numerous medications (e.g. aspirin, ciprofloxacin).

Drug distribution

The volume of distribution (V_d) of a drug is defined as the volume of fluid that the drug would need to be distributed in to produce the measured plasma concentration. It is calculated as follows:

$$V_d = \frac{\text{dose of drug administered}}{\text{plasma concentration}}$$

The volume of distribution for a drug exclusively confined to the plasma approximates the plasma volume.

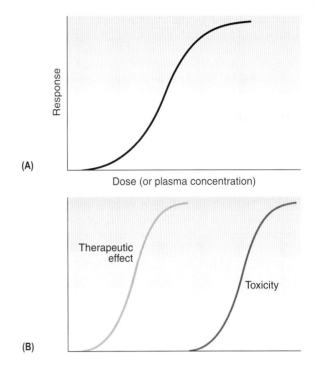

(A)

Dose (or plasma concentration)

(B)

Therapeutic effect

Toxicity

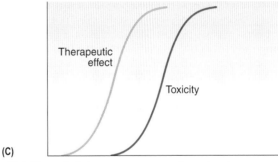

(C)

Therapeutic effect

Toxicity

Fig. 14.1 Theoretical dose–response curves for a drug (response on *y*-axis as percentage of maximum effect, dose on *x*-axis as log drug concentration). (A) Basic dose–response relationship; (B) dose–response relationship for the therapeutic effect and the toxic effect of a particular drug (no overlap, i.e. wide therapeutic index); (C) dose–response relationship for the therapeutic and toxic effects of another drug (with overlap, i.e. narrow therapeutic index).

This is likely to be the case for drugs that are very highly protein-bound. If a drug is very water-soluble, then the volume of distribution approximates body water (approximately 60% of body weight in men and 55% in women). The volume of distribution may be altered in people with kidney disease because of fluid retention and expansion of the circulating volume. For water-soluble drugs with low protein binding, this may reduce the effective drug concentration.

Kidney disease results in the accumulation of organic acids that compete with drugs for binding onto albumin and other plasma proteins. As serum albumin may be low in kidney impairment, an increased proportion of free drug may be available. However, the changes in protein binding rarely require a change in the loading dose of drugs, nor in the interpretation of steady state plasma drug levels, with the exception of phenytoin. In this instance, the therapeutic range for total plasma concentration needs to be adjusted downward to take into account increased free drug availability.

Renal excretion

The excretion of a drug (and its clearance) is related to the volume of distribution of the drug and its half-life ($t_{1/2}$), which is the time for its plasma concentration to half after absorption and distribution of the drug are complete. The $t_{1/2}$ of a drug may help in determining dosage intervals and predicting drug accumulation. It is often important to know how long it will take before a drug reaches its full effect, i.e. its steady state concentration. The time required for any drug to achieve this steady state is four to five times its $t_{1/2}$ (Fig. 14.2A).

If the half-life of a drug is prolonged in kidney impairment because of a reduction in clearance, then a widening of the dosage interval is required, and the time to reach a steady state may be prolonged (Fig. 14.2B). This has implications for drugs such as digoxin, which normally has a $t_{1/2}$ of 36 h, and thus the steady state is reached after 1 week. However, in renal impairment, the $t_{1/2}$ is prolonged, and steady state may not be reached for several weeks. A corollary of this is that, where the dosing interval is not altered, administration of the usual dose of the drug will rapidly lead to the accumulation of high serum concentrations (Fig. 14.2C). This may have serious clinical consequences for drugs such as digoxin, which have a narrow therapeutic index, and both the effective dose and toxicity correlate closely with the steady state plasma concentration.

The renal excretion of a drug is determined by filtration and the net effect of tubular secretion and reabsorption.

The filtration of a drug into the urine depends largely on its molecular weight and the degree to which it is protein-bound. In general, filtration is increased with a lower molecular weight and a lesser degree of protein binding. Once filtered, lipid-soluble drugs may be passively reabsorbed from the tubular fluid down a concentration gradient to the plasma. Water-soluble drugs may be 'trapped' in the tubular fluid and excreted if no specific reabsorptive mechanism exists.

Some drugs undergo active secretion into the urine by facilitated (carrier-mediated) transport mechanisms that normally transport organic acids or bases across the proximal tubular wall. The basic cellular mechanisms involved in this secretory process are illustrated in Fig. 14.3. It has been established that, for organic acids (including many anionic drugs), the initial step in secretion is the uptake of the anion into the cell across the basolateral membrane by cotransport with sodium, which enters the cell down its electrochemical gradient (generated by the action of the basolateral Na,K-ATPase). The anion then reaches a relatively high intracellular con-

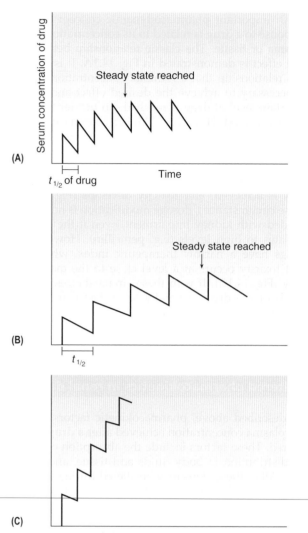

Fig. 14.2 Time course of plasma drug concentrations after repeated oral administration of the same dose at constant time intervals. (A) Drug administered at an interval corresponding to its half-life of elimination ($t_{1/2}$); steady state reached in approximately five half-lives. (B) Same drug with prolonged half-life caused by reduced drug excretion in renal impairment; when the dose is given every (new) half-life, the time to steady state is greatly prolonged; (C) same drug given in renal impairment at an interval corresponding to half-life in normal renal function, resulting in rapid accumulation of drug to excessively high levels.

centration and leaves the cell down its concentration gradient into the lumen, exchanging via a countertransport carrier with another anion such as chloride. The secretory mechanism for organic bases and cationic drugs is less well defined but probably involves a primary secretory step across the apical cell membrane, with a secondary increase in uptake across the basolateral membrane. A representative list of drugs undergoing secretion by one or other of these pathways is given in Table 14.1.

Drugs undergoing transport across the tubular epithelium may be affected by the pH of the tubular fluid. This is because the charged form of the drug (an organic acid

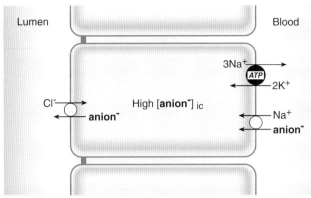

Fig. 14.3 Schematic of proximal tubular cell showing the mechanism for transepithelial secretion of an organic acid (e.g. anionic drug).

Table 14.1 Drugs that are actively secreted by the proximal tubule	
Organic acids	*Organic bases*
Penicillin	Amiloride
Cephalosporins	Quinidine
Sulphonamides	Tetracycline
Furosemide (frusemide)	
Thiazides	
Salicylates	
Probenecid	
Tenofovir	

in a high luminal pH environment or an organic base in a low luminal pH environment) is more water-soluble, favouring excretion (Fig. 14.4). Excretion of acidic drugs is therefore increased by raising the urinary pH, and the excretion of basic drugs is favoured by the excretion of acidic urine. This may be important when facilitating drug excretion following overdosage, e.g. alkalinisation of the urine with bicarbonate infusion to enhance aspirin excretion.

Finally, some drugs prevent the tubular secretion of other drugs by competing for binding to common transporters in the proximal tubule. This may be used therapeutically to enhance the desired effect of the drug and extend its half-life, e.g. treatment with the organic acid probenecid can cause an increase in serum penicillin concentrations and hence allow a reduced frequency of administration.

See Case 14.1: 2.

Drug dosing in kidney impairment

It is clear that Mrs. Johnson had pre-existing kidney impairment. Although her baseline serum creatinine was only just outside the normal range, her estimated GFR (see Chapter 5) was considerably reduced, at around 29 mL/min, when she first presented to hospital. Thus the dose and/or dosage interval of drugs such as digoxin (that are very largely excreted by the kidney) should

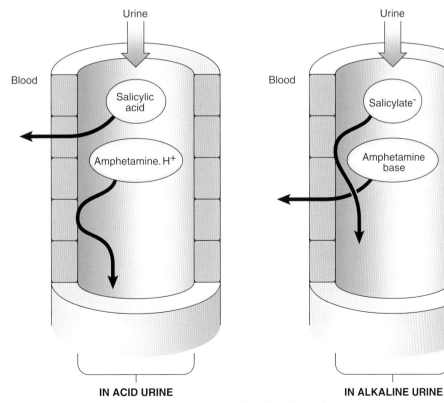

Fig. 14.4 Schematic of the effect of altering urine pH on the excretion of acidic and basic drugs.

Drugs and the kidney: 2

Follow-up on Mrs. Johnson

The results of Mrs. Johnson's blood tests come back, indicating that the serum digoxin level (taken some 8 h after the last dose) is 3.9 nmol/L. This is well outside the recommended therapeutic range (0.6–2.3 nmol/L) and, taken in conjunction with her clinical features, is indicative of digoxin toxicity.

Furthermore, her plasma biochemistry results now show some further deterioration in renal function, with the urea being *12.1 mmol/L and the creatinine *160 μmol/L. These results suggest that her poor fluid intake (because of nausea), in addition to her vomiting, have led to plasma volume contraction with a fall in renal blood flow and hence in GFR. This worsening renal impairment, in turn, would have led to further digoxin accumulation, setting up a vicious cycle of deterioration in her condition. Apart from the unpleasant gastrointestinal features experienced by this patient, other toxic effects of digoxin include visual disturbances and cardiac arrhythmias. The latter may be quite serious and are exacerbated by low plasma potassium levels, which may occur because of diuretic therapy and/or vomiting in this setting.

Fortunately, with temporary cessation of digoxin and restoration of her hydration state, Mrs. Johnson's digoxin toxicity state subsided, and she was later stabilised on a smaller daily dose of the drug (0.0625 mg).

It is now worth reviewing some of the factors which led Mrs. Johnson into so much trouble.

*Values outside the normal range; see Appendix.

Table 14.2 Characteristics of drugs that predict that a dosage adjustment should be made in kidney disease

1. Primary urinary excretion of the parent drug or metabolites
In general, if greater than 50% of a drug or its active metabolites is normally excreted in the urine, a dosage reduction will be necessary to prevent accumulation and potential toxicity (e.g. gentamicin, allopurinol).

2. Low therapeutic index
Because of a narrow therapeutic range of efficacy of the drug, accumulation will result in significant toxicity (e.g. digoxin).

3. High protein binding
Accumulation of organic acids in chronic kidney disease will displace acidic drugs from albumin and increase the free drug in the plasma so that the target therapeutic concentration range (measuring total drug) should be adjusted downwards (e.g. phenytoin).

4. A small volume of distribution of the drug
Changes in body water that occur in kidney disease are more likely to impact drugs that are distributed in smaller volumes (e.g. highly protein-bound drugs).

weight heparin. This is because safety studies of these drugs in renal impairment were performed using C-G calculated GFR, not CKD-EPI.

Drugs and the kidney: 1

A predictable reaction

Roger Woodruffe is a 60-year-old man who presents with recent pain in his left knee joint that has limited his golfing activities. He has a history of hypertension, well controlled on a combination of an angiotensin-converting enzyme (ACE) inhibitor (perindopril 4 mg/d) and a loop diuretic (furosemide (frusemide) 40 mg/d). He is otherwise well. His blood pressure at the time he is seen is 145/95 mmHg. His serum biochemistry was last measured 6 months ago with the following results:

- Sodium 140 mmol/L
- Potassium 5.0 mmol/L
- Chloride 105 mmol/L
- Bicarbonate 23 mmol/L
- *Urea 12.1 mmol/L
- *Creatinine 160 μmol/L.

His doctor prescribes a non-steroidal anti-inflammatory drug (NSAID), diclofenac, 50 mg twice daily.

Mr. Woodruffe returns for review in 10 days complaining of ankle swelling and mild dyspnoea on exertion. His blood pressure is now 175/105 mmHg, and he has pitting oedema bilaterally. His doctor orders a new serum biochemical profile which shows the creatinine has risen to *240 μmol/L, and the potassium is now elevated at *6.6 mmol/L. The serum albumin is normal at 41 g/L. Urinalysis shows only a trace of protein, and a midstream urine specimen reveals no increased excretion of cells and no bacterial growth.

have been modified to avoid accumulation and the attendant risk of toxicity. This risk should be considered before the administration of any drug to a patient with kidney impairment, and any adverse reaction occurring in temporal relationship to a drug being started should be considered as being caused by the drug unless another explanation can be found.

Several characteristics of a drug suggest that there is a need for dosage adjustment and an increased risk of toxicity when the drug is prescribed for patients with kidney impairment (Table 14.2). Some of these points have already arisen in the discussion about the case of Mrs. Johnson.

Numerous published tables and algorithms are available to guide the therapeutic use of a wide variety of drugs in patients with different degrees of renal impairment. Some examples are given in this chapter, but further details can be obtained from reference texts. An important aspect of drug dosing to be aware of is that dose calculations for some drugs are based on GFR calculated using the Cockcroft–Gault equation rather than CKD-EPI or the modification of diet in renal disease. Examples include aminoglycosides and low molecular

A full blood count is normal, with no increased eosinophil count to suggest that an allergic reaction is involved.

This case raises the issues associated with prescribing drugs with predictable effects on renal haemodynamics and transport for patients with already impaired kidney function. By understanding the relevant physiology and pharmacology, it will become clear that Mr. Woodruffe was at high risk of kidney functional deterioration from the prescription of the NSAID diclofenac.

*Values outside the normal range; see Appendix.

Part B

Renal impairment induced by drugs

Renal actions of non-steroidal anti-inflammatory drugs

Non-steroidal anti-inflammatory drugs (NSAIDs) inhibit the formation of prostaglandins through the inhibition of cyclo-oxygenase (COX). Prostaglandins have a vasodilatory effect in the kidney, which is of particular significance in the presence of kidney impairment. In this situation, glomerular filtration is maintained by increasing renal blood flow through afferent arteriolar vasodilatation (mediated by prostaglandins) and efferent arteriolar vasoconstriction (mediated by angiotensin II). Blockade of these compensatory mechanisms to maintain renal blood flow and GFR will be reflected by an increase in serum creatinine. Thus, prescription of NSAIDs in the presence of pre-existing kidney impairment will commonly aggravate the degree of renal impairment. This effect is exacerbated by the concomitant use of angiotensin-converting enzyme (ACE) inhibitors and diuretics, which will further reduce the glomerular pressure and thus the driving force for glomerular filtration (see Chapter 5).

As prostaglandins also promote natriuresis by interfering with tubular sodium reabsorption and blunt the effects of antidiuretic hormone on the tubular reabsorption of water, inhibition of prostaglandin production by NSAIDs results in salt and water retention, with resultant hypertension and oedema. Inhibition of prostaglandin synthesis also secondarily inhibits renin release, causing hyporeninaemic hypoaldosteronism, which results in the impairment of distal tubular potassium secretion and hence hyperkalaemia. As these effects are caused by alterations in 'normal' physiological function, the urinalysis is unremarkable (minimal proteinuria or haematuria), and the urinary sediment is bland. In general, the abnormalities are corrected by the withdrawal of the NSAID and any additional drugs affecting plasma volume and glomerular haemodynamics.

In summary, it is likely that all of Mr. Woodruffe's problems at his second presentation – the worsening of kidney function and hypertension, fluid retention and hyperkalaemia – are caused by the inhibition of renal COX by the NSAID diclofenac (See Case 14.2: 1 and 2).

COX exists in two isoforms. COX 1 is constitutively expressed in the kidney and gastrointestinal tract, whilst COX 2 is expressed in inflamed tissues. Recently, drugs that selectively inhibit COX 2 have been developed for use in inflammatory conditions with the expectation that the side effect profile will be better than the previously available non-selective COX 1 and 2 inhibitors. However, experience to date suggests that, whilst gastrointestinal side effects with the selective COX 2 inhibitors are somewhat reduced, the effects on kidney function and electrolyte homeostasis are comparable to the non-selective agents.

| Case 14.2 | Drugs and the kidney: 2 |

Course and outcome

Mr. Woodruffe is advised to cease the diclofenac, furosemide (frusemide), and perindopril, and is changed to sustained-release verapamil 240 mg/d as a replacement antihypertensive, in the short term.

After 1 week, his oedema has largely resolved, the blood pressure has improved to 150/90, and his serum creatinine has fallen to *170 µmol/L, with normal electrolytes.

*Values outside the normal range; see Appendix.

Mechanisms of nephrotoxicity

It is clear from the above case that drug-induced nephrotoxicity may be mediated by alterations in renal haemodynamics via an effect on humoral systems within the kidney. However, drugs may also be directly nephrotoxic to renal cells (largely affecting the tubular cells) or cause immunologically mediated damage. Thus a drug may directly induce acute tubular necrosis (although haemodynamic influences may also be involved) or trigger interstitial nephritis or, occasionally, glomerular injury.

Both of these latter mechanisms may be invoked in different patients in the nephrotoxicity observed with NSAIDs, in addition to the physiologically predictable haemodynamic and tubular transport effects noted above. In particular, NSAID-induced interstitial nephritis is seen relatively commonly, partly because of the high prevalence of usage in the community.

Drug-induced interstitial nephritis

Idiosyncratic responses to many drugs may include acute interstitial nephritis. Because of the inflammatory nature of the condition, characterised by an interstitial inflammatory response with eosinophilic infiltration (Fig. 14.5), the urinalysis will generally show sterile pyuria, occasionally eosinophiluria and often granular casts on urine microscopy. Renal function will generally deteriorate because of interstitial inflammation and oedema, causing a reduction in renal blood flow and GFR. The inflammatory cell infiltrate consists of a variety of cells, including

B and T lymphocytes, plasma cells, eosinophils, natural killer cells, and macrophages. In the majority of instances where T cell subsets have been studied in drug-induced interstitial nephritis, the CD4+ population predominates. Peripheral eosinophilia is often present, and, in occasional cases, a more systemic 'allergic' response will result in skin rashes and arthralgia. NSAIDs have been well documented to cause interstitial nephritis up to 6 months after stable therapy. However, in Mr. Woodruffe's case, the diagnosis of interstitial nephritis is not supported, as the urinalysis and urine sediment were not abnormal and systemic features were not prominent.

Many drugs have been implicated as a cause of acute interstitial nephritis (Table 14.3), which can arise within a variable period from the commencement of the drug. Thus, a deterioration in kidney function in this setting should alert the clinician to the possibility of this diagnosis.

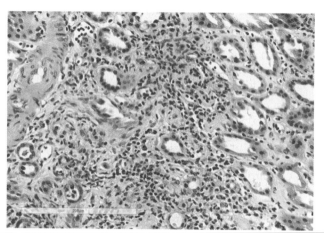

Fig. 14.5 Micrograph (stained with haematoxylin and eosin) showing acute interstitial nephritis. Note the intense inflammatory infiltrate and oedema in the interstitium; numerous eosinophils can be detected under high power.

Table 14.3   Drugs frequently implicated in acute interstitial nephritis

Antibiotics	Others
Penicillin (especially methicillin)	Phenytoin
Cephalosporins	Allopurinol
Sulphonamides	Aspirin
Rifampicin	Methyldopa
Quinolones	Carbamazepine
	Valproic acid
Diuretics	Diazepam
Thiazides	Interferon
Furosemide (frusemide)	Beta-blockers
	Quinine
NSAIDs	Doxepin
Proton pump inhibitors	Azathioprine
Checkpoint inhibitors	

NSAIDs, non-steroidal anti-inflammatory drugs.

An improvement in kidney function will generally follow the withdrawal of the offending agent. The time to recovery may vary from days to months. Renal biopsy is usually performed to confirm the diagnosis where there is severe kidney impairment or because of systemic features, which raise the question of another pathologic condition such as **vasculitis**. In these cases, short-term treatment with corticosteroids may be of benefit in shortening the natural course of the illness. Although in the majority of cases, GFR returns to baseline values, there is a loss of functional renal tissue in many cases, characterised histologically by interstitial fibrosis and sometimes glomerulosclerosis. Factors associated with a greater loss of kidney functional capacity include more severe initial kidney impairment, a slower rate of recovery after withdrawal of the offending agent, greater histological damage, older age group, and lack of initial steroid therapy.

Drug-induced glomerular pathologic conditions

Glomerular pathologic conditions are less common than tubulointerstitial injury in drug-induced nephrotoxicity. In general, glomerular damage presents as proteinuria and the most frequently observed pathologic condition is membranous nephropathy. The frequency with which glomerular injury occurs in patients treated with certain drugs, notably gold and penicillamine (used mainly in rheumatoid arthritis), is high enough to warrant routine surveillance by urinalysis. In general, the prognosis of the glomerular lesion is favourable after withdrawal of the drug, with an improvement in proteinuria generally observed. The occurrence of **glomerulopathy** in this setting is not clearly dose-related, and the cause remains unclear.

NSAIDs may also induce glomerulopathy, with minimal change nephropathy being the most widely recognised pathological lesion. However, this is rare and is unlikely to be implicated in the deteriorating renal function in the case reviewed in the current chapter, as proteinuria was not present on urinalysis.

Rarely drugs can be causally implicated in glomerulonephritis. An example is alemtuzumab, a monoclonal antibody used in multiple sclerosis, which is uncommonly associated with a clinical picture of anti-GBM disease.

Important causes of nephrotoxicity

In the case of some drugs, nephrotoxicity may be dose-related and predictable, whilst in other cases, the condition is an uncommon side effect but may be frequently observed if there is a high usage of the particular agent in the community. Some examples of common or important causes of nephrotoxicity are discussed below.

Gentamicin

Gentamicin (and other aminoglycosides) requires specific mention because of the serious and avoidable nature of the toxicity associated with this class of antibiotics. Aminoglycosides are almost entirely excreted by the kidney. Thus, in kidney impairment, excretion of the drug is reduced and, unless dosage modification is made, toxicity is likely to occur, affecting both the kidney and inner ear. The effectiveness of an aminoglycoside in killing bacteria correlates with its peak concentration rather than with its steady state concentration, whereas the nephrotoxicity correlates with the steady state accumulation of the drug into proximal tubular cells. Thus, in kidney impairment, the drug dosage remains the same, but the dose interval should be increased. In patients with kidney failure, where the only clearance is through the dialysis process, the dose interval may be up to every 3 days. This contrasts with agents such as digoxin (and cyclosporin, discussed below), where a therapeutic effect requires a defined steady state concentration to be maintained. In these cases, the dose is reduced, but the dosage interval remains constant.

In patients with any degree of renal impairment, the clearance of a renally excreted drug may be hard to predict. Thus, whenever accumulation of a drug poses a predictable risk of toxicity, serum concentrations of the drug just before the next scheduled dose (trough level) should be used to guide either the dose or the dosage interval, as appropriate.

Cyclosporin

Cyclosporin A is an immunosuppressive drug that is largely metabolised in the liver, but the main clinical manifestation of toxicity is renal injury. Several mechanisms of toxicity are recognised. Cyclosporin A induces marked intrarenal vasoconstriction and a fall in GFR, with acute damage to the proximal tubules and ischaemic nephropathy in the longer term. A classic histological appearance of 'striped fibrosis' occurs in chronic cyclosporin nephrotoxicity. An **arteriopathy** is also well recognised with a syndrome consistent with haemolytic uraemic syndrome, characterised by activation of the coagulation system and intravascular haemolysis, resulting in anaemia, **thrombocytopaenia,** and impaired renal function.

As cyclosporin A is metabolised by the cytochrome-dependent mixed function oxidases in the liver, drugs which interact with this system may impair its metabolism, thus precipitating significant toxicity or, alternatively, accelerate metabolism resulting in loss of the immunosuppressive effect. As cyclosporin is widely used in renal transplantation, drug levels are closely monitored as fluctuations in renal function in this circumstance are common, and a high cyclosporin level

may provide evidence suggesting the development of nephrotoxicity.

Kidney disease induced by non-prescription medicines

Epidemiological studies have clearly identified the ingestion of aspirin, phenacetin, and caffeine in over-the-counter compound analgesic medications as a cause of characteristic interstitial nephritis with **papillary necrosis**, associated with an increased propensity to uroepithelial carcinoma. This clinical entity of *analgesic nephropathy* has been the most prevalent clearly recognised cause of drug-induced kidney failure within defined demographic populations (including Australia). Although analgesic nephropathy accounted for up to 22% of patients entering dialysis programmes in the early 1980s, its incidence has steadily declined since the withdrawal of these medications in combination form from over-the-counter sale. Long-term ingestion of NSAIDs has been implicated in the pathogenesis of some cases of interstitial nephritis and papillary necrosis. However, the incidence is relatively low compared with the former usage of the compound agents.

'Natural' therapies are increasingly being used for a variety of conditions in both western and eastern cultures. The constituents of such therapies are often poorly documented, and they may result in either dose-dependent or idiosyncratic side effects. One reported form of so-called 'Chinese Herb Nephropathy' related to the use of *Aristolochia fangchi* for weight reduction. This has been causally demonstrated to induce a rapidly progressive non-inflammatory interstitial fibrosis in the kidney, resulting in kidney failure. Follow-up investigations in these patients have revealed an increased risk of uroepithelial cancer, high enough to justify the recommendation of prophylactic nephrectomy before consideration of transplantation and immunosuppression. More recent cases of 'Balkan' nephropathy have been linked to aristolochic acid found in seeds in the local wheat fields of Serbia.

Contrast agents

Intravenous administration of iodinated radiological contrast agents has been reported to be nephrotoxic, particularly in patients with volume depletion, pre-existing renal disease, diabetes mellitus, or multiple myeloma. In general, an acute reversible decline in renal function is observed, and in severe cases, the underlying pathological lesion is acute tubular necrosis. The newer non-ionic compounds are less nephrotoxic and are preferred, particularly in high risk patients. It is recommended that intravenous saline loading be undertaken in these patients before the procedure since this measure has been found to be protective in laboratory and clinical studies. Furthermore, agents that may exacerbate renal haemodynamic injury, such as NSAIDs and ACE inhibitors, should be ceased. In many instances, alternative means of imaging can now be undertaken, and these should be carefully considered in patients with advanced renal disease.

Checkpoint inhibitors

Interactions between T lymphocytes and antigen-presenting cells (APCs) are key to the body's immune response against cancer cells, such as those found in malignant melanoma and lung cancer. Drugs that block inhibitory co-stimulatory pathways between T lympho-cytes and APCs augment the body's immune response against these cancers. These drugs are monoclonal antibodies against targets such as cytotoxic T lymphocyte-associated protein 4 (CTLA-4), programmed cell death protein 1 (PD-1), and PD-ligand 1 (PD-L1). These same drugs can, however, cause a variety of off-target immune diseases, including interstitial nephritis and, less commonly, glomerulonephritis. The incidence is low (<5%), and cessation of these drugs usually leads to improvement of kidney function. Diagnosis is usually made based on the temporal nature of drug use (usually months after commencement) and bland urinary sediment except for sterile pyuria. Treatment consists of cessation of drugs and glucocorticoids in severe cases. Deciding which patients should be rechallenged with these drugs is a difficult decision because of the implications on overall survival.

Summary

1. Drugs are excreted by the kidney through glomerular filtration, tubular secretion, or a combination of these processes. Impaired kidney function leads to the accumulation of drugs and their metabolites and affects the distribution of the drug by altering total body water or altering its protein binding.
2. Dosage of many drugs should be modified in light of kidney disease, changes in total body water or protein binding, which will affect the distribution or toxicity of the drug.
3. Mechanisms that underlie nephrotoxic insults to the kidneys include acute tubular necrosis, tubulointerstitial nephritis, or glomerular injury.

Self-assessment case study

A 68-year-old man with diet-controlled type II diabetes develops hypotension and fever 16 h after the removal of an obstructing renal calculus using an endoscopic approach. The last serum creatinine available 1 month previously is 130 μmol/L, with urea of 6.8 mmol/L and a serum potassium of 5.2 mmol/L. His past history includes mild-moderate cardiac failure treated with a combination of ramipril and spirono-lactone. Doses of both of these drugs have been lowered recently because of hyperkalaemia. His additional medical problems include arthritis of both knees, for which he takes regular non-steroidal anti-inflammatory drugs (NSAIDs). In an attempt to control his arthritis, he has recently lost a significant amount of weight and now weighs 62 kg. Because of the risk of Gram-negative sepsis following urological intervention, treatment with gentamicin is recommended. He is commenced on 240 mg by intravenous injection (IVI) daily.

After studying this chapter, you should be able to answer the following questions:

Q1. What factors indicate that this man is likely to develop gentamicin nephrotoxicity?

Q2. What factors should guide the prescription dosing schedule of gentamicin?

Q3. List this patient's comorbidity and drug use which predispose him to hyperkalaemia.

Q4. Briefly indicate the mechanisms whereby drugs may result in acute kidney injury.

Self-assessment case study answers

A1. Gentamicin nephrotoxicity is likely to develop because a serum creatinine of 130 umol/L probably represents a mild-moderate reduction in renal function in a 68-year-old man. As gentamicin is entirely excreted by the kidney, a reduction in renal function causes an accumulation of the drug, and the main toxicity manifests as acute tubular necrosis.

A2. The dosage of gentamicin should be guided by trough levels of the drug. As the peak concentration of the drug correlates with efficacy and the trough level with toxicity, a small reduction in drug dose is recommended, with a significant increase in dosage interval.

A3. Factors that predispose him to hyperkalaemia include:

- Impaired renal function.
- Diabetes with the potential for impaired renal renin production and hyporeninaemic hypoaldosteronism.

- Concomitant use of ACE inhibitors, spironolactone and NSAIDs, all of which inhibit tubular potassium secretion by reducing aldosterone action in the kidney.

A4. Mechanisms of drug-induced nephrotoxicity:

- Haemodynamic change (fall in GFR caused by reduced glomerular capillary pressure).
- Immune injury (interstitial nephritis).
- Glomerular injury.
- Tubular cell injury.
- Tubular crystallisation.
- Multiple/uncertain.

Self-assessment questions and answers

Q1. Define the elimination half-life of a drug and explain how this may be altered in kidney impairment.

A1. The half-life of a drug is the time it takes for the plasma concentration of the drug to halve after absorption is complete. If renal excretion is responsible for the clearance of the drug, then a reduced renal clearance will prolong the half-life, and thus plasma concentrations of the drug are likely to be higher for an extended period. If the dosage schedule is not altered, then the drug will accumulate in the plasma, and drug toxicity may supervene.

Q2. What factors determine whether a drug is excreted by the kidney?

A2. Excretion of a drug by the kidney depends upon:

- Filtration of the drug into the urine. In general, if a drug has a lower molecular weight and is less protein-bound, filtration is enhanced.
- Lipid solubility. In general, water-soluble drugs will be excreted, but lipid-soluble drugs may be passively reabsorbed into the plasma.
- The presence of active transport processes that enhance the secretion or (less commonly) reabsorption of the com-

pound. This is more likely to occur with anionic and cationic drugs where carrier-mediated mechanisms in the proximal tubule facilitating secretion into the tubular fluid exist.

Q3. Describe the clinical and laboratory findings that differentiate interstitial nephritis from a haemodynamically mediated reduction in kidney function.

A3. Interstitial nephritis is often characterised by systemic features of rash and, occasionally, arthralgia and lymphadenopathy. Peripheral blood examination often shows eosinophilia and an elevated erythrocyte sedimentation rate. Urinalysis often reveals sterile pyuria and blood pressure may be elevated. In contrast, haemodynamic injury is characterised by hypotension and other features of tissue ischaemia, such as mild abnormalities in liver function. Urinalysis and urine microscopy are unremarkable, and clinical and laboratory features of systemic inflammation are absent. In general, it occurs in closer temporal relation to the introduction of a drug than does interstitial nephritis and responds more quickly to drug withdrawal.

The ranges shown are for adults unless otherwise stated.

	Range	Units
Haematology		
Haemoglobin (males)	130–180	g/L
(females)	115–165	g/L
White cell count	4.0–11.0	$\times 10^9$/L
Platelet count	150–400	$\times 10^9$/L
Packed cell volume (haematocrit)	0.38–0.52	
Erythrocyte sedimentation rate	3–15	mm/h
Biochemistry		
Venous plasma or serum		
Sodium (Na)	135–145	mmol/L
Potassium (K)	3.5–5.0	mmol/L
Chloride (Cl)	95–110	mmol/L
Bicarbonate (HCO_3^- or 'total CO_2')	22–30	mmol/L
Urea	3.0–8.0	mmol/L
Creatinine (adults)	60–120	µmol/L
(children)	30–80	µmol/L
Osmolality	280–300	mosm/kg water
Glucose ('BSL') (fasting)	3.0–5.4	mmol/L
(random)	3.0–7.7	mmol/L
HbA_{1C}	3.5–6.0	%
Total protein	62–80	g/L
Albumin	35–45	g/L
Total calcium (Ca)	2.10–2.60	mmol/L
Phosphate (PO_4)	0.8–1.5	mmol/L
Magnesium (Mg)	0.8–1.0	mmol/L
Urate	0.2–0.4	mmol/L
Total cholesterol	<5.5	mmol/L
Triglycerides (fasting)	<2.0	mmol/L
Arterial blood		
pO_2 Trigly	80–105	mmHg
pCO_2	35–45	mmHg
pH	7.36–7.44	
HCO_3^-	22–30	mmol/L
Urine		
Protein	<150	mg/24h
Urate	2.0–6.6	mmol/24h
Calcium	2.5–7.5	mmol/24h
Creatinine (depends on muscle mass)	6–16	mmol/24h
Sodium (depends on intake)	50–200	mmol/24h
Potassium (depends on intake)	40–100	mmol/24h
Osmolality (depends on hydration)	50–1200	mosm/kg water
Immunology		
Antinuclear antibodies (ANA)	1:80 or less	
dsDNA antibodies	<7	IU/mL
Complement:		
C3	0.75–1.75	g/L
C4	0.10–0.40	g/L
Microbiology		
Midstream urine – microscopy and culture		
White blood cells	<10	$\times 10^6$/L
Red blood cells	<10	$\times 10^6$/L
Epithelial cells	<10	$\times 10^6$/L
Bacterial colony count	$<10^7$	/L

adrenocortical hormones – steroid hormones produced by the adrenal cortex, including cortisol and aldosterone.

amyloidosis – a systemic disease in which a waxy, starch-like glycoprotein (amyloid) accumulates in tissues and organs.

anorexia – loss of appetite.

antinuclear antibodies – auto-antibodies that react with nuclear material.

arteriovenous nipping – narrowing of the venules in the retina at the point where they are crossed by arterioles, seen on fundoscopy of the eye in states of hypertension.

arteriopathy – any pathological condition affecting the arteries.

asterixis – a coarse flapping tremor seen in the limbs during severe metabolic disturbances.

atherosclerosis – a degenerative disease affecting arteries, characterised by deposition of lipid plaques in the inner layers of the walls of medium- and large-sized arteries.

atrial fibrillation – a cardiac arrhythmia characterised by disorganised electrical activity in the atria accompanied by a rapid, irregular ventricular response.

auscultation – the process of listening for sounds within body organs (especially the heart and lungs) to assess normality or signs of disease.

bipolar affective disorder – a psychiatric condition characterised by episodes of excitement, depression, or mixed mood, usually associated at some time with delusions or other major thought disorder.

bruit – an abnormal sound or murmur heard whilst auscultating over a blood vessel or organ.

cirrhosis – chronic liver disease involving fibrosis (scarring) and nodular regeneration.

claudication – cramp-like pains felt typically in the calves during walking, caused by inadequate arterial circulation.

complement – a series of enzymatic serum proteins involved in mediating the inflammatory consequences of antigen-antibody reactions.

crepitations (crackles) – crackling noise heard during auscultation of the lung in conditions involving fluid exudation into the alveolar airspaces.

dialysis – procedure for altering the chemical composition of the blood, particularly in renal failure, involving the diffusion of solutes through a semi-permeable membrane, either externally (in the case of haemodialysis) or internally (in the case of peritoneal dialysis).

differential diagnosis – the consideration of several alternative diseases as the cause for a patient's presentation.

diverticular disease – a condition of the colon involving the development of pouch-like herniations through the muscular layer of the bowel wall, prone to local rupture resulting in inflammation and abscess formation (diverticulitis).

DMSA – dimercaptosuccinic acid, a chemical used for radionuclide studies of the integrity of the renal parenchyma.

DTPA – diethylene triamine penta-acetic acid, a chemical used for radionuclide studies of organ function, particularly blood flow through the kidney.

end-stage kidney disease – chronic kidney disease (reduction in glomerular filtration rate) so advanced as to be incompatible with life without the institution of a form of renal replacement therapy (dialysis or transplantation).

fenestrated – (of a membrane) characterised by the presence of numerous small holes or openings.

glomerulopathy – any pathological condition affecting the glomeruli of the kidney.

glycoside – a chemical often of plant origin that yields sugar and non-sugar on hydrolysis (e.g. digitalis).

glycosuria – the presence of glucose in the urine.

Goodpasture's syndrome – an inflammatory condition involving the lungs (causing pulmonary bleeding) and the kidneys (causing glomerulonephritis), characterised by autoimmune antibody formation to basement membrane antigens.

habitus (bodily) – the overall bodily appearance or physique.

hyperglobulinaemia (polyclonal) – an increase in the concentration of globulin proteins in the plasma (with different antigenic specificities).

metastatic calcification – deposition of calcium salts in previously healthy soft tissues.

microscopic polyangiitis (polyarteritis) – an inflammatory condition of the walls of small-sized arteries, producing focal ischaemia in the affected tissues.

myeloma (multiple) – a plasma cell tumour arising in the bone marrow (in multiple sites).

osteitis fibrosa cystica – pathological changes of bone in severe hyperparathyroidism, involving replacement of normal bone by cysts and fibrous tissue.

osteomalacia – a condition of reduced calcification of the matrix of lamellar bone, resulting in bone weakness and predisposition to fracture.

osteoporosis – a condition of reduced bone density, occurring most frequently in post-menopausal women and in catabolic states.

papillary necrosis – death of the renal papillae, the innermost segment of the medullary pyramids.

paraprotein – an immunoglobulin of a single type, over-produced during a plasma cell disorder.

parenchyma – the specialised tissue of a particular organ (e.g. kidney).

parenteral nutrition – provision of nutritional requirements by a route other than the digestive tract (typically intravenously).

pericarditis – inflammation of the pericardial sac surrounding the heart.

rigor – an episode of coarse shivering that may be associated with chills and fever.

stent – a cylindrical device made of artificial material used to maintain the patency of a vessel or tubular structure in the body.

syndrome – a combination of symptoms (complaints) and signs (physical features), which characterise a particular disease or inherited condition.

systemic lupus erythematosus (SLE) – an autoimmune inflammatory disorder affecting multiple body systems.

thrombocytopenia – an abnormally low platelet count in the blood.

tubulo-interstitium – the component of the kidney parenchyma consisting of the tubules and interstitial tissue.

tumour lysis syndrome – a condition resulting from the rapid breakdown of malignant tissue, typically after chemotherapy.

uraemia (uraemic syndrome) – a biochemical and clinical state associated with the presence of large amounts of urea and other nitrogenous waste products in the blood, as occurs in advanced renal failure.

urinalysis – a chemical examination of the urine, most commonly performed using a dipstick containing reagents impregnated on paper squares.

Index